Adrian Lussi and Markus Schaffner (eds)
ADVANCES IN RESTORATIVE DENTISTRY

Advances in Restorative Dentistry

Edited by
Adrian Lussi and Markus Schaffner

With contributions from:
Adrian Lussi, Brigitte Zimmerli, Klaus Neuhaus,
Matthias Strub, Stefan Hänni, Markus Schaffner, Svante Twetman,
Martina Eichenberger, Simon Flury, Philippe Perrin, Rainer Seemann,
Philip Ciucchi, Anne Grüninger, Daniel Jacky, Thomas Jaeggi,
Franziska Jeger, Karin Kislig, Domenico Di Rocco, Jonas Rodrigues,
Benjamin Schüz, and Beat Suter

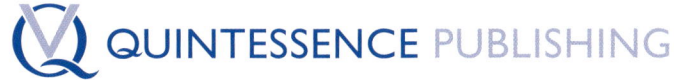

London, Berlin, Chicago, Tokyo, Barcelona, Beijing, Istanbul, Milan,
Moscow, New Delhi, Paris, Prague, São Paulo, Seoul, Singapore and Warsaw

Acknowledgements

Thanks go to Ueli Iff and Anne Seeger (Department of Multimedia and Computer Science, University of Bern) for the production of the graphical figures, as well as to Herrmann Stich (Department of Preventive, Restorative and Pediatric Dentistry, University of Bern) for the histology pictures.

British Library Cataloguing in Publication Data
Lussi, Adrian.
   Advances in restorative dentistry.
   1. Dentistry, Operative. 2. Dentistry, Operative--
   Technological innovations.
   I. Title II. Schaffner, Markus.
   617.6'05-dc23

ISBN-13: 978-1-85097-228-0

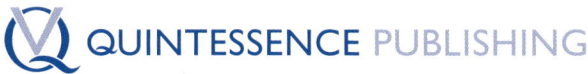

Quintessence Publishing Co. Ltd,
Grafton Road, New Malden, Surrey KT3 3AB,
United Kingdom
www.quintpub.co.uk

Copyright © 2012 Quintessence Publishing Co. Ltd
All rights reserved. This book or any part thereof may not be reproduced, stored in a retrieval system, or transmitted in any form or by any means, electronic, mechanical, photocopying, or otherwise, without prior written permission of the publisher.

Editing: Quintessence Publishing Co. Ltd, London, UK
Layout and Production: Walburga Rothenhagen, Falkensee, Germany and
Quintessenz Verlags-GmbH, Berlin, Germany
Printed and bound in Germany

Preface

Dentistry has undergone a major transformation over recent years and decades. New technologies have been developed and a better understanding of biological principles and processes has been gained. This book sheds light on these new aspects in preventive dentistry and restorative dentistry.

Advances in Restorative Dentistry gives an overview of current trends in this diverse and important specialist field for dental practitioners. The broad scope of restorative and preventive dentistry is examined in 25 chapters. The following subjects are discussed:

- Structure and pathology of the tooth
- Aspects of prevention
- Caries
- Magnification aids in restorative dentistry
- Damage to adjacent teeth and minimally invasive preparation
- Yesterday retention – today adhesion?
- Bleaching
- Dental erosion
- Endodontology
- Halitosis

The wealth of illustrations and highlighted key sentences make it easy to incorporate current knowledge into daily practice as well as into teaching and study activities.

Adrian Lussi
Markus Schaffner

Authors and contributors

Prof. Dr. med. dent. Adrian Lussi
Executive Director and Head of Department
Department of Preventive, Restorative and
Pediatric Dentistry
University of Bern
E-Mail: *adran.lussi@zmk.unibe.ch*

Dr. med. dent. Markus Schaffner
Senior Lecturer
Department of Preventive, Restorative and
Pediatric Dentistry
University of Bern
E-Mail: *markussch@bluewin.ch*

Dr. med. dent. Philip Ciucchi
Research Associate
Department of Preventive, Restorative and
Pediatric Dentistry
University of Bern
E-Mail: *Philip.ciuchhi@zmk.unibe.ch*

Dr. med. dent. Martina Eichenberger
Lecturer
Department of Preventive, Restorative and
Pediatric Dentistry
University of Bern
E-Mail: *martina.eichenberger@zmk.unibe.ch*

Dr. med. dent. Simon Flury
Research Associate
Department of Preventive, Restorative and
Pediatric Dentistry
University of Bern
E-Mail: *simon.flury@zmk.unibe.ch*

Dr. med. dent. Anne Grüninger
Senior Lecturer
Department of Preventive, Restorative and
Pediatric Dentistry
University of Bern
E-Mail: *amvv@bluewin.ch*

Dr. med. dent. Stefan Hänni
Senior Lecturer
Department of Preventive, Restorative and
Pediatric Dentistry
University of Bern
E-Mail: *stefan.haenni@zmk.unibe.ch*

Dr. med. dent. Daniel Jacky
Lecturer
Department of Preventive, Restorative and
Pediatric Dentistry
University of Bern

Dr. med. dent. Thomas Jaeggi
Senior Lecturer
Department of Preventive, Restorative and
Pediatric Dentistry
University of Bern
E-Mail: *thomasjaeggi@bluewin.ch*

Dr. med. dent. Franziska Jeger
Senior Lecturer
Department of Preventive, Restorative and
Pediatric Dentistry
University of Bern
E-Mail: *franziska.jeger@zmk.unibe.ch*

Dr. med. dent. Karin Kislig
Senior Lecturer
Department of Preventive, Restorative and
Pediatric Dentistry
University of Bern
E-Mail: *karin.kislig@zmk.unibe.ch*

Dr. med. dent. Klaus W. Neuhaus
Senior Lecturer
Department of Preventive, Restorative and
Pediatric Dentistry
University of Bern
E-Mail: *klaus.neuhaus@zmk.unibe.ch*

Dr. med. dent. Philippe Perrin
Senior Lecturer
Department of Preventive, Restorative and
Pediatric Dentistry
University of Bern
E-Mail: *perrins@bluewin.ch*

Dr. med. dent. Domenico Di Rocco
Senior Lecturer
Department of Preventive, Restorative and
Pediatric Dentistry
University of Bern
E-Mail: *domenico@dirocco.ch*

**Dr. med. dent. Jonas de Almeida Rodrigues
MSc, PhD**
Research Associate
Department of Preventive, Restorative and
Pediatric Dentistry
University of Bern
E-Mail: *jorodrigues@hotmail.com*

PD. Dr. med. dent. Rainer Seemann
Senior Lecturer
Department of Preventive, Restorative and
Pediatric Dentistry
University of Bern
E-Mail: *rainer.seemann@zmk.unibe.ch*

Benjamin Schüz, Dipl.-Psych.
Lecturer
School of Psychiatry
University of Tasmania
E-Mail: *Benjamin.Schuez@utas.edu.au*

Dr. med. dent. Matthias Strub
Senior Lecturer
Department of Preventive, Restorative and
Pediatric Dentistry
University of Bern
E-Mail: *mathias.strub@zmk.unibe.ch*

Dr. med. dent. Beat Suter
Senior Lecturer
Department of Preventive, Restorative and
Pediatric Dentistry
University of Bern
E-Mail: *bs@endodontic-bern-ch*

Prof. Svante Twetman
Head of Department
Department of Cariology and Endodontics
Faculty of Health Sciences
University of Copenhagen
E-mail: *stw@odont.ku.dk*

Dr. med. dent. Brigitte Zimmerli
Senior Lecturer
Department of Preventive, Restorative and
Pediatric Dentistry
University of Bern
E-mail: *brigitte.zimmerli@zmk.unibe.ch*

Contents

I Structure and pathology of the tooth — 1

1. Structure and pathology of the tooth — 3
   Markus Schaffner and Adrian Lussi

II Aspects of prevention — 17

2. Motivation and action – two aspects of oral hygiene at home — 19
   Benjamin Schüz and Rainer Seemann
3. Cariostatic mechanisms of action of fluorides — 25
   Adrian Lussi
4. The role of xylitol in caries prevention — 33
   Svante Twetman
5. Probiotics – a new approach in caries prevention? — 39
   Svante Twetman
6. Novel methods of promoting remineralization — 45
   Klaus Neuhaus and Adrian Lussi
7. Antibacterial agents for the prevention of caries — 53
   Svante Twetman and Klaus Neuhaus

III Caries — 63

8. Diagnosing caries and caries activity — 65
   Adrian Lussi, Markus Schaffner, Jonas Rodrigues, and Klaus Neuhaus
9. Sealing and infiltration of caries – is this the future? — 79
   Brigitte Zimmerli and Simon Flury

IV Magnification aids in restorative dentistry — 85

10. Utility and futility of magnification aids in restorative dentistry — 87
    Martina Eichenberger, Philippe Perrin, Daniel Jacky, and Adrian Lussi

V Damage to adjacent teeth and minimally invasive preparation — 95

11. Damage to adjacent teeth and minimally invasive preparation — 97
    Martina Eichenberger, Philippe Perrin, and Adrian Lussi
12. Novel preparation and excavation methods — 105
    Klaus Neuhaus, Franziska Jeger, Philip Ciucchi, and Adrian Lussi

VI	**Yesterday retention – today adhesion?**	**113**
13	Adhesive techniques for dental restorations
Brigitte Zimmerli and Matthias Strub	115
14	Direct restorative technology
Brigitte Zimmerli, Matthias Strub, and Simon Flury	123
15	Restoration repairs
Brigitte Zimmerli and Matthias Strub	137
16	Post systems
Brigitte Zimmerli and Matthias Strub	143
17	The CEREC system
Domenico Di Rocco and Adrian Lussi	151

VII	**Bleaching**	**161**
18	Bleaching
Brigitte Zimmerli and Anne Grüninger	163

VIII	**Dental erosion**	**173**
19	Dental erosion
Adrian Lussi and Thomas Jaeggi	175

IX	**Endodontology**	**191**
20	Root canal preparation
Beat Suter	193
21	Root canal irrigation
Stefan Hänni	207
22	Root canal filling
Stefan Hänni	215
23	Cracked tooth syndrome
Stefan Hänni and Adrian Lussi	223
24	Endodontology in the primary dentition
Markus Schaffner, Klaus Neuhaus, and Adrian Lussi	233

X	**Halitosis**	**243**
25	Halitosis
Rainer Seemann and Karin Kislig	245

	Index	**261**

Structure and pathology of the tooth

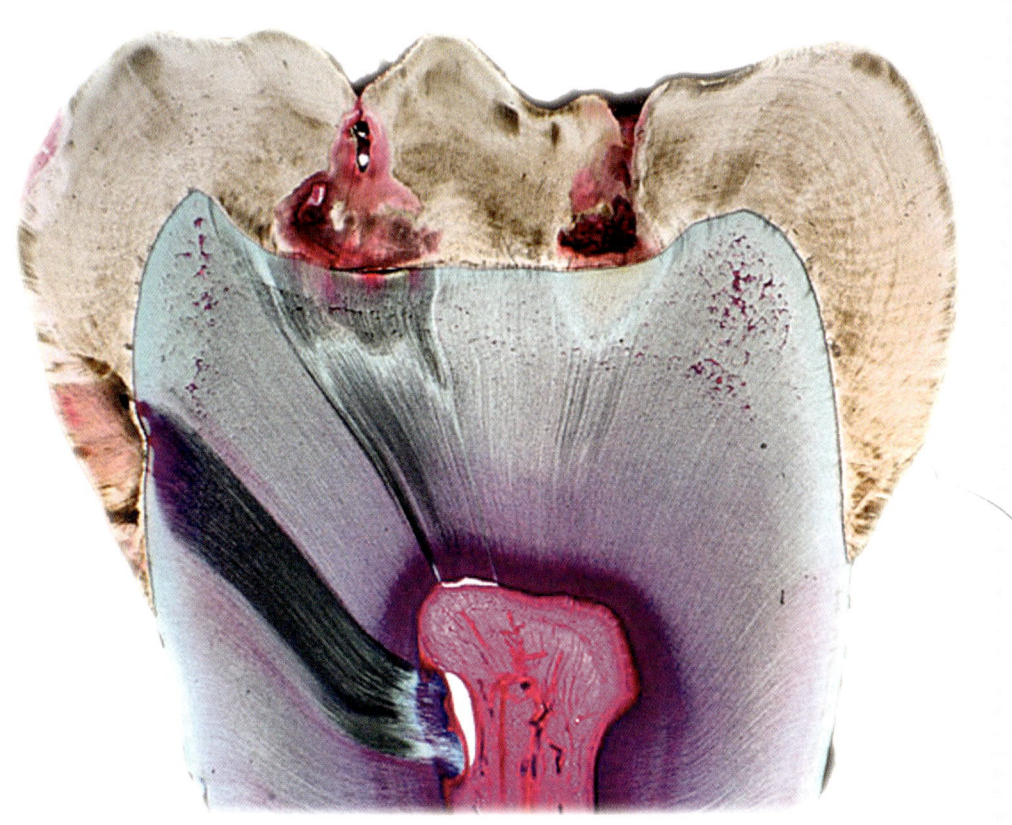

1 Structure and pathology of the tooth

Markus Schaffner and Adrian Lussi

■ Development of the teeth

Development of the teeth (odontogenesis) starts in the human embryo 28 to 40 days after ovulation. Epithelial cells grow into the ectomesenchymal parts of the jaw. This gives rise to an epithelial bulge. The dental papilla is formed by the continued penetration of epithelial cells into the ectomesenchyme.

At this stage the cells destined for the formation of hard dental tissue are differentiated: the ameloblasts arise from the ectodermal cells and the odontoblasts from the adjacent ectomesenchymal cells of the dental papilla, in which a mutual induction chain exists. Formation of the dental hard tissue starts at the same time on the whole area of contact between the ectodermal parts and the dental papilla. In the case of the anterior teeth, the first enamel and dentin layers originate in the middle of the eventual incisal margin; in the posterior teeth, they originate in the area of the eventual cusp tips. With increasing growth, the various centers involved in the formation of dental hard tissue merge and thereby form the occlusal surface.

Hertwig's epithelial root sheath, which is only two layers thick, results from the continued penetration of epithelial cells into the ectomesenchyme. It determines the size, form, and number of tooth roots that are formed. For multiple-root teeth, tongue-like processes grow out of the circular border of Hertwig's epithelial sheath over the apical edge of the dental papilla. These processes merge to form the bifurcation or trifucation. The dentin layers arising here will form the eventual floor of the coronal pulp chamber. The epithelial root sheaths proliferate apically and form the tooth roots (Figs 1-1 to 1-4).

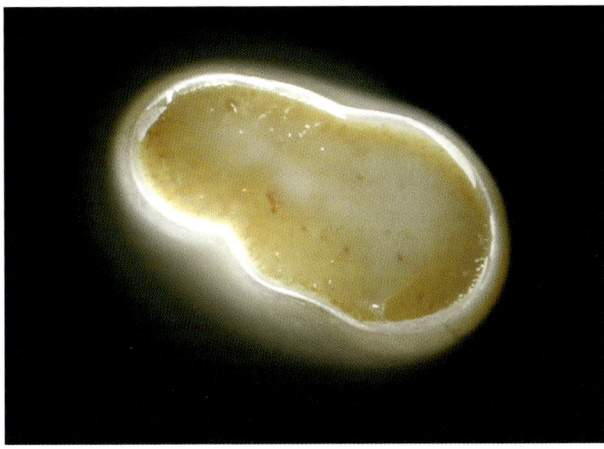
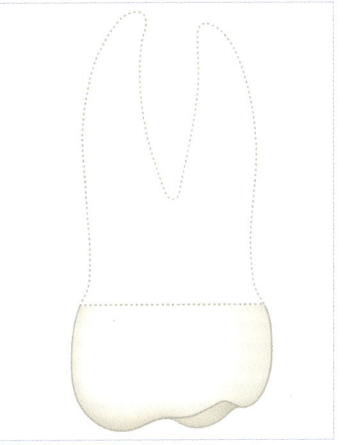

Fig 1-1 **Formation of the root** *Left and right: apical view of the developing tooth roots. Tooth development has advanced as far as the eventual cementoenamel junction.*

Fig 1-2 **Formation of the root**
Left and right: the tongue-like processes meet in the area of the eventual bifurcation, where they merge and form new epithelial sheaths for the development of two tooth roots.

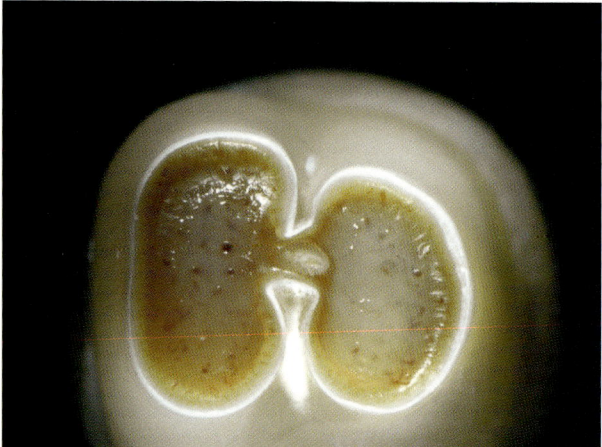
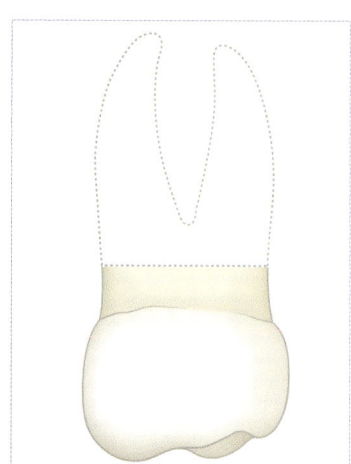

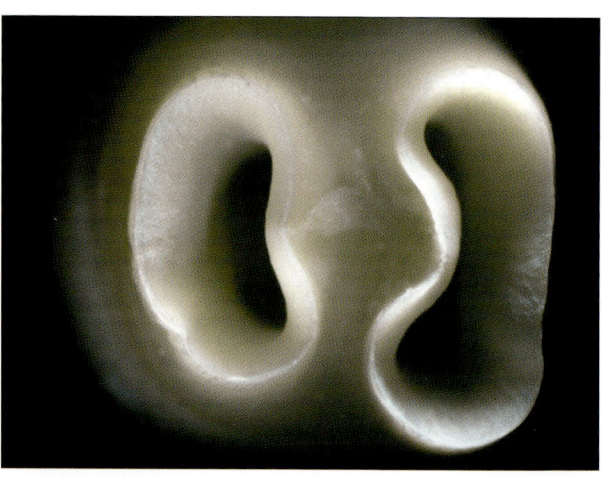
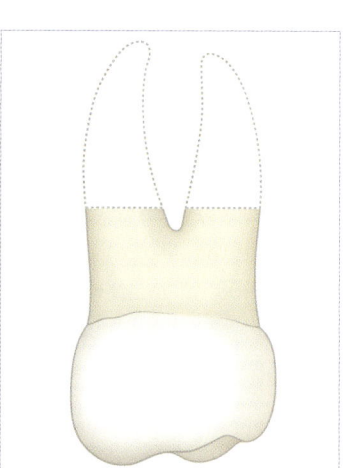

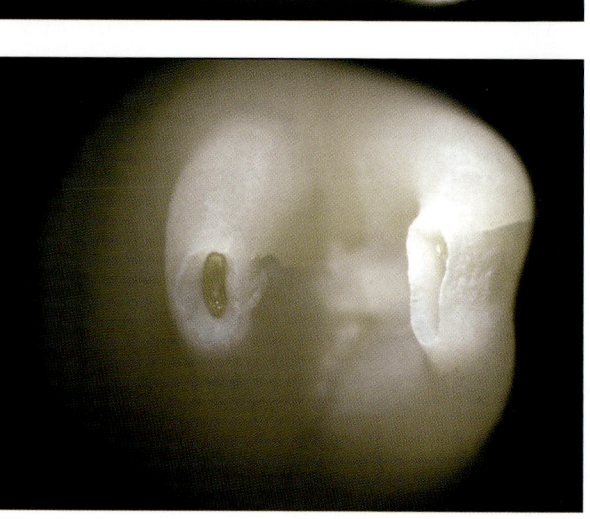
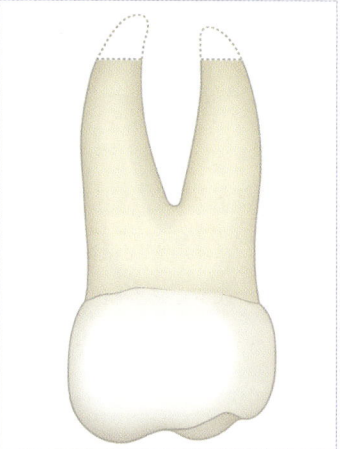

Figs 1-3 and 1-4
Formation of the root
Left and right: with increasing apical root development, the root canals narrow until the apex is reached. Root growth accelerates tooth eruption.

Structure and pathology of the tooth

The remnants of Hertwig's epithelial root sheath are responsible for the development of enamel pearls (see Fig 1-10) or cementum-free root parts. As epithelial rests of Malassez, they play an important role in the formation of cysts.

■ Enamel

The ameloblasts with their Tomes' processes are responsible for the formation of the prism rod and the interprismatic (inter-rod) enamel (Figs 1-5 and 1-6). The formation of enamel (amelogenesis) starts with the secretion of enamel matrix by the ameloblasts. The average rate of amelogenesis is 4 μm per day. However, it varies widely, depending on the tooth and tooth surface that is being formed. The enamel prisms run from the dentoenamel junction as far as the enamel surface. Their arrangement is not linear. They can be interwoven in a kind of spiral or arranged in a wavelike fashion. The wave movement of the prism rods disappears in the outer third of the enamel. The periodic formation of enamel matrix by the ameloblasts, the variable production of enamel matrix in the area of the Tomes' process, and the three-dimensional arrangement of the enamel prisms lead to the different structural characteristics of enamel seen under light and electron microscopy.

Structural characteristics of enamel

Under light microscopy, brown lines can clearly be seen in the enamel zone, which in longitudinal section run obliquely from the dentoenamel junction in an occlusal direction. These are the lines of *Retzius*, which result from the periodic laying down of enamel. In horizontal section, these lines or striae resemble the growth rings of a tree. Where the lines of Retzius emerge at the enamel surface, the imbrication lines are formed. The perikymata lie between the imbrication lines and are clearly visible on newly erupted teeth (Figs 1-7 and 1-8).

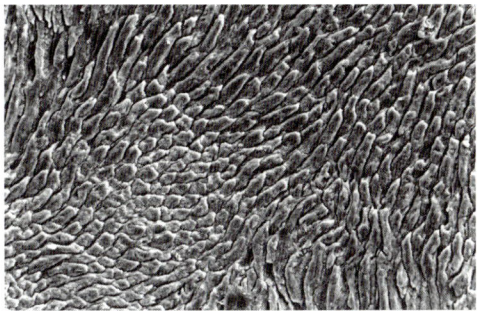

Fig 1-5 Enamel under scanning electron microscope (SEM)
Etched human enamel. Within only 100 μm the enamel prisms were longitudinally and transversally sectioned.

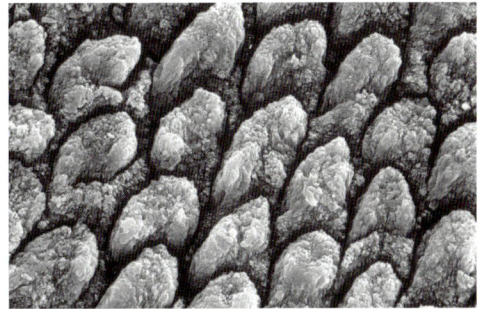

Fig 1-6 Enamel under scanning electron microscope (SEM)
The etching here attacked the interprismatic enamel more markedly than the prism rod.

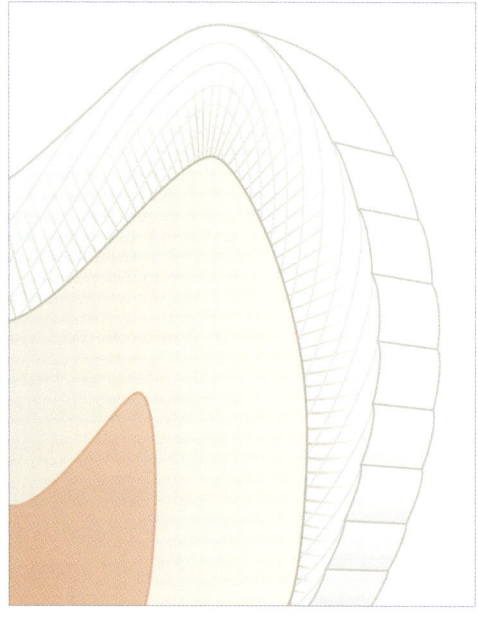
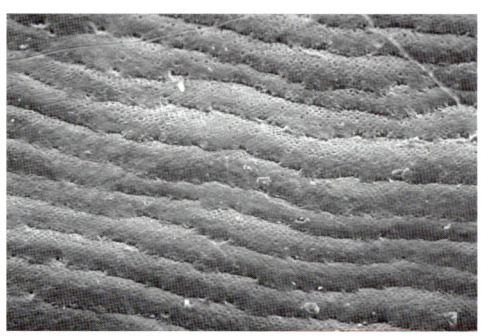

Fig 1-7 **Structural characteristics – enamel**
The periodic laying down of enamel is expressed in the lines of Retzius. Where these lines reach the surface, the perikymata are visible. Viewing the longitudinal and transverse sections of enamel by light microscopy reveals light and dark striae in the inner two-thirds. These Hunter-Schreger bands are caused by the wavelike path of the enamel prisms.

Fig 1-8 **Perikymata under scanning electron microscope (SEM)**
The magnification clearly shows not only the perikymata but also the lines of imbrication running between them.

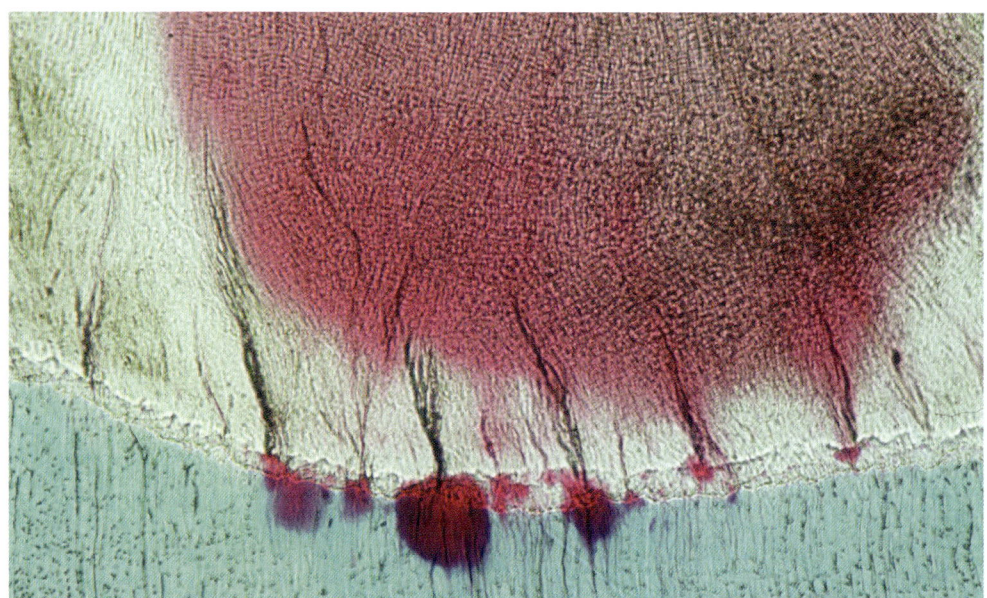

Fig 1-9 **Enamel tuft**
Enamel tufts are hypomineralized areas of enamel which look like tufts of grass under light microscopy. Enamel tufts can provide a location favourable to bacteria in the event of carious attack. Caries is clearly visible in the histologic image.

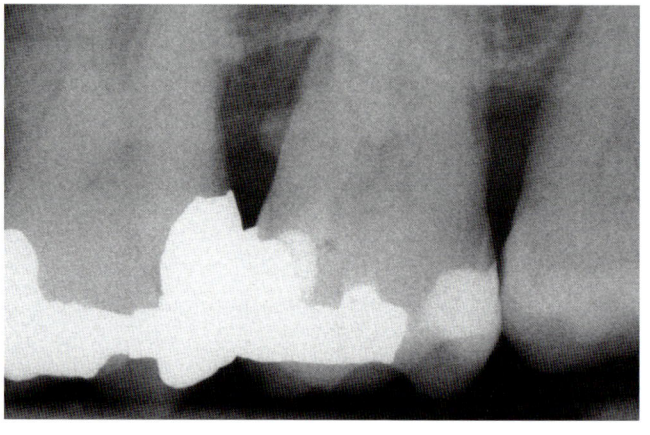
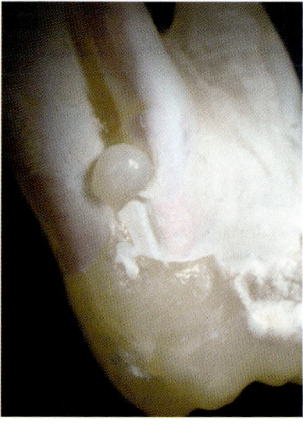

Fig 1-10 **Enamel pearl**
Left: radiograph of an enamel pearl in the interproximal area of a maxillary molar.
Right: enamel pearl in the bifurcation of a molar.

Structure and pathology of the tooth

Structural defects and paraplasias of the enamel
In most teeth, enamel structural defects can be identified by light microscopy. A large proportion of these defects arise during amelogenesis. These include enamel tufts (Fig 1-9) and enamel lamellae. Enamel tufts and lamellae can prove to be the line of least resistance in respect of the spread of caries.

The enamel pearl is a paraplasia of the enamel. This means the formation of enamel in an atypical localization. Enamel pearls can cause isolated periodontitis in the area of the furcation (Fig 1-10).

Dysplasias of the enamel (and dentin)
Dysplasia of enamel and/or dentin can be caused by defects of genes that are responsible for odontogenesis. However, traumatic, inflammatory, and chemical processes as well as metabolic disorders and systemic diseases can also cause malformations of the enamel and/or dentin.

In enamel and/or dentin dysplasias of genetic origin, all the teeth of one or both dentitions are usually affected to a varying degree. They can be inherited from generation to generation, so that similar disorders of odontogenesis can be found in siblings, parents, and grandparents (Figs 1-11 to 1-13, see also Fig 1-19).

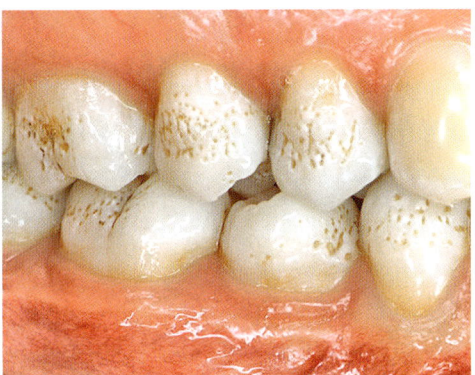

Fig 1-11 **Amelogenesis imperfecta, hypoplastic form (pitting type)**
Deposition of exogenous dyes makes the enamel pits in the area of the vestibular surface clearly visible.

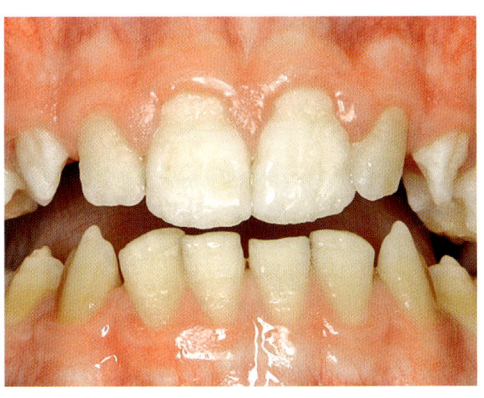 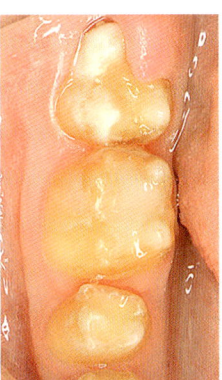 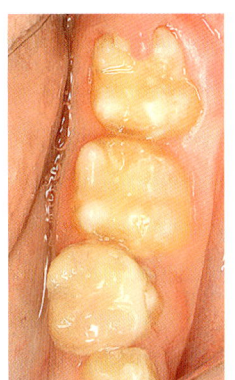

Fig 1-12 **Amelogenesis imperfecta, hypomatured form**
Left and right: the enamel is incompletely mineralized. White, opaque enamel areas are visible in the area of the cusp tips and incisal margins.

Fig 1-13 **Amelogenesis imperfecta, hypocalcified form**
The enamel is very soft. Severe loss of hard dental tissue occurs as a result of abrasion and attrition.

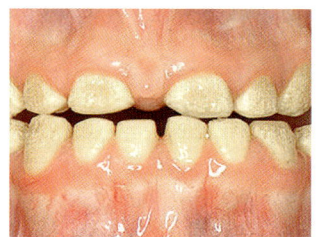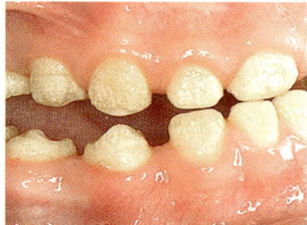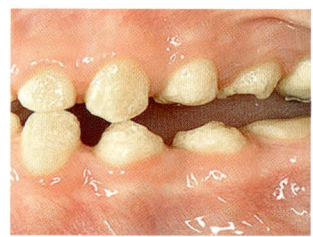

Fig 1-14 **Enamel hypoplasias in maxillary central incisors**
A local infection in the apical region of the primary maxillary central incisors led to extensive enamel defects in the permanent teeth with cementum deposits in the incisal area. Such teeth are referred to as Turner's teeth.

Fig 1-15 **Enamel hypoplasias in mandibular central incisors**
A local trauma to a primary tooth during development of the permanent central incisors led to these form and colour changes in the coronal area (yellow-brown enamel stains and ring-shaped pits apical to the enamel stains).

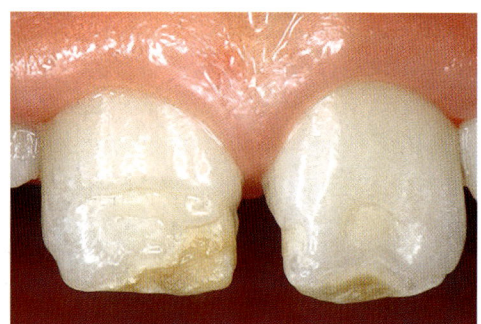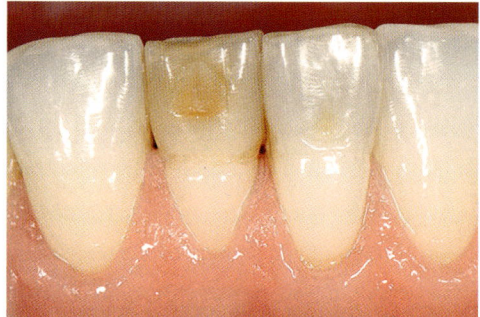

Enamel/dentin dysplasias caused by environmental factors (trauma, infection, drugs, etc) or systemic diseases are far more common and can vary in severity. They range from white or yellowish-brown discolorations through to severe surface and form defects of the dental crowns (Figs 1-14 and 1-15).

■ Dentin

The mature odontoblast is a long, columnar cell with a process on the secretory side. Predentin is secreted around the odontoblast process and later calcifies at the mineralization front. The odontoblast processes and the dentinal tubules grow longer with advancing dentin formation (Figs 1-16 to 1-18).

The development of circumpulpal dentin, which forms the main part of dentin, is a periodic process with secretory and resting phases. This periodic laying down of dentin can be detected by light microscopy. The incremental lines of *von Ebner* develop during the resting phases. They are equivalent to the lines of Retzius in the enamel. Widened and hypomineralized incremental lines are known as contour lines of *Owen*. They are caused by disruption of dentin mineralization. These disruptions can occur because of birth trauma or in systemic diseases affecting the child.

Mineralization of the circumpulpal dentin starts from centers in the area of the mineralization front, known as calcospherites. These can be detected by electron microscopy after removal of the predentin (Fig 1-18). They partly persist in the coronal dentin as interglobular dentin.

Structure and pathology of the tooth

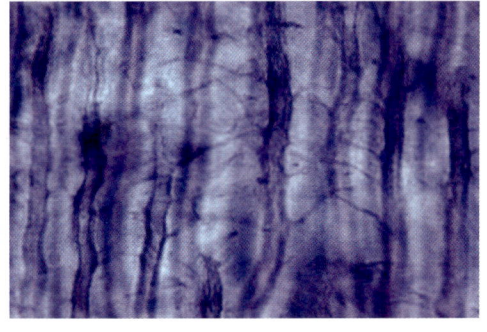

Fig 1-16 **Tubules with odontoblast processes**
The branches and communicating side-branches of the odontoblasts are clearly visible.

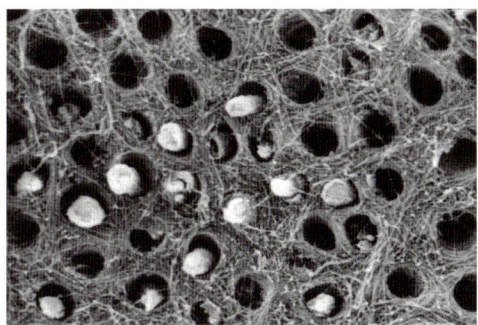
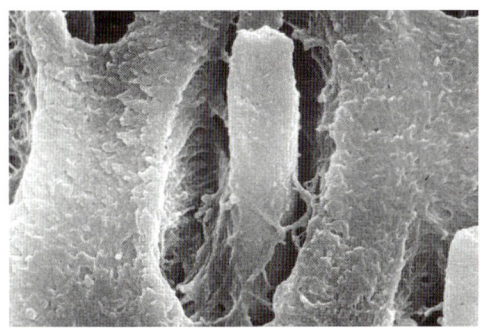

Fig 1-17 **Dentinal tubules with odontoblast processes under scanning electron microscope (SEM)**
Left: SEM image of transversely sectioned dentinal tubules with and without odontoblast processes. The collagen network is still clearly visible after decalcification.
Right: odontoblast process in a dentinal tubule.

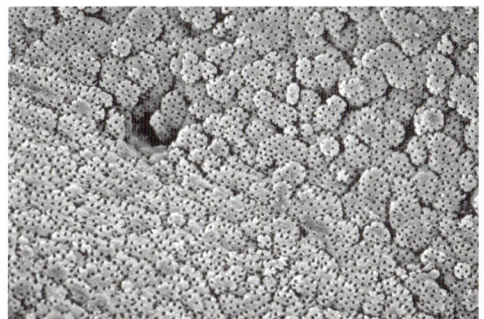
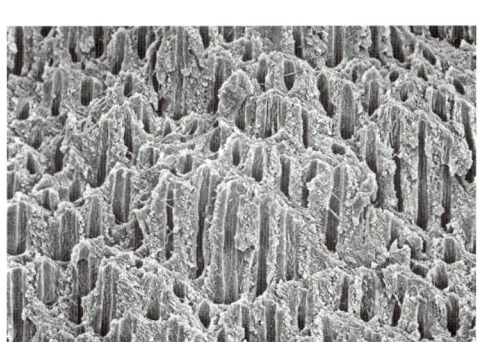

Fig 1-18 **Mineralization front**
(left) Due to removal of the pre-dentin, the calcospherites facing the pulp wall and the numerous openings to the dentinal tubules are clearly visible by SEM. The entrance to an accessory canal can be seen in the middle of the image.
Dentinal tubules *(right)*
SEM image of broken dentin with dentinal tubules.

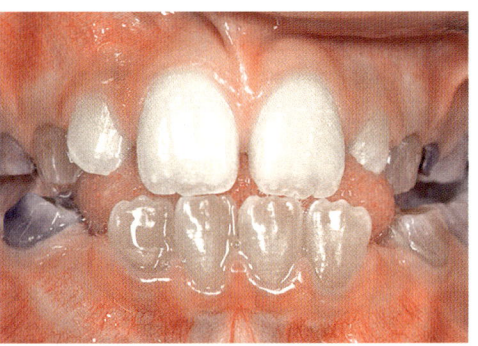

Fig 1-19 **Dentinogenesis imperfecta**
Disturbed tooth development led to blue-brown discoloration of primary molars and to brownish discoloration of permanent mandibular anterior teeth (amber/pearlescent tooth discolorations) (image: P. Hotz).

If the broad-spectrum antibiotic tetracycline is administered during tooth formation, tetracycline becomes irreversibly deposited in the tooth. Prolonged tetracycline treatment gives rise to extensive grey-bluish discoloration of the dental crowns; the depositions resulting from short-term treatments during odontogenesis can only be detected histologically.

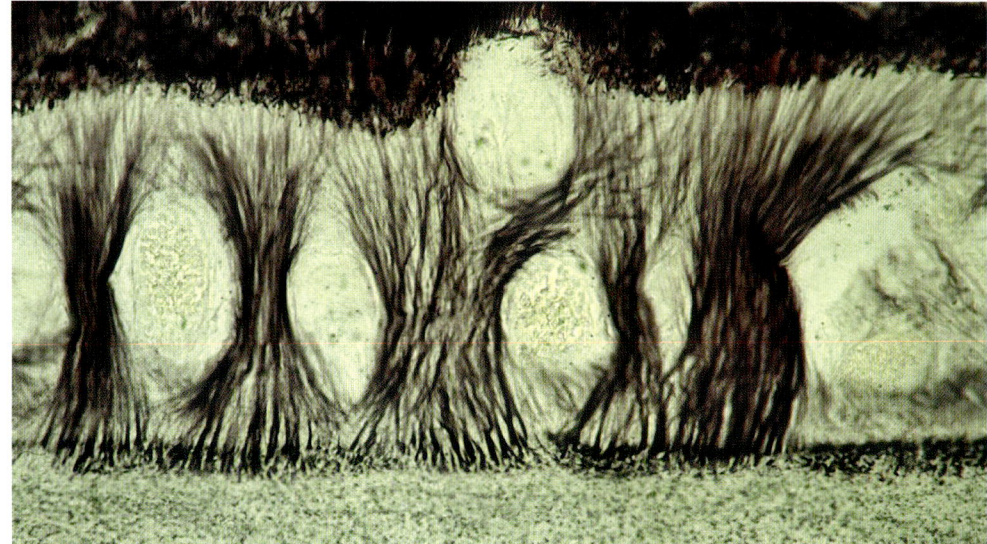

Fig 1-20 **Sharpey's fiber bundles**
Sharpey's fiber bundles, which are anchored in the acellular area of the cellular mixed fiber cementum.

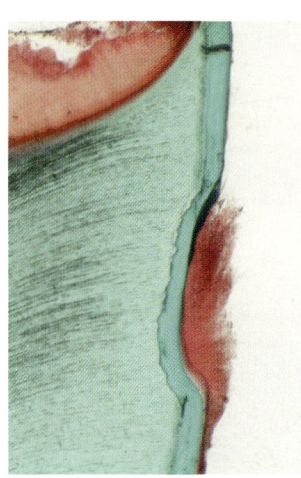 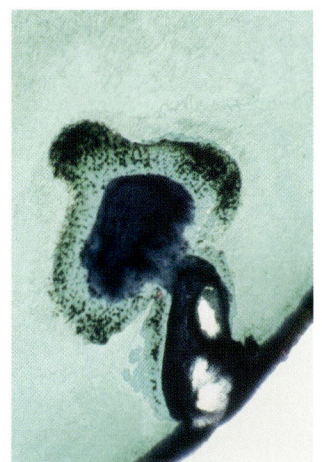 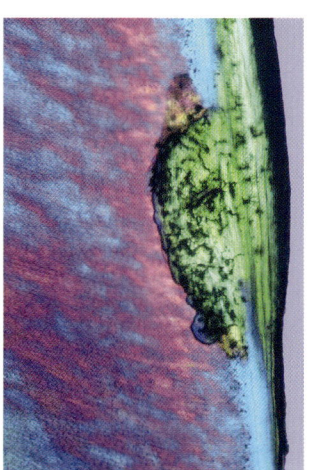

Fig 1-21 **Cementum repairs**
Left: repair of surface root resorption in the area of the coronal third of the root by acellular extrinsic fiber cementum.
Middle and right: repair of root resorptions by cellular intrinsic fiber cementum.

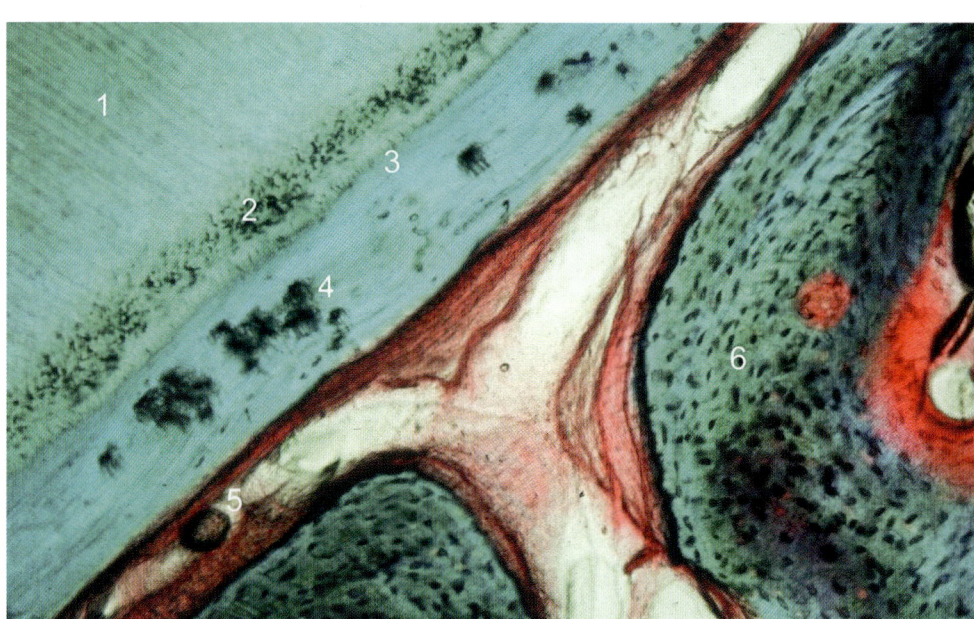

Fig 1-22 **Periodontal ligament**
1. Dentin with tubules
2. Tomes' granular layer
3. Acellular layers of cellular of cellular mixed fiber cementum
4. Cellular layers of cellular mixed fiber cementum
5. Periodontal space with blood vessels
6. Alveolar bone

The irreversible deposition of tetracycline in enamel, dentin, and cementum comes about because of complexing of the antibiotic with calcium. In children aged over seven years, the administration of tetracycline for dental traumas does not result in coronal discolorations until the first molars because the crown formation of these teeth is already completed by this stage.

■ Cementum

The cementum is a mineralized connective tissue that covers the entire surface of the tooth root. Its job is to anchor the periodontal fibers to the tooth (Fig 1-20). Cellular cementum has a certain similarity to bone. However, bone is vascularized, cementum is not. Cementum continues to be formed after eruption has taken place. Cementum therefore has reparative properties, which can be significant in the event of dental trauma or root resorption (Fig 1-21).

The cementoblasts, cementocytes, and fibroblasts of the periodontal ligament are responsible for the formation of cementum (Fig 1-22). These are cells of the ectomesenchyme. The cementoblasts form and secrete the cemental matrix. Cementocytes originate from cementoblasts which are laid down in the cementum during cementogenesis. Fibroblasts which lie against the cemental layer form the acellular extrinsic fiber cementum. Their structure very closely resembles that of the cementoblasts.

Types of cementum

Four types of cementum can be distinguished from each other:

1. Acellular afibrillar cementum (AAC), which contains neither cementocytes nor fibers. This type of cementum is found in the cervical area of the tooth.
2. Acellular extrinsic fiber cement (AEFC), which is mainly made up of *Sharpey's* fibers radiating from the outside inwards (Fig 1-21). This type of cementum is largely to be found in the coronal third of the root surface.
3. Cellular intrinsic fiber cementum (CIFC), which can contain cementocytes in varying numbers. It possesses fibers that run parallel to the root surface. Cellular intrinsic fiber cementum is formed during repair of root resorptions and root fractures (Fig. 1-21).
4. Cellular mixed stratified cementum (CMSC), which comprises alternating layers of acellular extrinsic and cellular intrinsic fiber cementum (Fig 1-22). Cementocytes, Sharpey's fibers radiating inwards from outside, and cemental fibers are found in this type of cementum. CMSC mainly occurs in the middle and apical thirds of the root. Above-average formation of cellular mixed stratified cementum in the periapical and/or interradicular root area is known as hypercementosis.

Pulp

The pulp arises from the dental papilla. The fibroblasts develop from the undifferentiated mesenchymal cells of the dental papilla. Various zones can be identified in the pulp:

1. Zone of odontoblasts.
2. Zone of *Weil* (cell-free zone). This zone lies below the odontoblast layer. It is more pronounced in the coronal pulp than in the root pulp. The nerve endings of the sensory and autonomic nerve fibers as well as vascular loops of the subodontoblastic capillary plexus, which extend up to the odontoblasts, lie in the cell-free zone of Weil.
3. Bipolar zone (cell-rich zone). This zone contains numerous fibroblasts and undifferentiated mesenchymal cells. These cells can transform into odontoblasts and replace dead cells of the odontoblast layer. The bipolar zone hardly exists in the apical third of the root.

After the bipolar zone, the central zone of the coronal and root pulp starts with the nerve plexus of *Raschkow* and the subodontoblastic capillary plexus. The main purpose of the zones of the coronal pulp containing vascular and nerve plexus as well as undifferentiated mesenchymal cells is defence against infection and repair in the area of the odontoblasts.

The shape of the pulp can vary very widely in the coronal and root areas. Formation of the apical foramen, in particular, is subject to enormous variability (Fig 1-23).

Accessory canals and denticles

The pulp can be linked to the periodontal ligament via accessory canals. A neurovascular bundle runs through each of these accessory canals (Fig 1-24).

Denticles (pulp stones) are often found in the pulp. These can occur either freely and unattached to the pulp wall (free denticles) or fused to the pulp wall (adherent denticles, Fig 1-25 right). A further distinction is made between true and false denticles. True denticles are rare and are usually to be found in the area of the root canals. They are often embedded in the pulp wall. False denticles are more common and are mainly located in the coronal pulp. They can occur freely or attached to the pulp wall. In rare cases they almost entirely fill the pulp or the root canal (Fig 1-25 left). This can make the preparation of a root canal difficult. Denticles are more common in old age and are often found in several teeth.

Structure and pathology of the tooth

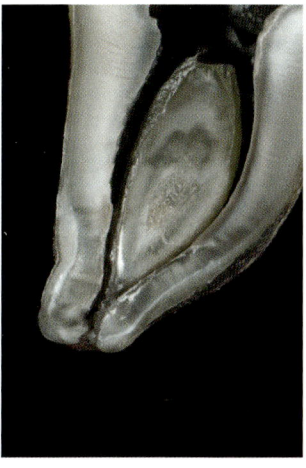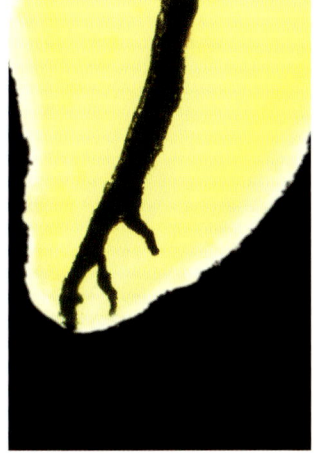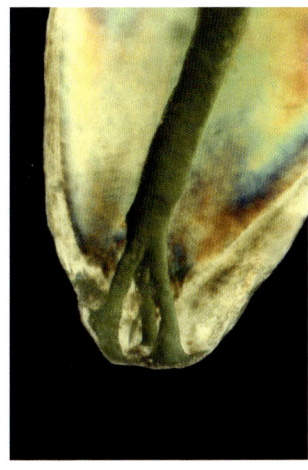

Fig 1-23 **Apical foramen**
Left, middle and right: differing formation of the apical foramen.

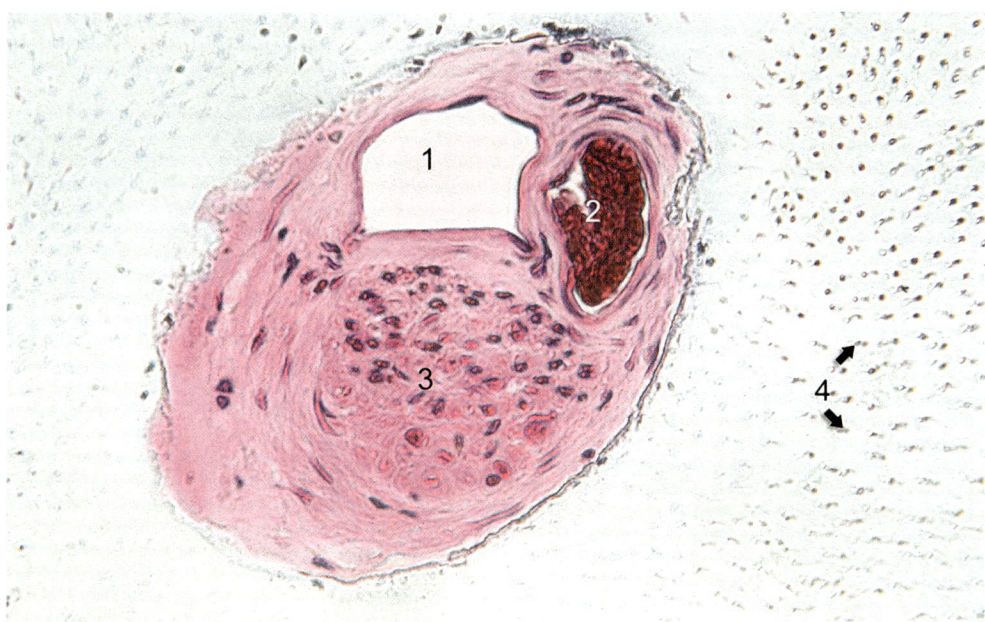

Fig. 1-24 **Cross-section through an accessory canal**
1. Venule
2. Arteriole
3. Nerve fiber bundle
4. Dentinal tubules

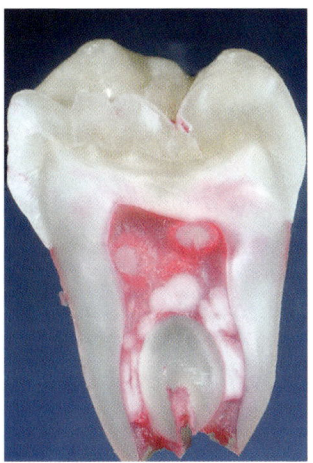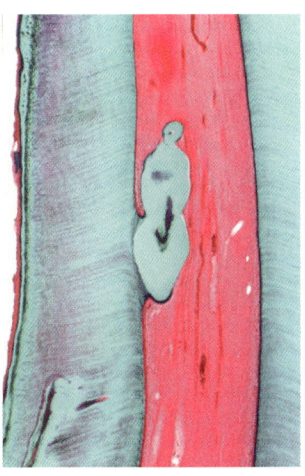

Fig 1-25 **Denticle**
Left: molar with multiple denticles that almost completely seal the root canals.
Right: the histologic image shows an adherent denticle, ie, a denticle which is fused to the dentin of the root wall. Adherent denticles often have an elongated form.

Structure and pathology of the tooth

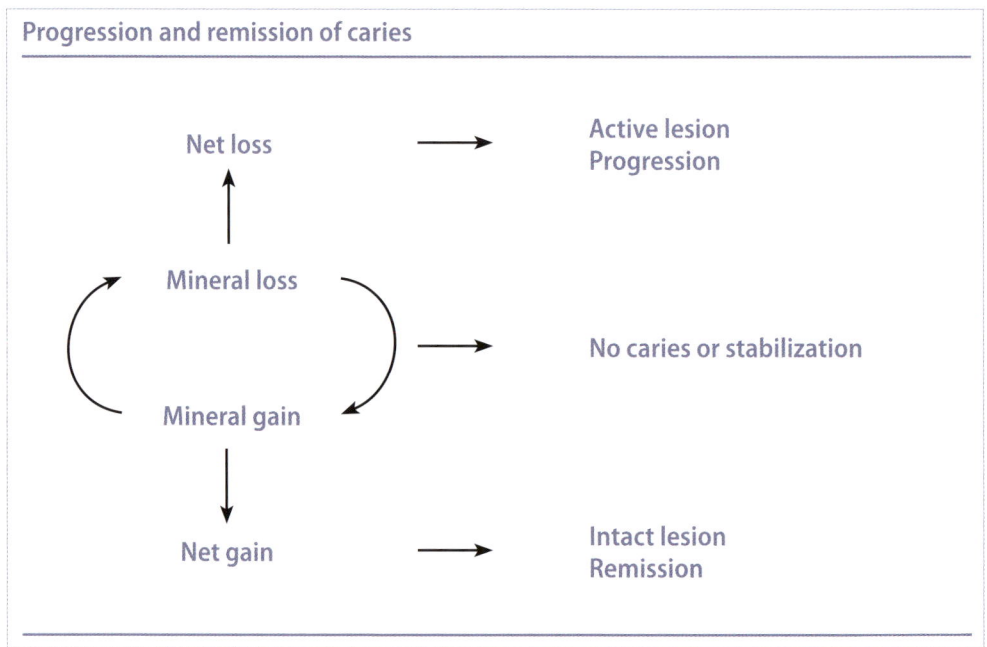

Progression and remission of caries

Net loss → Active lesion / Progression

Mineral loss ⇄ Mineral gain → No caries or stabilization

Net gain → Intact lesion / Remission

Fig 1-26 **Progression and remission of caries**

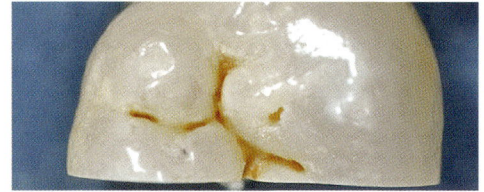 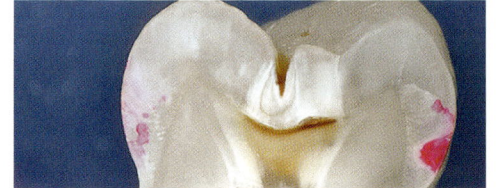

Fig 1-27 **Fissure caries**
Left: discolorations in the fissure area with intact surface.
Right: the cut surface shows enamel and dentin caries.

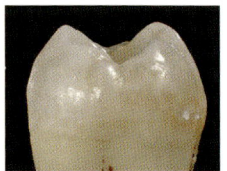 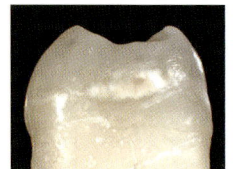 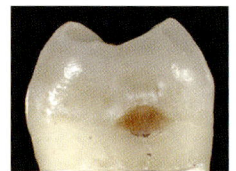 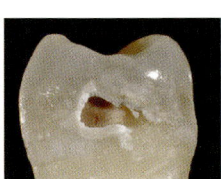

Fig 1-28 **Appearance of interproximal caries**
From left to right: caries-free interproximal surface. Interproximal initial lesion (white spot). The interproximal enamel surface starts to break down. Massive breakdown of the interproximal tooth surface.

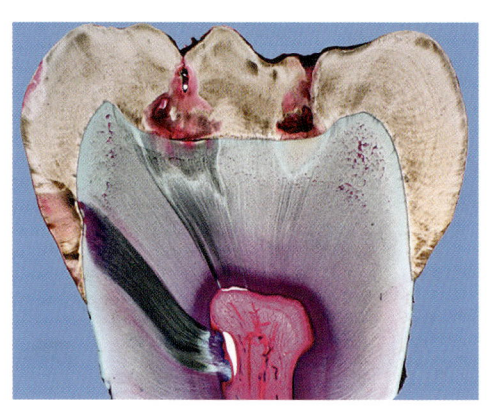

Fig 1-29 **Molar with interproximal and fissure caries**
In the area of the carious lesions, changes extending into the pulp are already visible histologically. The caries led to sclerosis of the dentinal tubules and to tertiary dentin formation in the pulp.

Structure and pathology of the tooth

■ Caries

Caries starts with local chemical demineralization of the tooth surface, caused by bacterial metabolic activities that take place in the biofilm over the tooth surface (Fig 1-26). Enamel, dentin, and cementum can be demineralized and destroyed if the carious process advances. Carious lesions arise where the biofilm is not removed and is able to develop over a prolonged period. The most common sites for caries to develop are embrasures, pits, and fissures on the occlusal surfaces (Fig 1-27), the interproximal tooth surfaces below the contact points (Fig 1-28), and the tooth surfaces in the region of the marginal gingival crest. These sites are largely protected against the mechanical cleaning effect of tongue, cheeks, abrasive food, and toothbrush.

The metabolic activities of bacteria cause wide pH fluctuations in the biofilm and at the tooth surface, above all during consumption of low-molecular-weight carbohydrates (sugars). These fluctuations then lead to demineralization or remineralization, depending on the degree of saturation of the biofilm relative to the chemical composition of the tooth surface. If the pH in the biofilm is frequently excessively low over weeks or months, the result is the loss or relocation of calcium and phosphate in the enamel surface, giving rise to a white spot.

If the biofilm is removed, the mineral loss in the enamel is halted, and because saliva is oversaturated with calcium, phosphate and, if present, fluoride relative to the white spot, remineralization of the enamel surface occurs. However, if the biofilm is not removed over a prolonged period, the mineral loss progresses and leads to breakdown of the tooth surface (Fig 1-26).

Where a white spot has developed but the enamel surface remains intact, there might, depending on extent, already be histologic changes extending into the dentin and the pulp (Fig 1-29). If the carious process advances, further inflammatory reactions rapidly ensue in the pulp without the patient necessarily having any pain. The reactions of the pulp-dentin complex to advancing caries are described below.

■ Pulpitis

Pulpitis can be triggered by bacteria and also by mechanical, thermal, and biochemical stimuli. The first signs of inflammation of the pulp can be seen in the odontoblast layer and the marginal zones of the pulp. The first pulp changes include the following: reduction of odontoblasts, increase in inflammatory cells in the subodontoblastic region, dilatation and proliferation of blood vessels, and edema.

A bacterial attack will result in sclerosis of the dentinal tubules, disruption of the dentinal tubule structures, and tertiary dentin formation (Fig 1-30). If the bacteria get close to the pulp margin, the inflammation becomes acute. The result is a pulpal abscess with pus and granulation tissue.

In the initial stages, the pulpal abscess comprises a central necrotic area with pus and a rim of neutrophilic granulocytes, surrounded by severely inflamed pulpal tissue (Fig 1-31). In older abscesses, the central necrosis is bordered by a macrophage rim with lots of lymphocytes and plasma cells. Old abscesses may be absorbed and replaced by connective tissue.

Fig 1-30 **Reaction of the pulp-dentin complex to a carious attack**
The root caries led to sclerosis of the dentinal tubules and tertiary dentin formation in the pulp. The free denticles are also probably a reaction to the carious process in the root area.

Fig 1-31 **Pulpal abscess**
The central necrosis of the pulpal abscess, which is surrounded by a rim of neutrophilic granulocytes, is clearly visible. The carious lesion led to destruction of the odontoblast layer and tertiary dentin formation in the pulp area.

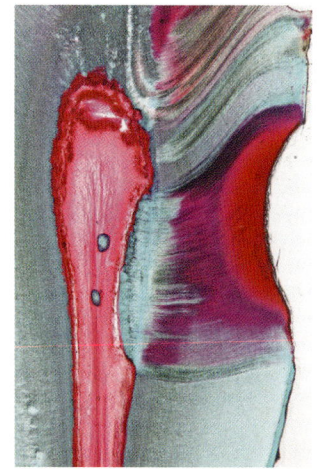
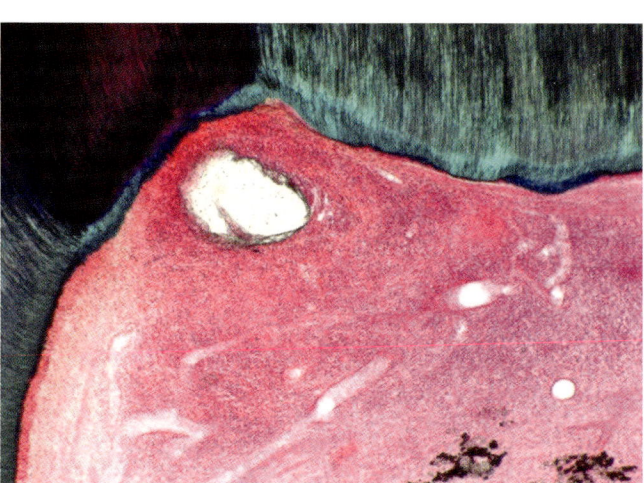

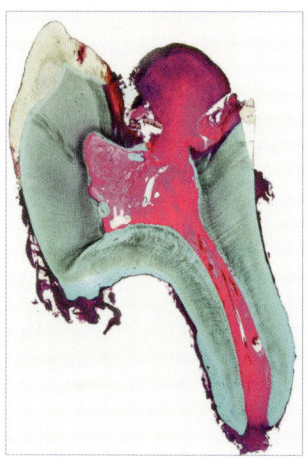

Fig 1-32 **Pulpal polyp**
After opening of the pulp chamber by the carious process, prolific growth of pulpal granulation tissue in the direction of the oral cavity led to a pulpal polyp. The surface of the pulpal polyp can be colonized by epithelial cells and epithelialized.

If the carious process results in opening of the pulp chamber, the purulent exudate drains off. If no dental treatment has yet taken place up to this point, a pulpal polyp may be formed if there is sufficient blood supply and proliferation of the pulpal granulation tissue in the direction of the oral cavity (Fig 1-32).

■ References

This chapter is based on the books *Oral Structural Biology* (Stuttgart: Thieme, 2000) and *Pathobiology of Oral Structures* (Basel: Karger, 1997) by *Hubert E. Schroeder* and other scientific publications.

Aspects of prevention

II

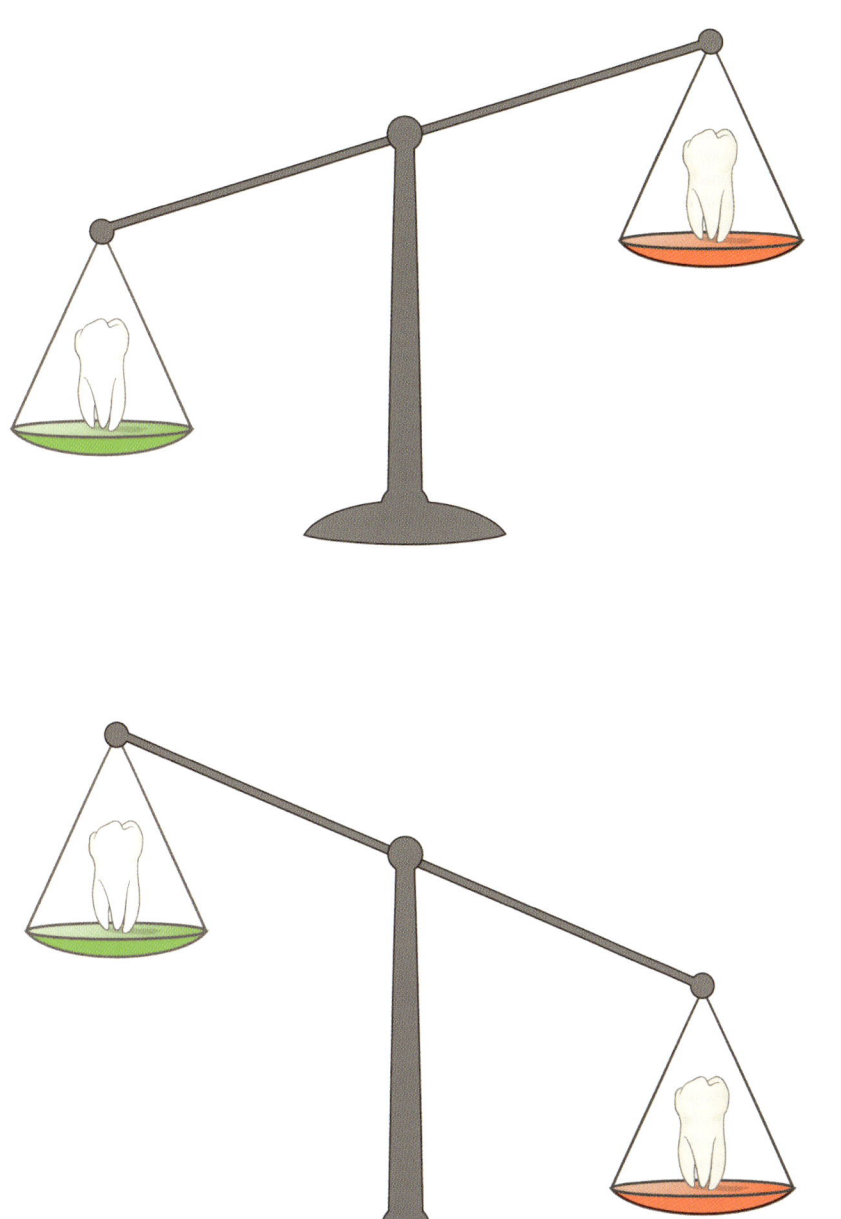

2 Motivation and action – two aspects of oral hygiene at home

Benjamin Schüz and Rainer Seemann

Pointing out to patients that their dental health depends heavily on their own behavior actually ought to be enough to get them to follow our advice on oral hygiene. But in fact that is not reality or this does not happen.

In this context, "behavior" includes not only classic oral hygiene with toothbrush and toothpaste but also interdental cleaning, the regular application of fluoride gel, denture cleaning, attending recall appointments, and much more.

Unfortunately, in reality these recommendations are followed nowhere near as thoroughly as we might wish. Consequently, figures concerning oral hygiene behavior in Switzerland and Germany show that, although most people do clean their teeth twice a day, only about 2 % carry out interdental cleaning as recommended.[8] Why is this so and how can dental practitioners get their patients to follow their advice on what to do? Psychology can provide answers to these questions.

■ Motivation and action – two aspects of regular oral hygiene

It is assumed that a change of behavior goes through two phases. The first phase is when people consider the pros and cons of behavior changes and resolve to make a change. The second phase is when they actually try to put that decision into action.

Motivation: the intention to take action

Psychology uses the terms "motivation" and "intention" largely interchangeably – someone who is motivated towards a certain behavior is therefore characterized by having formed intentions to adopt that behavior.

Whether and to what extent such intentions are formed will depend on various determining factors, but essentially on the individual's convictions:

- The conviction that the behavior adopted generally makes sense.
- Whether a person feels capable of carrying out the behavior.
- Whether the behavior is relevant to the person concerned.

For example, someone who has become convinced that interdental hygiene is ideally suited to removing plaque and thereby preventing caries, who also knows how to use the appropriate products (dental floss, interdental brushes), and has furthermore realized that he or she personally might be affected by caries, is more likely to form such a conviction than someone who is not yet so convinced of those points.

However, the fact that such personal convictions are crucial to people's intentions to make behavioral changes also shows that how well the information underlying those convictions is communicated is a determining factor. This poses a major challenge to the dental team. Studies from general medicine and also from orthodontics show that immediately following a conversation with their medical practitioner patients can only remember about 50% of the information given to them. This underlines how important it is to prepare and convey information in such a way that it is well received by the patients.

An interesting approach from psychology is based on the assumption that the decision for or against a health-related behavior, eg, regular oral hygiene, follows convictions derived from general knowledge ("common sense"), which are then implemented in the form of health-related concepts. For an understanding of caries and periodontitis, information about the following five aspects would thus be required for a patient to form an intention to practice daily oral hygiene:[2]

1. **Understanding symptoms of the disease**
   Patients encounter advanced caries as toothache and periodontitis as gingival bleeding.
2. **Understanding causes of the disease**
   Caries and periodontitis are caused by relevant microorganisms in plaque (biofilm) and their metabolic products. How long plaque remains on the teeth is dependent on a patient's behavior.
3. **Assessing progression of the disease**
   Caries and periodontitis are rather chronic conditions, but their progression can be altered through a patient's cooperation.
4. **Understanding consequences of the disease**
   Caries as well as periodontitis can cause a reduction in quality of life – not only in terms of health but also socially.
5. **Acknowledging manageability of the disease**
   Professional and personal oral hygiene measures can have a beneficial effect on caries and periodontitis, and oral hygiene measures can be carried out by patients at home without any great effort.

If the information arising from these five aspects is prepared systematically in a clearly understandable way and made available to patients, even patients with chronic periodontal disease can be encouraged to perform better interdental hygiene and improve their oral health.[2]

The challenge lies in preparing and communicating the information so that patients understand what is required. It is important to ensure that the information, whether in written or verbal form, is explained as basically and unambiguously as possible. It is vital to avoid unnecessary technical language (eg, refer to "spaces between the teeth" instead of "interdental spaces") and vague expressions (eg, state "daily in the morning after cleaning your teeth" instead of "regularly"). The more concrete these instructions are, the better patients are able to remember them. For example, a patient consultation might be initiated as follows:

> "Today you have come to me because your gums have been bleeding a lot, which you are concerned about. Unfortunately, I have to tell you that this bleeding can be a sign of periodontitis; in other words, the breakdown of the periodontal tissue that supports the teeth. The bleeding is a perfectly normal inflammatory reaction by your body to toxins that are secreted by bacteria in dental plaque. But your periodontal tissue does not necessarily have to continue breaking down because, fortunately, you can do something to stop it. You simply have to remove the bacterial deposits by cleaning your teeth and, above all, cleaning the spaces between the teeth. Therefore, in addition to cleaning your teeth, you should clean between the teeth with dental floss every night. I will just show you exactly how it works: take out around 50 cm of dental floss..."

Acting on intentions

An intention does form the foundation for a behavioral change, but current psychological research results show that motivation (or intention) alone is unfortunately not enough to really alter behavior permanently.[7] Forming an intention based on sound information is one thing – actually changing behavior is regrettably something else. The best-known example in this connection is undoubtedly the way that people make New Year's resolutions ("good intentions"), most of which are either not acted upon or are not kept for very long. From the psychological point of view, this discrepancy between intention and action is entirely understandable because the two processes are subject to different laws and different influencing factors.

People who have already formed an intention to practice interdental hygiene need no additional information about the pros and cons of this measure, but they do need information that can help them carry it out. To be specific: the patient has already come to realize that daily cleaning of the interdental spaces has more advantages than disadvantages. Similarly, the patient is already convinced that they can manage this form of teeth cleaning – they are familiar with the technique. Thus the patient is no longer in the deliberative phase (before the intention) but already in the volition phase, when they have to put that intention into practice. What is needed here is information, strategies, and techniques that help the patient to do so. The psychologist Heinz Heckhausen likened this point to the "crossing of the Rubicon" because a lot changes once an intention is formed.[1] Once a person has formed an intention, he or she mainly seeks and processes information that conforms to that intention and is aimed at its realization. Hence there is basically an information deficit in the deliberative phase, whereas there is basically an implementation deficit in the volition phase.

Most of our patients are likely to have less of an information deficit leading to a lack of intention, but more of an implementation deficit preventing them from realizing their intentions in terms of oral hygiene.

■ Overcoming implementation deficits

Implementation deficits can have a whole range of causes: good opportunities for behavior are missed; behavior is simply forgotten; behavior is displaced, especially when a person is tired or exhausted. In recent years psychological research has concerned itself with measures designed to aid realization of intentions. According to these studies, structured plans and systematic self-observation seem to be particularly helpful with respect to oral hygiene. Hence people are more likely to act in accordance with their good intentions when their implementation is well planned and they notice for themselves whether and how they fulfill their intentions. Furthermore, both can be put into practice with relatively little effort.

Planning

A good plan comprises very precise descriptions of both a situation and the action to be taken in that situation. Good plans also follow a when-where-how pattern: "Every night, before going to bed (when) in my bathroom, in front of the mirror (where), I will clean the spaces between my teeth with dental floss, as demonstrated to me at the dental practice (how)."

By means of this when-where-how structure, patients create a vivid image of themselves in a concrete situation performing a concrete action. This leads to a cognitive association which means that, in the described situation (at bedtime before the bathroom mirror), it is more probable that the action will be performed. A study involving students in Scotland showed that more dental floss was used if such a concrete plan existed,[6] and a study from Germany showed that these plans not only lead to better interdental cleaning, but also work especially well for people who have already formed the appropriate intentions.[3,5] Such plans are ideally produced with the involvement of the patient: a template is issued to the patient who notes precisely when, where, and how he or she intends to carry out the planned behavior (Fig 2-1).

Motivation and action – two aspects of oral hygiene at home

A plan for your teeth
Regular cleaning between your teeth works best if you plan exactly when, where, and how you are going to do it. Enter in the columns below when, where, and how you clean the spaces between your teeth. The more precise, specific, and personal you make your plan, the more it will help you! Visualize yourself in this situation as clearly as possible.

When? When do you clean your interdental spaces?	Where? Where do you clean your interdental spaces?	How? How do you clean your interdental spaces?
At night before cleaning my teeth.	In the bathroom in front of the mirror.	I use 50 cm of dental floss between all my teeth.

Fig 2-1 Example of a planning form.

Self-observation

Systematic self-observation can also help to convert intentions into actual behavior. Systematic self-observation means that the patient documents what they have done every time. Any kind of calendar is suitable for the purpose. An ideal solution is a calendar that is hung up in the place where the event takes place, eg, by the bathroom mirror, because it will simultaneously act as a memory aid. A monthly calendar, as shown in Fig 2-2, can be created with little effort and can be provided at the same time as the relevant instructions in the dental practice. As with the planning, calendars used for self-observation have been shown to work particularly well for people who have already formed the necessary intentions.[4]

Your interdental calendar
On this calendar mark with a cross (X) every day when you have used dental floss or interdental brushes, then bring the calendar with you to your next appointment.

Monday	Tuesday	Wednesday	Thursday	Friday	Saturday	Sunday

Fig 2-2 Example of an interdental calendar.

■ Conclusions and practical implications for the dental team

Generally understandable information that has been written with the actual patient in mind is necessary to motivate people to practice regular oral hygiene. In other words, many patients require more information and others need less, while some patients require less complex and others more complex information. The primary aim of this information should be to convince patients that oral hygiene generally makes sense, that they will benefit from it themselves, and that it is practical for them to manage their oral hygiene personally. The five areas of symptoms, causes, progression, consequences, and manageability of the disease can be used as the basis for drawing up the information.

However, information and education are primarily effective with patients who have not yet formed any intentions to change their behavior. Once the intention is formed, it is largely pointless and, strictly speaking, a waste of time. The patient hears what he or she has known for a long time and the dental practitioner might be frustrated that, despite the best information, the patient still does not clean their teeth as required.

Motivated patients require assistance to overcome a possible implementation deficit. This is ideally done by concrete planning of the desired behavior (when-where-how) and by appropriate self-observation (eg, using a monthly plan hung up in the bathroom).

The skill of the dental team lies in distinguishing an information (motivation) deficit from an implementation deficit and compensating for it accordingly.

■ References

1. Heckhausen H. Motivation und Handeln. Berlin, Heidelberg, New York: Springer 1980.
2. Philippot P, Lenoir N, Hoore W, Bercy P. Improving patients' compliance with the treatment of periodontitis: a controlled study of behavioural intervention. J Clin Periodontol 2005;32:653–658.
3. Schüz B, Sniehotta FF, Wiedemann A, Seemann R. Adherence to a daily flossing regimen in university students: effects of planning when, where, how and what to do in the face of barriers. J Clin Periodontol 2006;33:612–619.
4. Schüz B, Sniehotta FF, Schwarzer R. Stage-specific effects of an action control intervention on dental flossing. Health Educ Res 2007;22:332–341.
5. Schüz B, Wiedemann A U, Mallach N, Scholz U. Effects of a brief behavioural intervention for dental flossing: RCT on planning when, where and how. J Clin Periodontol 2009;36:498–505.
6. Sniehotta FF, Soares VA, Dombrowski SU. Randomised controlled trial of a one-minute intervention changing oral self-care behaviour. J Dent Res 2007;86:641–645.
7. Sniehotta FF. Towards a theory of intentional behaviour change: Plans, planning, and self-regulation. Br J Health Psychol 2009;14:261–273.
8. Staehle HJ. Das aktive Mundgesundheitsverhalten in Deutschland und in der Schweiz [Active oral health behavior in Germany and Switzerland]. Schweiz Monatsschr Zahnmed 2004;114:1236–1251.

3 Cariostatic mechanisms of action of fluorides

Adrian Lussi

■ Introduction

Various authors have shown that the decrease in caries observed in the industrialized countries during the past few decades is due to the use of fluorides. The most significant factor is local fluoride application, in particular the use of fluoride dentifrice. These studies have shown that local fluoridation is far more important than systemic fluoridation. Other protective and promoting factors have also been identified as significant in the development of caries (Fig 3-1).

The mechanism of action of local fluoridation was investigated by Ogaard et al[12] on sharks' teeth, which are composed of almost pure fluorapatite (FAP) but which nevertheless display only limited resistance to caries. The addition of small quantities of dissolved fluoride to the solution surrounding the tooth significantly inhibited the demineralization. It was concluded from this and other studies that the bound fluoride in the form of fluoride apatite has only minimal caries-protective potential, yet the dissolved fluorides surrounding the crystals are effective in both promoting remineralization and inhibiting demineralization.

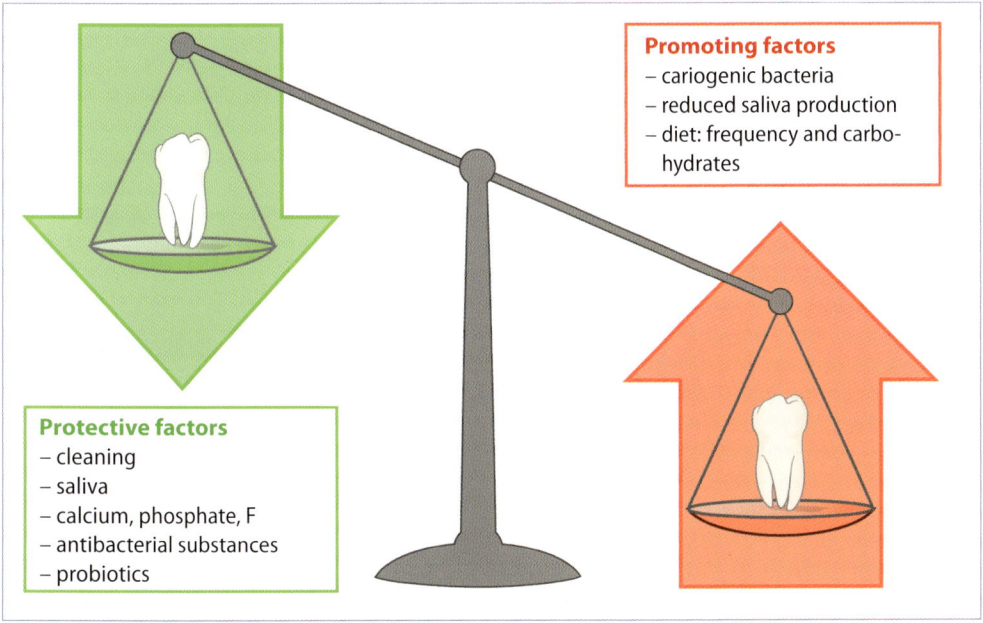

Fig 3-1 **The caries balance:** *protective and promoting factors that influence the balance between demineralization and remineralization (adapted from Featherstone[5]).*

Aspects of prevention

Chemical properties of enamel and dentin

Dental enamel consists of (by volume) 86% mineral, 12% water, and 2% organic matrix or proteins;[16] dentin comprises 45% mineral, 30% organic matrix, and 25% water. The larger part of the inorganic, crystalline phase of dental enamel is formed by calcium phosphates, which can exist in various forms. Hydroxyapatite (HAP) is the lowest-energy and most stable form of calcium phosphate and is characterized by a relatively high level of hardness and low solubility.

Enamel is not a pure HAP. The nature of the variation is dependent on the ionic composition and the degree of saturation of the fluid surrounding the tooth. Ion exchange can take place pre-eruption with tissue fluid, and also posteruption with oral and plaque fluid. These variations from pure HAP result in changes in important characteristics of enamel, such as solubility and crystal size. The incorporation of hydrogen phosphate, carbonate, or magnesium ions into the HAP mesh leads, for example, to a less stable, more readily soluble apatite. Enamel is a calcium-deficient HAP modified with other ions (Fig 3-2). In this connection, the increased carbonate content of dentin (5.5%) compared with enamel (3%) is worth mentioning because it results in crystals in the dentin that are more vulnerable to acid. Fluoride ions can be incorporated into the crystalline mesh to a small extent instead of OH groups and bring about a certain stabilization of the apatite structure.

In healthy human dental enamel, fluoridated hydroxyapatite (FHAP) is present alongside HAP. By contrast, there is virtually no FAP present. Studies have shown that on average less than 10% of OH groups are substituted by fluoride in the outermost layer of enamel. This proportion falls when a depth of 50 μm is reached.

Hydroxyapatite:	$Ca_{10}(PO_4)_6(OH^-)_2$
Enamel:	$Ca_{10-x}Na_q(PO_4)_{6-y}(CO_3)_z(OH^-)_{2-u}F_u$
Dentin:	like enamel but higher proportion of carbonate, which results in smaller crystals more vulnerable to acid

Fig 3-2 Formulae of hydroxyapatite and the crystals of enamel and dentin.

Acid attack

In a stable state, there are sufficient Ca^{2+}, PO_4^{3-} and OH ions in the immediate vicinity of the crystals to ensure that the enamel crystals are in balance with the surrounding fluid. During cariogenic acid attack, organic acids are formed from sugars by plaque bacteria, and H^+ ions are released as a result of their dissociation. Owing to the increased H^+ concentration (low pH) in the plaque fluid surrounding the tooth, the OH^- concentration falls, which leads to dissolution of the crystal, for reasons of homeostasis. Furthermore, the H^+ ions protonize phosphate ions (PO_4^{3-}) in the plaque fluid to HPO_4^{2-} and to $H_2PO_4^-$, which results in a lower PO_4^{3-} concentration. To establish homeostasis, phosphate ions (PO_4^{3-}) are released from the tooth. This process – also in order to maintain neutrality – leads to the release of calcium from the dental hard tissue; the tooth dissolves.

The dynamics of this dissolution process depend on the composition of the enamel, dentin, and cementum crystals, but the fluid surrounding the tooth also plays an important role. This situation explains the differing critical pH values for enamel (approx. 5.5) and dentin (approx. 6.3) for caries, and also the variations between patients because the calcium and phosphate concentrations in plaque can differ from patient to patient. In the case of direct dissolution of the teeth in terms of erosion, it is not the pH and the calcium or phosphate content of the plaque fluid that matters but the pH and the calcium and phosphate content of the drink. This is why the "critical" pH in erosion may be significantly lower if, for example, calcium is added to the drink or food (see chapter 19).

■ Promotion of remineralization by fluoride

At a neutral pH of 7, relatively low concentrations of calcium ions or phosphate ions are enough to keep the calcium phosphate phases stable. If the pH falls, for instance due to acid production by plaque, higher calcium ion concentrations are required to prevent dissolution. At a pH of approximately 5.5 and a calcium concentration in the plaque of around 3.5 mmol/l, the solution is undersaturated with respect to enamel, ie, the calcium ion and phosphate ion concentrations in the plaque fluid are not sufficient to maintain enamel in a stable state of homeostasis; dissolution of enamel therefore ensues (Fig 3-3, yellow and red zones). FHAP, on the other hand, still remains stable at lower pH levels; here the undersaturation and the resulting dissolution start at a lower pH of about 4.7. If the pH of plaque fluid is below (Fig 3-3, red zone), supersaturation will appear again as the pH increases, firstly with respect to FHAP; this means that during remineralization, FHAP is re-formed as the first calcium phosphate phase. In the yellow zone (Fig 3-3), enamel continues to dissolve as before, whereas FHAP is formed in the presence of fluoride. Consequently, redistribution of mineral phases takes place during remineralization after an acid attack as the proportion of stable FHAP in enamel is increased at the expense of carbonate-rich HAP. The proportion of readily

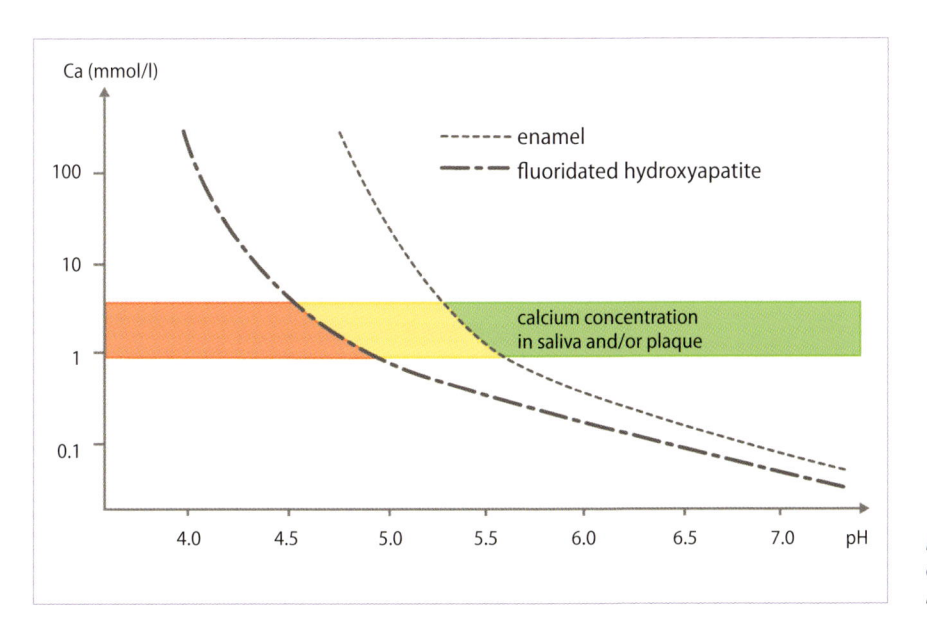

Fig 3-3 **Solubility curves:** *enamel and fluoridated hydroxyapatite.*

Aspects of prevention

soluble calcium phosphate phases is reduced. A demineralized then remineralized enamel is thus slightly more acid resistant than intact enamel. In the remineralization stage, the entry of saliva that contains the remineralizing ions Ca^{2+} and PO_4^{3-} and the presence of dissolved F^- at the enamel surface are particularly important.

In summary it can be stated that, because of its low solubility product even in a slightly acidic pH range, FHAP is re-formed earlier than the other calcium phosphate phases of enamel, which means that fluoride accelerates and promotes remineralization.

The fluoride content is lower in native enamel than in enamel that has been demineralized and subsequently remineralized. This has been demonstrated by the example of the white spot (initial lesion).[19] Figure 3-4 shows the different areas of a white spot. In the surface area (B) Weatherell et al[19] found greatly increased F^- concentrations of over 1,100 ppm, whereas a concentration of 450 ppm was measured in the area of the healthy enamel surface (A). Towards the center of the lesion (C) the fluoride concentration fell to around 150 ppm, as it did in the deeper layers of enamel, where it was only around 100 ppm. This means that healthy enamel compared with pure fluoride apatite has around 2% bound fluoride. Under ideal remineralization conditions this percentage can rise to around 10% in the surface of an initial lesion.

The increased fluoride concentration in the superficial area of the white spot is partly due to the promotion of remineralization by fluoride, ie, due to the formation of the fluoride-rich apatite FHAP (see Fig 3-4), and partly to increased F^- absorption caused by the porous surface of the white spot.[7] Remineralization is enhanced by partially demineralized crystals which, in the presence of fluoride, act as a nucleus for the deposition of new mineral. As outlined above, fluoride speeds up this process because remineralization is possible even at a lower pH level. The consequence is a surface mineral layer that is fluoride-rich, low in carbonate, and acid resistant (Fig 3-5). This is why cleanable initial lesions should not be treated operatively (see chapter 3).

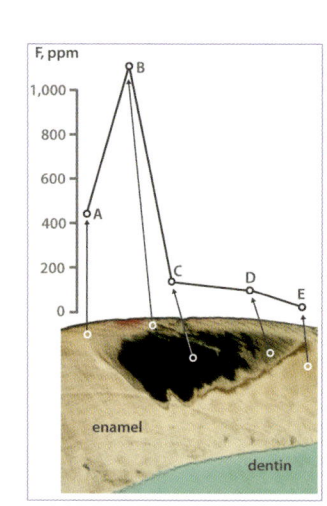

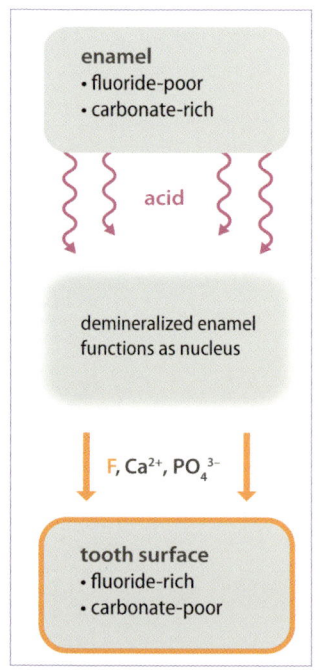

Fig 3-4 Fluoride content of healthy enamel and different areas of a white spot (initial lesion) (adapted from Weatherell et al[19]).

Fig 3-5 Overview of demineralization and remineralization processes (adapted from Featherstone[5]).

■ Inhibition of demineralization by fluoride

Based on numerous studies, it has been fully documented that the incorporation of fluorides into the mineral portions of enamel only reduces the solubility by a minimal amount.[1,18] Small amounts of dissolved fluorides in the vicinity of a tooth inhibit demineralization more effectively than a high FHAP content in the enamel.

Ogaard et al[12] showed that the presence of dissolved fluorides in the vicinity of the enamel crystals has a far greater caries-protective potential than a high FAP content in the enamel mineral. The authors used shark tooth enamel, which is almost pure FAP. By comparison, healthy human dental enamel contains far less F-, which is found predominantly in the outermost layer. In shark tooth enamel, for a fluoride content of 32,000 ppm, over 90% of the OH- sites are substituted by F-, whereas in human enamel only about 2% of the OH- sites are substituted by fluoride. Despite this wide difference in the content of the two types of enamel, their caries resistance does not differ significantly in response to acid attack. In an in-vivo part of the above study,[12] shark and human dental enamel was mounted in a removable appliance which was additionally fitted with plaque-retentive components. Carious lesions were formed in both shark and human enamel, and while the lesion depth was smaller in the shark tooth enamel, the difference was clinically insignificant. In another part of the study it was shown that the mineral loss was even less in human enamel than in shark enamel when the test subjects with the human enamel samples were rinsed daily with a 0.2% NaF solution. The theory that the dissolved fluorides in the solution surrounding the tooth play a far more important role in caries prevention than the fluorides incorporated into enamel crystal was thereby proven (Fig 3-5).

In this connection, it is worth mentioning the fact that dentin requires a markedly higher fluoride concentration in the surrounding fluid than enamel if equivalent inhibition of demineralization is to be achieved. This is significant for the prophylaxis of root caries. Baysan and coworkers[2] showed that a highly concentrated dentifrice (Duraphat® 5,000 ppm), if used at least daily, remineralizes initial root caries (Fig 3-6).

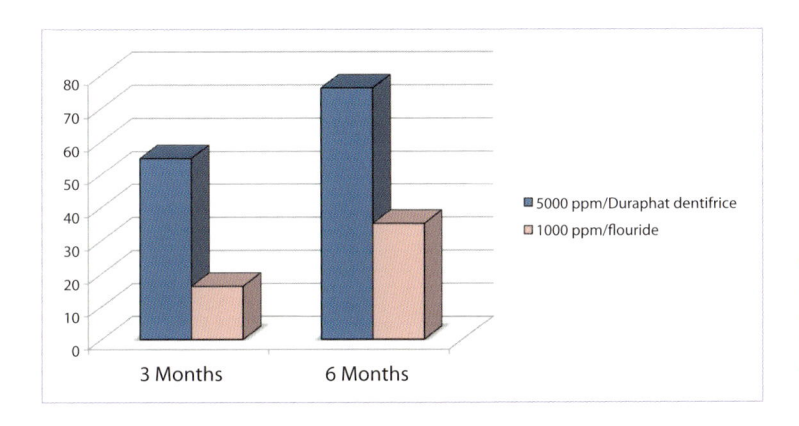

Fig 3-6 Hardness of initial root caries lesions after 3 and 6 month's use of Duraphat® fluoride 5,000 ppm dentifrice compared with a cosmetic dentifrice with 1,100 ppm fluoride[2].

■ Adsorbed and incorporated fluorides

The fluorides adsorbed on the surface of the enamel crystals are held to be mainly responsible for caries prevention. The ionic processes during caries are comparable to a dynamic balance between the fluorides adsorbed on the crystal surface and the dissolved fluorides. If the surface of the enamel crystals is completely covered with adsorbed fluorides, inhibition of demineralization is maximized. In the uncovered areas, on the other hand, the enamel crystal may be locally dissolved if subjected to acid attack. The destruction due to acid attack depends on the pH, the concentration of adsorbed fluorides, and the degree of saturation of the solution. By contrast, the quantity of fluoride incorporated into the enamel crystal plays only a minor role. These small fluoride concentrations are also important after consumption of foods prepared with salt, although the fluoride content in saliva is only increased for about 30 minutes.

■ Calcium fluoride (CaF_2)

CaF_2 is today regarded as another significant factor in caries prevention. Human saliva is usually saturated with calcium. This means that when topicals containing F^- are used, CaF_2 is precipitated and a precipitate is formed on the tooth surface. Many authors talk about CaF_2-like material because it is not pure CaF_2 but also contains phosphates, proteins, and other constituents which stabilize the precipitate and make it more resistant to acid.

This stability is based on the adsorption of hydrogen phosphate ions (HPO_4^{2-}) on the surface of the CaF_2 crystals, giving rise to a protective layer that inhibits solubility. In the case of carious attack, F^- ions are released from the CaF_2 depot because of the reduced HPO_4^{2-} ion concentrations in the surrounding solutions at acidic pH levels. CaF_2 consequently functions as a pH-regulated F^- reservoir which releases F^- in the presence of carious acid attack or low pH, and it remains stable on the enamel surface in the neutral pH range. As a result of these mechanisms, CaF_2 is regarded as the main supplier of free F^- ions during carious attack. The released F^- ions inhibit demineralization on the one hand and have a promoting effect on remineralization on the other. These results clearly show that the ion activity of free F^- ions during carious attack is of far greater significance than a high F^- content in enamel crystal.[6] These findings explain the intention of wanting to increase CaF_2 formation on the tooth surface after relatively brief contact with topicals. A reduced pH, increased F^- concentrations, and lengthened exposure times have proved effective measures in increasing the deposition of CaF_2.[14,15]

Under scanning electron microscopy, CaF_2 has the appearance of globules which can vary in terms of size and quantity. It has been shown that slightly acidic dentifrices with a reduced F^- content have just as good a clinical effect as neutral dentifrices with a higher fluoride content. By contrast, CaF_2 formation on healthy enamel after application of neutral F^--containing rinses is low.[3,8] In clinical trials Ogaard et al[10,11] investigated the retention of CaF_2 on healthy enamel after use of conventional fluoride preparations. After a single application of 2% NaF, a 142% increase in deposited fluoride was found after 15 minutes and this was still 33% 2 weeks after the treatment. The highest F^- content on the enamel surface was observed after application of Duraphat varnish; F^- retention after rinsing with 0.05% NaF solutions was lower.

Rinsing and teeth cleaning

Studies in the 1990s showed that around 20% more caries was found when copious rinsing took place after teeth cleaning than with other rinsing methods.[4,13,17] It was later demonstrated in a prospective study with supervised teeth cleaning that rinsing does not have the adverse effect that was previously suspected.[9] The same facts were also demonstrated with respect to prevention of interproximal caries. The recommendation to rinse thoroughly with just a little water means that a caries-reducing effect is achieved and, at the same time, the majority of the dentifrice with its numerous additives is spat out.

Recommendations on the use of fluoride
- Clean the teeth twice a day with a fluoride dentifrice (before going to bed and after eating).
- Use a little water to rinse out dentifrice after teeth cleaning.
- If there is an increased risk of caries, use fluoride varnishes or a more highly concentrated dentifrice (5,000 ppm).
- If erosion rather than caries is the main problem, see chapter 19.

Conclusions

The cariostatic action of fluorides is based on the effects of the free fluoride ions in solution, which bring about inhibition of demineralization and promote remineralization while also performing an important function in the formation of CaF_2. As topically applied fluoride (eg, F^- dentifrices, F^- rinses, fluoridated salt) can only work for a limited period of time, life-long continuous F^- supply is important.

Bearing in mind that the decrease in the incidence of caries occurred at the same time as the use of F^- dentifrices became widespread, it seems reasonable to conclude that optimum caries inhibition can be achieved by regular F^- application, which intervenes in the demineralization and remineralization involved in the carious process.

References

1. Arends J, Christoffersen J. The nature of early caries lesions in enamel. J Dent Re 1986;65:2–11.
2. Baysan A, Lynch E, Ellwood R, Davies R, Petersson L, Borsbomm P. Härtung initialer Wurzelkariesläsionen nach Anwendung zweier Zahnpasten mit 5000 ppm oder 1100 ppm Fluorid. Caries Res 2001;35:41–46.
3. Bruun C, Givskov H. Formation of CaF on sound enamel and in caries-like lesions after different forms of fluoride application *in vitro*. Caries Res 1991;25:96–100.
4. Chesters RK, Huntington E, Burchell CJ, Stephen KW. Effect of oral care habits on caries in adolescents. Caries Res 1992;26:299–304.
5. Featherstone JDB. The science and practice of caries prevention. JADA 2000;131:887–889.
6. Fejerskov O, Thylstrup A, Larsen MJ. Rational use of fluorides in caries prevention. A concept based on the possible cariostatic mechanisms. Acta Odontol Scand 1981;39:241–249.
7. Hallsworth AS, Weatherell JA, Robinson C. Fluoride uptake and distribution in human enamel during caries attack. Caries Res 1975;9:294–299.
8. Harding AM, Zero DT, Featherstone JDB, McCormack SM, Shields CP, Proskin HM. Calcium fluoride formation on sound enamel using fluoride solutions with and without lactate. Caries Res 1994;29:1–8.
9. Machiulskiene V, Richards A, Nyvad B, Baelum V. Prospective study of the effect of post-brushing rinsing behavior on dental caries. Caries Res 2002;36:301–307.
10. Ogaard B, Rölla G, Helgeland K. Uptake and retention of alkali soluble and alkali insoluble fluoride in sound enamel *in vivo* after mouthrinses with 0.05% or 0.2% NaF. Caries Res 1983;17:520–524.
11. Ogaard B, Rölla G, Helgeland K. Fluoride retention in sound and demineralized enamel *in vivo* after treatment with a fluoride varnish (Duraphat). Scand J Dent Res 1984;92:190–197.
12. Ogaard B, Rölla G, Ruben J, Dijkman T, Arends J. Microradiographic study of demineralization of shark enamel in a human caries model. Scand J Dent Res 1988;96:209–211.
13. O'Mullane DM. The changing patterns of dental caries in Irish schoolchildren between 1961 and 1981. J Dent Res 1997;90 (Spec Iss):1317–1320.
14. Saxegaard E, Rölla G. Fluoride acquisition on and in human enamel during topical application *in vitro*. Scand J Dent Res 1988a;96:523–535.
15. Saxegaard E, Rölla G. Dissolution of calcium fluoride in human saliva. Acta Odontol Scand 1988b;46:355–359.
16. Schroeder HE. Orale Strukturbiologie, 4. überarbeitete Aufl. Thieme, Stuttgard/New York, 1992; pp 73ff.
17. Sjörgen K, Birkhed D. Factors related to fluoride retention after tooth-brushing and possible connection to caries activity. Caries Res 1993;27:474–477.
18. ten Cate JM, Duijsters PPE. Influence of fluoride in solution on tooth demineralization. I. Chemical data. Caries Res 1983;17:193–199.
19. Weatherell JA, Deutsch D, Robinson C, Hallsworth AS. Assimilation of fluoride by enamel throughout the life of the tooth. Caries Res 1977;11 (suppl 1):85–89.

4 The role of xylitol in caries prevention

Svante Twetman

■ Introduction

Xylitol is a naturally occurring 5-carbon sugar alcohol that has become the subject of controversy in caries prevention (Fig 4-1). Although positive results have been achieved worldwide in a number of field trials, the acceptance of its effectiveness is not universal. In fact, two systematic reviews of the literature have concluded that the evidence for a caries-preventive effect is insufficient or inconclusive.[2,7] It is however important to keep in mind that lack of evidence is not the same as lack of effect. Inconclusive or insufficient evidence is most often due to the fact that studies are lacking or that the existing research is compromised by bias or confounders. Moreover, results based on group levels are not directly applicable on the individual patient. The "best available evidence" is only one of the cornerstones in evidence-based medicine, which should always be weighed together with the clinician's skill and experience as well as the patient's needs and demands. This section reviews the evidence for the role of xylitol in the non-surgical management of dental caries.

■ The role of xylitol in the caries balance

It is well known that sucrose is a major player in caries aetiology, driving the oral biofilm to an ecological collapse with a subsequent overgrowth of acidogenic and acid-tolerating bacteria. Since the per capita consumption average of sugar is approximately 40 to 60 kg per year in industrialized countries, it could be beneficial to replace some of the sugar with a non-cariogenic substitute. Xylitol may influence the oral ecology through a different chain of antibacterial events:[14]

1. Xylitol hampers bacterial metabolism and diminishes the pH drop in the dental plaque. The polyol is incorporated by oral bacteria through the fructose-specific phosphotransferase system and phosphorylated to xylitol-5-phosphate, which is a toxic end-product. Only very few oral species can use this substance for energy production.
2. Xylitol reduces the volume and amount of supragingival plaque due to a reduced production of extracellular polysaccharides and biofilm matrix.
3. Xylitol promotes the selection of xylitol-resistant mutans streptococci which are thought to be less virulent and adherent than xylitol-susceptible strains.
4. Xylitol exerts a stimulating effect on saliva secretion.

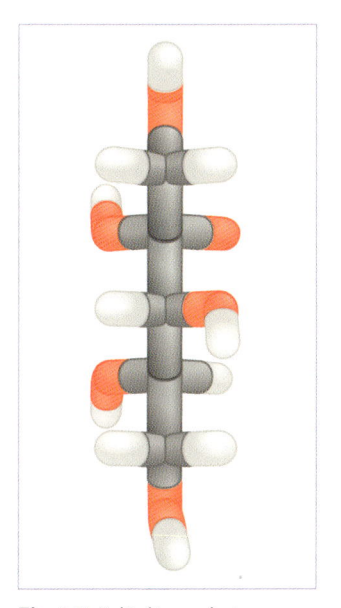

Fig 4-1 *Xylitol is a caloric 5-carbon sugar (sugar alcohol) with similar sweetness to sucrose.*

Collectively, these properties suggest that xylitol may have a unique and dual impact on the caries balance by decreasing the acid challenge on the pathological side and by enhancing the antibacterial action on the protective side.[5]

■ What is the clinical evidence?

There are several reviews available on the caries-preventive efficacy of xylitol, but the conclusions differ in substantial ways. While some conclude that xylitol is superior to other polyols and has an important role in caries prevention,[3,10] others claim that the beneficial effects are primarily based on saliva stimulation.[11] The conflicting statements can be traced to different opinions on how findings from non-randomized or quasi-randomized investigations should be graded. Many of the initial xylitol studies were field projects based on cohorts with quite remarkable results. For example, the pioneering trial "The Turku Sugar Studies" in 1975 presented an almost complete eradication of caries increment over 25 months after "total" sugar replacement. Likewise, later studies conducted in high caries populations in developing countries indicated that caries lesions actually could be reversed. Thus, when the results from the early randomized controlled and observational studies are compiled, a caries prevention proportion of almost 60 % is calculated.[4] A somewhat more cautious figure emerges however when data from the major clinical trials from the present decade are taken into account (Fig 4-2). All trials presented results in favor of xylitol, although the difference between test and control groups was not always statistically significant. The mean prevented proportion was 35 %. However, few studies were placebo-controlled and as comparisons between intervention and no-treatment groups have a tendency to overestimate the treatment effect, it is likely that the true caries preventive effect is lower. Nevertheless, a very conservative conclusion from the recent trials would be that a beneficial effect of xylitol on caries development in children and young adults cannot be excluded. Notably, few studies have been conducted in adults or elderly, which means that there is a lack of knowledge on the efficacy of xylitol regimes in those age groups.

■ Side effects of xylitol

It is commonly established that very high single doses (50–60 g/day) of xylitol can result in osmotic diarrhea, which can be prevented through a slow and step-wise introduction together with fractioned doses. Reports on adverse effects from clinical trials are however

Table 4-1 Dose response to xylitol consumption. MS = mutans streptococci

Desired clinical effect	Daily xylitol dose
Affects vertical mother-child transmission of MS	3–5 g/day
Affects MS metabolism and colonization	6–10 g/day
Reduces the volume of plaque	10–15 g/day

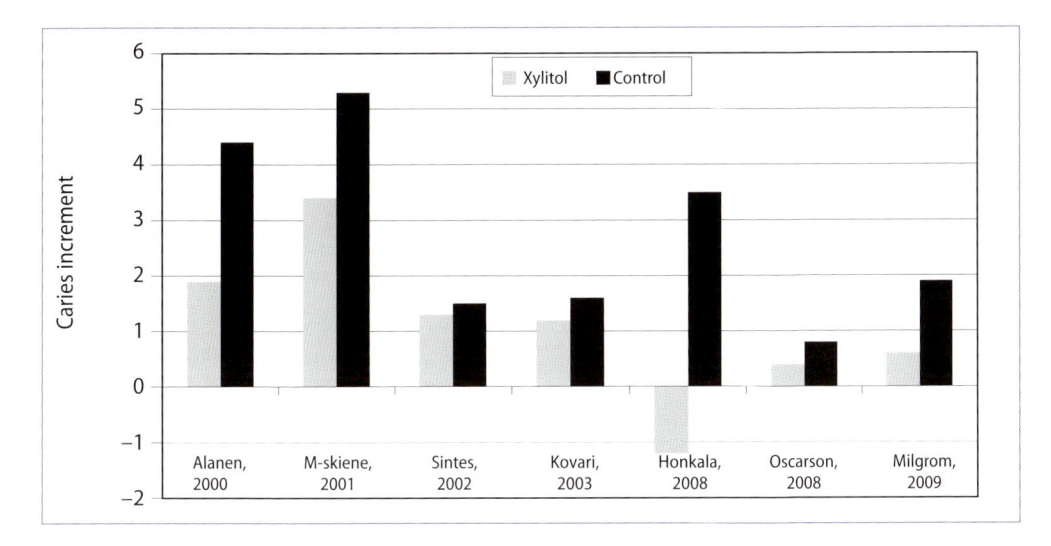

Fig 4-2 Caries increment in recent clinical trials comparing xylitol intervention with a control group. For more detail, see Twetman[16].

very scarce, indicating that xylitol is well accepted by the patients. However, according to EU regulations, xylitol should be avoided in small children since bulk sweeteners, among them sugar alcohols, in food and drinks are not recommended for children under the age of 3 years.

■ How much xylitol is needed to control caries?

The pioneering studies with xylitol utilized high daily doses but the trend has moved to lower amounts. From recent studies it has become evident that a dose-response relationship exists and that the frequency of administration could affect the outcome.[12] Moreover, different daily doses may exert different clinical effects as shown in Table 4-1. Thus, the recommended daily dose may vary from 3 to 15 g per day. It is possible that a frequent low dose of xylitol, such as from dentifrice, may be beneficial, but it is not possible to conclude definitively based on the existing literature. It is recommended that xylitol be administered in 3 or 4 doses per day in order to decrease the risk of possible adverse effects.

■ Is the use of xylitol feasible from a cost-benefit perspective?

In evidence-based medicine it is common to calculate the "number needed to treat" (NNT) from randomized controlled trials in order to compare the outcome of various studies. The value is a measure that indicates how many patients need to undergo a defined intervention over a period of time in order to gain one patient free from the disease. For example, the NNT value was 4 in a double-blind randomized trial carried out on the Marshall Islands in which a topical oral syrup containing xylitol was compared with placebo syrup in infants.[13] However, such figures are seldom available from xylitol trials and instead, the number of pieces of chewing gum needed to avoid one cavity can be estimated. Such a calculation based on the 3-year chewing gum trial by Machiulskiene et al[9] revealed that approximately 3,000 pieces of chewing gum would be needed to avoid one cavitated lesion. The direct cost for the gum alone would therefore exceed €250 according to average chewing gum prices. Whether or not the price is affordable can only be decided by the individual patient. As a comparison, one study found that the cost for xylitol-based caries prevention was equal to that of fissure sealants.[1]

■ Which patients benefit from xylitol?

A common recommendation is that xylitol-containing oral products should be included in the armamentarium for preventing caries in patients with high risk or active caries,[8] but there are actually few studies to support this. One recent randomized controlled trial included xylitol among other preventive measures in a 3-year intensive targeted program for adolescents with active caries.[6] The efforts were focused on self-empowerment and healthy behavior. The program resulted in significantly less decay, but the relative impact of the various components of the program remained unclear. A common problem with at-risk patients is that they have a tendency to "not follow the protocol," and studies in caries-susceptible groups often suffer from poor compliance and high dropout rates. Individuals lacking confidence and motivation are probably unlikely to comply with any treatment regimen, and in this aspect xylitol products seem to be no exception.

Other suggested target groups for xylitol-based interventions include frail elderly patients as well as those with mental retardation or a physical disability.[15] In such vulnerable groups, the daily oral care may be difficult to perform adequately and the saliva-enhancing and plaque-reducing properties of xylitol can be a valuable adjunct to other preventive measures. Studies have also indicated that adolescents undergoing treatment with fixed orthodontic appliances may benefit from habitual intake of xylitol-containing lozenges or gum in order reduce risk for white spot lesion development adjacent to the fixed appliances.[15] Xylitol-based interventions have also proven successful in clinical trials with the aim to diminish and delay the early transmission of mutans streptococci from highly colonized mothers to their children.[14] This concept is further elaborated in chapter 7.

■ Are some xylitol products better than others?

Xylitol is available in a wide range of commercial products such as dentifrice, chewing gum, slow-melting tablets, syrup and candy. Although there are no direct head-to-head comparisons available, the current thinking seems to favor chewing gum due to its superior saliva-stimulating capacity. As all self-administered interventions are heavily dependent on compliance, the challenge for dental professionals is to advocate a convenient way to administer xylitol in sufficient amounts. These amounts should be adjusted for different

Table 4-2 Proposed guidelines for patient-based caries management with xylitol products

Patients with an increased risk of caries may be advised to use products containing xylitol in addition to their daily fluoride dose.
At least 3–5 g xylitol per day are required to optimize the beneficial effects on the oral flora in school children and adolescents.
The daily quantity should be divided into three or four doses, eg, morning, mid-day, evening. The exposure time should not be less than 5–10 minutes.
Xylitol products that actively stimulate the secretion of saliva should be recommended.
Recommended products should contain as much xylitol as possible and xylitol as the sole sweetener.

age groups and also realistic from a financial point of view. Products with a high amount of xylitol and with xylitol as the single sweetener should be preferred since a high intake frequency may be a barrier for patients to follow a given recommendation. Unfortunately, there are many low-xylitol products with mixed sweeteners out on the market that are less suitable for clinical use, eg, more than 20 pieces of gum per day would be needed to obtain an appropriate dose.

■ Conclusions and clinical recommendations

There is a good body of evidence that xylitol has antibacterial properties that may alter the oral ecology and reduce caries risk. Recent studies indicate that preventive programs should include as many complementary strategies as possible, especially when directed towards patients with active caries. Therefore, xylitol should be considered as an adjunct to other measures such as fluoride exposure, fissure sealants and dental health education in individuals assessed as being at risk for future caries development or with a proven caries activity. The evidence-based clinical guidelines are summarized in Table 4-2.

■ References

1. Alanen P, Holsti M-L, Pienihäkkinen K. Sealants and xylitol chewing gum are equal in caries prevention. Acta Odontol Scand 2000;58:279–258.
2. Bader JD, Shugars DA, Bonito AJ. A systemic review of selected caries prevention and management methods. Community Dent Oral Epidemiol 2001;29:399–411.
3. Burt BA. The use of sorbitol- and xylitol-sweetened chewing gum in caries control. J Am Dent Assoc 2006;137:190–196.
4. Deshpande A, Jadad AR. The impact of polyol-containing chewing gums on dental caries: a systematic review of original randomized controlled trials and observational studies. J Am Dent Assoc 2008;139:1602–1614.
5. Featherstone JDB. The science and practice of caries prevention. JADA 2000;131:887–899.
6. Hausen H, Seppä L, Poutanen R, Niinimaa A, Lahti S, Kärkkäinen S. Non-invasive control of dental caries in children with active initial lesions. A randomized clinical trial. Caries Res 2007;41:384–391.
7. Lingström P, Holm AK, Mejàre I, Twetman S, Söder B, Norlund A, Axelsson S, Lagerlöf F, Nordenram G, Petersson LG, Dahlgren H, Källestål C. Dietary factors in the prevention of dental caries: a systematic review. Acta Odontol Scand 2003;61:331–340.

8. Ly KA, Milgrom P, Rothen M. Xylitol, sweeteners and dental caries. Pediatr Dent 2006;28:154–163.
9. Machiulskiene V, Nyvad B, Baelum V. Caries preventive effect of sugar-substituted chewing gum. Community Dent Oral Epidemiol 2001;29:278–288.
10. Maguire A, Rugg-Gunn A. Xylitol and caries prevention – is it a magical bullet? Br Dent J 2003;194:429–436.
11. Mickenautsch S, Leal SC, Yengopal, Bezerra AC, Cruvinel V. Sugar-free chewing gums and dental caries – a systematic review. J Appl Oral Sci 2007;15:83–88.
12. Milgrom P, Ly KA, Rothen M. Xylitol and its vehicles for public health needs. Adv Dent Res 2009a;21:44–47.
13. Milgrom P, Ly KA, Tut OK, Mancl L, Roberts MC, Briand K, Gancio MJ. Xylitol pediatric topical oral syrup to prevent dental caries: a double-blind randomized clinical trial of efficacy. Arch Pediatr Adolesc Med 2009b;163:601–607.
14. Söderling EM. Xylitol, mutans streptococci, and dental plaque. Adv Dent Res 2009;21:74–78.
15. Twetman S. Current controversies-is there merit? Adv Dent Res 2009a;21:48–52.
16. Twetman S. The role of xylitol in patient caries management. Oralprophylaxe und Kinderzahnheilkunde 2009b;32:122–127.

Probiotics – a new approach in caries prevention?

Svante Twetman

■ Introduction

Oral infections are among the most common pathological conditions in humans. The oral cavity is sterile at birth and a number of various factors govern the early establishment of the oral biofilm. The decisive factors are genetic disposition, mode of delivery, breeding habits, the type of bacteria that the child is exposed to, and in which order the different types of bacteria are introduced. The composition of the mature and stable plaque is complex and over 900 different species are identified in the oral cavity. The presence of a diversified biofilm is in fact protective against invasions of pathogens and essential for the maintenance of well-being and good health. Many infections in the mouth and in the digestive, urinary, and respiratory tracts are the result of a reduced diversity caused by an uncontrolled overgrowth of pathogenic bacteria. Caries is actually a disease in which aciduric (acid tolerating) microorganisms (eg, mutans streptococci) have an ecological advantage and grow at the expense of non-aciduric strains during periods of low pH in the environment. This shift in the stability of the microflora is usually described by the ecological plaque hypothesis.

Traditionally, interventions against oral infections are based on methods that reduce the amount of pathogenic bacteria, and antibiotics and chlorhexidine are typical examples. The weaknesses of such strategies are that they have a broad-spectrum and non-selective effect with a risk of developing resistant strains. In recent years, an increasing interest has therefore been focused on finding new and complementary techniques. One possible way to influence the formation and composition of the biofilm could be to bring in non-pathogenic bacteria in order to promote and maintain the diversity. In principle, a harmless effector strain is implanted in the host's microflora to maintain or restore a natural microbiome by interference and/or inhibition of other microorganisms. As the oral biofilm composition in infants is immature, it has been suggested that an intake of probiotic bacteria early in life could lead to a permanent colonization, but there are still no good quality studies with a dental focus that supports this hypothesis. In adults, any permanent probiotic biofilm colonization seems unlikely.

Definition and safety

The first probiotic bacteria discovered, *Lactobacillus bulgaricus*, was described by the "father of immunology" *Élie Metchnikoff* in the early 1900s. Probiotics is an antonym of antibiotics and derived from the Greek *pro bios* (for life). The term was first used by Lilly and Stilwell, and since then various definitions have been proposed over the years. The WHO defines probiotics as "live microorganisms which when administered in adequate amounts confer a health benefit on the host".[10] Prebiotics are food additives containing substances that favor the growth of probiotics (eg, fibers and oligosaccharides). There is also a concept called synbiotics, which means food containing a mixture of pro- and prebiotics.

A regular intake of probiotics is classified as safe (GRAS = Generally Regarded As Safe) by food and drug agencies around the world.[2] This is supported by the fact that lactobacilli have been used to preserve and flavor food as long as humanity can be traced back in time. Fermented products have been consumed daily by generations of people without negative side effects. Furthermore, the currently used probiotic strains have been tested for virulence and other risk factors and found to be absolutely safe. No health risks have been linked to overconsumption or during long-term use among immune compromised patients. Certain restrictions, however, are recommended for severely ill patients with a depressed immunologic response, as in the case of HIV and leukemia.

What are the most common probiotic bacteria?

The most common probiotic bacteria belong to the lactobacilli and bifidobacteria groups, which are naturally present in the intestinal flora. Some strains of streptococci and fungi can also be defined as probiotic (Table 5-1). With few exceptions, probiotics are human isolates from healthy individuals and not genetically modified bacteria. A characteristic property is that they are strongly aciduric in order to survive passage through the stomach. For dental applications, strains with a proven efficacy on gastrointestinal conditions are more or less "inherited," and it's unclear if these strains are optimal to combat oral diseases, especially since lactobacilli and bifidobacteria are non-dominant species in the oral cavity. Therefore, intensive research is under way to find the most suitable probiotic candidates for the oral cavity.

Mechanisms of action

Despite intensive research over the years, a detailed understanding of the mechanisms of action is still incomplete. Three main routes can be distinguished:
1. Probiotic bacteria compete for nutrients and binding sites in the biofilm.
2. Probiotic bacteria can produce bacteriocins (eg, hydrogen peroxide and reuterin) that may hamper and inhibit growth of a variety of bacteria.
3. Probiotic bacteria stimulate the specific and non-specific immune response through activation of T-cells and production of cytokines that mediate the inflammatory process.

Table 5-1 Some of the probiotic strains commonly used in commercial and experimental products

Lactobacilli	Bifidobacteria	Others
L. acidophilus	B. longum	Streptococcus thermophilus
L. paracasei	B. bifidum	Streptococcus salivarius
L. plantarum	B. animalis	Saccharomyces boulardii*
L. rhamnosus	B. breve	
L. reuteri		

*also classified as S. cerevisiae

Probiotics can thus influence the ecology of the oral cavity, both locally and systemically; locally through direct contact with the oral mucosa and systemically ("indirectly") via the gastrointestinal tract. In this context it should be noted that approximately 70% of the human immune system is regulated via the intestines. In many cases the term "replacement therapy" is used a synonym of probiotics, but as indicated above, a direct colonization of the oral biofilm is not a prerequisite for probiotic action.

■ Effect on general health

In the commercial marketing of probiotic products, general health-promoting claims such as "increased well-being," "facilitates digestion," "strengthens the immune system," or "reduces allergy risk" are commonly seen. In the scientific community however, the effects are widely debated. It is more or less generally accepted that a daily intake of dairy products with live lactobacilli and bifidobacteria reduces the risk of certain gastrointestinal problems.[3] In addition, a wide range of health effects have been suggested, eg, reduced susceptibility to infections, reduced prevalence of allergies, and lactose intolerance (Table 5-2). The strongest evidence for a therapeutic effect is presently related to infant diarrhea and for the management of diarrhea during treatment with broad-spectrum antibiotics. The potential applications include rheumatoid arthritis, cancer prevention, and irritable bowel syndrome as well as chronic conditions associated with a metabolic syndrome (diabetes, high blood pressure, and elevated levels of blood lipids). However, it is important to stress that probiotic therapy should be regarded as an adjunct rather than an alternative to conventional pharmaceutical treatment.

■ Effects on oral health

The research on probiotics and oral diseases is focused on caries and periodontitis, albeit potentially beneficial effects on halitosis and hyposalivation are also suggested. Studies from Finland have shown that probiotic bacteria can survive and grow in saliva and attach to the oral biofilm.[4] However, it is unlikely that a permanent colonization occurs. Therefore, daily

Table 5-2 Medical applications for different probiotics and their evidence levels

Illness	Probiotic	Evidence level
Acute diarrhea	LAB, bifidobacteria, S. boulardii	High
Antibiotic-induced diarrhea	LAB, v	High
Tourist diarrhea	LAB	Moderate
Allergies, atopic dermatitis	LAB, bifidobacteria	Moderate
Lactose intolerance	LAB, S. salivarius	Moderate
Chronic gastrointestinal infection	LAB	Low
Urinary tract infections	LAB	Low
Otitis media	LAB	Low

LAB = Lactobacilli

and regular consumption of probiotic products is needed in order to maintain the preventive and therapeutic levels that are obtained after 4 to 5 days of ingestion. The optimal dosage to prevent oral disease is not known, so the recommendations from general medicine have simply been transferred to dentistry. Probiotics are commonly available in dairy products but is also marketed in tablets, capsules, and chewing gum. A daily intake of 1 to 2 dl of fluid (eg, yogurt) with approximately 100 million live bacteria per ml is advocated. The corresponding recommendation for lozenges would be two pieces per day. Unfortunately, the term probiotics is loosely defined so there are several products on the market with very limited clinical documentation and only a minute quantity of active bacteria.

Caries

There is evidence to suggest that naturally occurring lactobacilli such as *L. acidophilus* and *L. reuteri* are associated with low caries prevalence in young children, while *Streptococcus mutans* and *Streptococcus sobrinus* are strongly linked to high caries incidence. As early as the 1950s, the Polish microbiologist *Polonskaya* showed that *L. acidophilus* can inhibit the growth of streptococci *in vitro*. Since then, a number of clinical trials have confirmed this event *in vivo*. Regular consumption of probiotic bacteria has been shown to lead to a reduction of mutans streptococci in saliva,[9] but, interestingly, no increase in the number of lactobacilli has been demonstrated. For example, a study by Caglar and co-workers[1] compared the effect of *L. reuteri* either as a lozenge for maximum contact with the oral tissues or through a straw to minimize contact with teeth. The study was placebo-controlled and both methods of administering *L. reuteri* reduced the amount of salivary mutans streptococci, but the inhibition was superior in the lozenge group as they were exposed both locally and systemically. Concerns have been raised that the introduction of homo- and hetero-fermentative lactobacilli could increase acid production in the biofilm, but studies have shown that *Lactobacillus rhamnosus* and *L. reuteri* have a very low metabolic activity when exposed to cariogenic sugars. It is clear that probiotics in dairy products is a successful combination from a cariological point of view because milk-derived products contain ingredients needed to stimulate remineralization (calcium, phosphate, and casein). Many probiotic over-the-counter drinks and yogurts contain excessive amounts of added sugars and should therefore be avoided.

There are still few clinical trials designed to evaluate the effects of probiotics on caries development. In a Finnish study, preschool children were served milk containing *L. rhamnosus* LGG over a period of 7 months, which reduced the risk for caries compared to a control group.[5] The caries incidence at the age of 3 to 4 years was 6% in the intervention group and 15% among children in the control group who received conventional milk. An interesting "side-effect" was that significantly fewer upper respiratory infections were reported as well as a reduced need for antibiotics. A similar study was recently completed in northern Sweden in which preschool children at risk were served milk supplemented by a combination of *L. rhamnosus* LB21 and 2.5 ppm of fluoride.[6] Caries increment was scored on the dentin level. After 21 months, the prevented fraction was 75% compared with a control group who received normal milk. It was also found in this study that significantly fewer antibiotic prescriptions were needed and that there was a lower incidence of middle ear infections. As the study only had two parallel arms due to limited access to potential participants, the beneficial effects of fluoride and probiotics could not be separated from each other.

Periodontitis

Tooth loss due to periodontitis is caused by a bacterial infection that induces chronic inflammation in tooth-supporting tissues. Studies with different probiotic strains, mainly *L. reuteri*, have been clinically proven to inhibit the occurrence of *Aggregatibacter actinomycetemcomitans* and *Porphyromonas gingivalis* in both rats and humans. Dutch researchers have also studied recolonization of pathogenic bacteria in periodontal pockets after surgery and root scaling in dogs. The findings indicated that a topical application of *L. reuteri* during the operation could delay and to some extent prevent the re-growth of bacteria associated with periodontitis.[7] The same probiotic bacterium has been used in a Danish study for the treatment of gingivitis in young adults.[8] Bleeding on probing and the amount gingival crevicular fluid decreased compared with a placebo group, and the levels of the pro-inflammatory cytokines TNF-a and IL-8 were significantly reduced. The study had few participants and a short follow-up, but was a proof of concept that the intake of probiotic bacteria can influence the immune response in the oral cavity.

■ Summary

The interest in probiotics for oral health is increasing because of the proven beneficial effects in the gastrointestinal tract. The results to date suggest that regular consumption or topical treatment with probiotic bacteria can reduce the incidence of caries-associated microorganisms and prevent recolonization by periodontal pathogens. Although the approach seems promising, many questions remain to be answered before any evidence-based clinical recommendations can be formulated.

References

1. Caglar E, Cildir SK, Ergeneli S, Sandalli N, Twetman S. Salivary mutans streptococci and lactobacilli levels after ingestion of the probiotic bacterium Lactobacillus reuteri ATCC 55730 by straws and tablets. Acta Odontol Scand 2006;64:314–318.

2. de Vrese M, Schrezenmeier L. Probiotics, prebiotics and synbiotics. Adv Biochem Engin/Biotechnol 2008;111: 1–66.

3. Doron S, Gorbach SL. Probiotics: their role in the treatment and prevention of disease. Expert Rev Anti Infect Ther 2006;4:261–275.

4. Haukioja A, Yli-Knuuttila H, Loimaranta V, Kari K, Ouwehand AC, Meurman JH, Tenovuo J. Oral adhesion and survival of probiotic and other lactobacilli and bifidobacteria *in vitro*. Oral Microbiol Immunol 2006;21:326–332.

5. Näse L, Hatakka K, Savilahti E, Saxelin M, Pönkä A, Poussa T, Korpela R, Meurman JH. Effect of long term consumption of a probiotic bacterium, Lactobacillus rhamnosus GG, in milk on dental caries and caries risk in children. Caries Res 2001;35:412–420.

6. Stecksén-Blicks C, Sjöström I, Twetman S. Effect of long-term consumption of milk supplemented with probiotic lactobacilli and fluoride on dental caries and general health in preschool children: a cluster-randomized study. Caries Res 2009;43:374–381.

7. Teughels W, van Essche M, Sliepen I, Quirynen M. Probiotics and oral healthcare. Periodontology 2000 2008;48:111–147.

8. Twetman S, Derawi B, Keller M, Ekstrand K, Yucel-Lindberg T, Stecksén-Blicks C. Short-term effect of chewing gums containing probiotic Lactobacillus reuteri on the levels of inflammatory mediators in gingival crevicular fluid. Acta Odontol Scand 2009;67:19–24.

9. Twetman S, Stecksén-Blicks C. Probiotics and oral health effects in children. Int J Paediatr Dent 2008;18:3–10.

10. WHO, http://www.who/int/foodsafety/fs_management/en/probiotic_guidelines.pdf

6 Novel methods of promoting remineralization

Klaus Neuhaus and Adrian Lussi

The term "remineralization" describes the restoration to the tooth of ions belonging to the hard dental tissue, which were previously dissolved out of the tooth in phases of demineralization. Whole saliva in itself has a remineralizing effect, being oversaturated with calcium and phosphate ions with respect to dental enamel. As described in chapter 3, in this dynamic balance fluoride acts as a catalyst for remineralization and as an inhibitor of demineralization. However, other substances can also have an influence on the ion balance. Milk proteins occupy a prominent position in this regard.

■ Milk proteins

Milk proteins (peptides) can have a bioactive effect at the tooth level in that they block bacterial deposition by competing for binding sites on the hydroxyapatite; they are responsible for improved buffer capacity in the pellicle; and they prevent demineralization and promote remineralization. Thus they even have a certain anticariogenic potential. Casein is the predominant protein found in milk, accounting for 80%. It is capable of stabilizing calcium phosphate in micelles so that milk can be oversaturated with calcium and phosphate without either being precipitated.

The main fractions of casein in cow's milk are alpha(s)-casein (54%), beta-casein (32%), and a smaller proportion of kappa-casein. These polypeptide chains differ in the arrangement of their amino acids. Alpha(s)-casein can be subdivided into further subtypes, depending on the degree of phosphorylation (presence of phosphate residues within the polypeptide chain). In relation to dentistry, it is worth noting that different caseins, such as alpha(s1)-casein, beta-casein, and kappa-casein, have a strong binding affinity for hydroxyapatite and are hence able to reduce the solubility of hydroxyapatite.[3,20]

Casein makes up the bulk of the protein contained in cow's milk. Casein exhibits strong binding affinity for hydroxyapatite and can reduce its solubility.

Casein phosphopeptide-amorphous calcium phosphate (CPP-ACP)

Although casein has been classified as anticariogenic in several studies, owing to its negative organoleptic properties it has not enjoyed widespread use (eg, in dentifrice), especially since a large amount is required for an anticariogenic effect. By contrast, casein phosphopeptide (CPP) is not subject to these limitations and also presents less allergizing antigens.[1]

CPP makes up about 10% by weight of casein, and as a colloidal complex is small enough to be able to diffuse through enlarged enamel pores, which includes into a white spot. CPP can be produced from casein easily and relatively cost-effectively by enzymatic splitting using trypsin. CPP is processed and obtained by selective precipitation with calcium in the presence of ethanol, by ion exchange, or by ultrafiltration.

Like all caseins, CPP contains Ser(P)–Ser(P)–Ser(P)–Glu–Glu as a characteristic phosphoseryl residue sequence. This amino acid sequence is a region with high negative charge and hence high calcium-binding capacity. As a result CPP displays the remarkable ability to stabilize calcium phosphate, which, as a rule, is practically insoluble. In this state a complex is formed out of CPP and amorphous calcium phosphate (ACP) (Recaldent™). CPP can bind 25 calcium ions, 15 phosphate ions and 5 fluoride ions per molecule.[10] This complex is an ACP nanocluster with four phosphorylated peptides. These prevent agglomeration of calcium phosphate to a critical size, which would be necessary for nucleation, transformation, and precipitation of calcium phosphate salts. Without stabilization of the ACP complex, the local calcium and phosphate ion concentration would induce the formation of tartar.

CPPs also have a systemic effect because, interestingly, they are formed *in vivo* during the digestion of casein in the gastrointestinal tract. Since these peptides are relatively resistant to further proteolytic degradation, they accumulate in the distal part of the small intestine. As a result of the marked increase in the solubility of calcium phosphate, the CPPs lead to improved calcium absorption irrespective of vitamin D status.

Reynolds and colleagues[21] reported that CPP-ACP easily undergoes binding to the tooth surface and the surrounding bacteria in plaque. By this means CPP-ACP leads to a high ACP concentration on the tooth surface. The authors suggested that this localized CPP-ACP can buffer free calcium and phosphate ions under acidic conditions and thereby greatly increase the quantity of calcium phosphate in plaque. As a result, the plaque is oversaturated with calcium and phosphate with respect to dental enamel that the concentration gradient inhibits demineralization of the enamel and promotes remineralization. In the presence of fluoride, CPP and amorphous calcium fluorophosphate (ACFP) are formed. An *in vitro* study recently demonstrated that, at a pH of 4.5 to 5.5, CPP-ACFP has markedly greater remineralization potential than CPP-ACP.[9]

CPP-ACP binds readily to dental enamel and to plaque. There it stabilizes high concentrations of calcium and phosphate ions without precipitation of crystals and tartar formation arising. In the demineralizing environment, the CPP-ACP nanocomplexes become unstable and thus increase the calcium phosphate content of the plaque. The resulting concentration gradient inhibits demineralization and promotes remineralization.

Use of CPP-ACP for caries prevention and treatment of white spot lesions

CPP-ACP nanocomplexes display the ability to promote remineralization and inhibit enamel demineralization *in situ*.[21] The results of *in situ* studies with chewing gum containing the active substance Recaldent™ prove the efficacy of CPP-ACP in respect of the remineralization of initial carious lesions. The addition of CPP-ACP to chewing gums containing sorbitol or xylitol led dose-dependently to remineralization of white spot lesions on palatally borne human enamel samples by as much as 152 % after 14 days' use at a rate of 4-hour daily exposure.[24] In an *in situ* study with Recaldent chewing gum, Iijima et al[13] showed that enamel areas remineralized by CPP-ACP were more resistant to acid attack than enamel areas which had only been remineralized by chewing gum without CCP-ACP. The addition of citric acid to a CPP-ACP chewing gum led *in situ* to significantly greater remineralization than sugar-free chewing gums with citric acid but without CPP-ACP or chewing gums without citric acid but with CPP-ACP.[8] Comparison of the results of a study by Shen et al,[24] in which the enamel samples were *in situ* for 160 minutes over a period of 10 days, with an older publication[14] reveals that the degree of remineralization of artificial initial lesions achieved by sorbitol chewing gums (without CPP-ACP) can be even higher if the samples are left in the mouth continuously for 21 days. This means that a study design with a shorter test period favors CPP-ACP chewing gums, but that a higher level of efficacy of CPP-ACP compared with remineralization by normal saliva is not proven. Another factor that is not sufficiently taken into account is the increase in the saliva flow rate caused by the action of chewing gum. Bots et al[4] measured approximate doubling of the saliva flow rate with eight different chewing gums. By contrast, it was reported by Shen et al[24] that chewing CPP-ACP chewing gums raised the saliva flow rate 4 to 7-fold in 10 test subjects. Bearing this in mind, it is reasonable to assume that CPP-ACP has an additional mechanism of action resulting from a relatively sharp increase in the saliva flow rate.

Other forms of administration of CPP-ACP (mouthwash, lozenge) are also capable of maintaining high concentrations of CPP not only in plaque on the bacterial membrane but also in the intercellular biofilm matrix, so that calcium and phosphate ions are able to diffuse into a white spot because of the increased concentration gradient.[22] The effect of CPP-ACP seems to be concentration-dependent, higher concentrations of CPP-ACP at the tooth surface clearly representing a diffusion barrier to further remineralization processes.[7]

The results of a placebo-controlled randomized study conducted in 47 patients with white spot lesions following orthodontic treatment revealed that there was markedly greater regression of these lesions in the 12-week period in the group who used Tooth Mousse with Recaldent™ in addition to their oral hygiene routine at home with fluoridated dentifrice and monthly prophylactic appointments.[2] The differences from the control group were significant. Particularly in the case of white spots that were clearly visible even without drying, the regression rate (white spots were no longer visible or only still visible after drying) and the conversion rate from active to inactive lesions were significantly higher. After 12 weeks, the proportion of unchanged and regressive white spots was 23% and 78% respectively in the group treated with Recaldent™, whereas it was 40% and 60% respectively in the control group.

There is increasing evidence from clinical trials that proves the efficacy of Recaldent™ in terms of faster and possibly even deeper penetrating remineralization of white spots. This effect also appears to exist as a complementary effect to existing fluoride regimens.

CPP-ACP for erosion

There are limitations to the efficacy of fluorides, especially regarding erosion. In a laboratory experiment, adding CPP-ACP to an erosive sports drink led to significantly less erosion than without the addition of CPP-ACP.[19] In this *in vitro* study, the concentration of CPP-ACP was only 0.09%. A rising pH and a decreasing quantity of titratable acid correlated with increasing CPP-ACP concentrations. Thus the results were comparable to results of other studies investigating the addition of calcium to experimental sports drinks. These drinks resulted in only minimal erosion compared with conventional, commercially available sports drinks.[25] Another casein-calcium phosphate complex (Topacal C-5) was compared with sodium fluoride (NaF, 250 ppm), Topacal and NaF, amine fluoride (AmF, 12,500 ppm), and a control group in an *in vitro* erosion model.[15] After 7 and 14 days, significantly less enamel loss was found by means of profilometry in the group with amine fluoride only, compared with all the other groups. It may be assumed that the affinity of the milk proteins for enamel was reduced because of the low pH of 2.3 in this investigation. This might be why Topacal, either alone or in combination with 250 ppm NaF, was unable to provide any protection against an erosive acid attack. In another *in vitro* study, the effect of GC Tooth Mousse on enamel surfaces previously eroded by apple juice was measured quantitatively by electron beam microprobe and qualitatively by scanning electron microscopy.[27] The CPP-ACP paste led to a minimal, non-significant improvement in the mineral content. After application of the CPP-ACP paste, there were hardly any differences in the erosion pattern compared with the control group using NaCl. By contrast, in an *in vitro* study on teeth treated with 10-times diluted Tooth Mousse, Oshiro et al[17] found markedly less pronounced demineralization patterns than in the control group. Unlike the previous study, in this case the teeth had been treated with Tooth Mousse before they were demineralized. This fact is more suggestive of a protective rather than a therapeutic effect of the CPP-ACP paste.

In contrast to the remineralization of initial lesions due to caries, a possible effect of CPP-ACP in areas of dental erosion is not adequately proven.

■ Other methods of promoting remineralization and inhibiting demineralization

Metallic ions, condensed phosphates

In situ studies have shown that iron can exert a protective effect against caries[16,18] and can prevent demineralization.[6] With regard to erosion, a 10 millimolar iron sulphate mouth rinse was tested on enamel and dentin *in vitro*.[23] While it caused a decrease in surface hardness in the enamel, in the dentin altered by erosion it led to significantly less toothbrush abrasion. Unfortunately, there was no control group receiving fluoride in this study design, which means the study results remain debatable.

Sodium hexametaphosphate, an inorganic condensed linear phosphate which is used as an antioxidant in many foods, also has the effect of inhibiting demineralization. A tin fluoride dentifrice with sodium hexametaphosphate was compared with a sodium fluoride dentifrice over 2 weeks in an *in situ* study.[12] The artificially produced erosion damage was far more pronounced in the group receiving sodium fluoride than in the test group. The binding of sodium hexametaphosphate to free calcium valences in enamel[11] and its deposition in the pellicle[5] might be responsible for some protection against demineralization. However, the extent to which sodium hexametaphosphate provides erosion protection in addition to tin fluoride is unclear.

Proteins with metallic ions can reduce the solubility of enamel. However, possible problems lie in their unpleasant taste and discoloration of teeth can be an adverse effect. Sodium hexametaphosphate might afford erosion protection over and above the effect of tin fluoride. Further studies need to be conducted.

Bioactive glass

Another novel approach to remineralization involves the use of the bioactive glass NovaMin®. This product, licensed by the FDA for the treatment of dentin hypersensitivity, basically comprises calcium sodium phosphosilicate (CSPS) and reacts with water to give off calcium and phosphate ions, which is supposed to stimulate the formation of hydroxycarbonate apatite. It was suggested that CSPS enhances remineralization but does not reduce solubility of hard dental substance *in vitro*.[11] However, there are not yet any published clncal study results on NovaMin that prove its efficacy against caries formation. Such publications should definitely be awaited before any decision is made on whether this material is a meaningful addition to the dental practitioner's arsenal of preventive measures.[26]

> Recommendations on the use of bioactive glass to promote caries-relevant remineralization cannot be made at the present time.

■ Conclusions

With a degree of caution, products containing CPP-ACP can be recommended as remineralizing (not caries-protective!) agents. For patients at risk of caries it therefore seems reasonable to expand the range of treatments by including CPP-ACP in addition to an existing fluoride regimen, dietary guidance, and frequent dental check-ups. In the case of erosion, apart from conventional fluoride applications, mouthwashes containing metallic ions seem to have a positive effect, although the question of permanent discoloration of the teeth has not yet been adequately investigated.

■ References

1. Ametani A, Kaminogawa S, Shimizu M, Yamauchi K. Rapid screening of antigenically reactive fragments of alpha s1-casein using HPLC and ELISA. J Biochem 1987;102:421-425.
2. Bailey DL, Adams GG, Tsao CE, Hyslop A, Escobar K, Manton DJ, Reynolds EC, Morgan MV. Regression of post-orthodontic lesions by a remineralizing cream. J Dent Res 2009;88:1148-1153.
3. Barbour ME, Shellis RP, Parker DM, Allen GC, Addy M. Inhibition of hydroxyapatite dissolution by whole casein: the effects of pH, protein concentration, calcium, and ionic strength. Eur J Oral Sci 2008;116:473–478.
4. Bots CP, Brand HS, Veerman EC, van Amerongen BM, Nieuw Amerongen AV. Preferences and saliva stimulation of eight different chewing gums. Int Dent J 2004;54:143–148.
5. Busscher HJ, White DJ, van der Mei HC, Baig AA, Kozak KM. Hexametaphosphate effects on tooth surface conditioning film chemistry -*in vitro* and *in vivo* studies. J Clin Dent 2002;13:38–43.
6. Buzalaf MA, de Moraes Italiani F, Kato MT, Martinhon CC, Magalhaes AC. Effect of iron on inhibition of acid demineralisation of bovine dental enamel *in vitro*. Arch Oral Biol 2006;51:844–848.
7. Cai F, Shen P, Morgan MV, Reynolds EC. Remineralization of enamel subsurface lesions *in situ* by sugar-free lozenges containing casein phosphopeptide-amorphous calcium phosphate. Aust Dent J 2003;48:240–243.
8. Cai F, Manton DJ, Shen P, Walker GD, Cross KJ, Yuan Y, Reynolds C, Reynolds EC. Effect of addition of citric acid and casein phosphopeptide-amorphous calcium phosphate to a sugar-free chewing gum on enamel remineralization *in situ*. Caries Res 2007;41:377–383.

9. Cochrane NJ, Saranathan S, Cai F, Cross KJ, Reynolds EC. Enamel subsurface lesion remineralisation with casein phosphopeptide stabilised solutions of calcium, phosphate and fluoride. Caries Res 2008;42:88–97.

10. Cross KJ, Huq NL, Palamara JE, Perich JW, Reynolds EC. Physicochemical characterization of casein phosphopeptide-amorphous calcium phosphate nanocomplexes. J Biol Chem 2005;280:15362–15369.

11. Diamanti I, Koletsi-Kounari H, Mamai-Homata E, Vougiouklakis G. *In vitro* evaluation of flouride and calcium sodium phosphosilicate toothpastes, on root dentin caries lesions. J Dent 2011;39:619–628.

12. Hooper SM, Newcombe RG, Faller R, Eversole S, Addy M, West NX. The protective effects of toothpaste against erosion by orange juice: studies *in situ* and *in vitro*. J Dent 2007;35:476–481.

13. Iijima Y, Cai F, Shen P, Walker G, Reynolds C, Reynolds EC. Acid resistance of enamel subsurface lesions remineralized by a sugar-free chewing gum containing casein phosphopeptide-amorphous calcium phosphate. Caries Res 2004;38:551–556.

14. Leach SA, Lee GT, Edgar WM. Remineralization of artificial caries-like lesions in human enamel *in situ* by chewing sorbitol gum. J Dent Res 1989;68:1064–1068.

15. Lennon AM, Pfeffer M, Buchalla W, Becker K, Lennon S, Attin T. Effect of a casein/calcium phosphate-containing tooth cream and fluoride on enamel erosion *in vitro*. Caries Res 2006;40:154–157.

16. Martinhon CC, Italiani Fde M, Padilha Pde M, Bijella MF, Delbem AC, Buzalaf MA. Effect of iron on bovine enamel and on the composition of the dental biofilm formed *"in situ"*. Arch Oral Biol 2006;51:471–475.

17. Oshiro M, Yamaguchi K, Takamizawa T, Inage H, Watanabe T, Irokawa A, Ando S, Miyazaki M. Effect of CPP-ACP paste on tooth mineralization: an FE-SEM study. J Oral Sci 2007;49:115–120.

18. Pecharki GD, Cury JA, Paes Leme AF, Tabchoury CP, Del Bel Cury AA, Rosalen PL, Bowen WH. Effect of sucrose containing iron (II) on dental biofilm and enamel demineralization *in situ*. Caries Res 2005;39:123–129.

19. Ramalingam L, Messer LB, Reynolds EC. Adding casein phosphopeptide-amorphous calcium phosphate to sports drinks to eliminate *in vitro* erosion. Pediatr Dent 2005;27:61–67.

20. Reynolds EC, Riley PF, Storey E. Phosphoprotein inhibition of hydroxyapatite dissolution. Calcif Tissue Int 1982;34 Suppl 2:S52–56.

21. Reynolds EC. Remineralization of enamel subsurface lesions by casein phosphopeptide-stabilized calcium phosphate solutions. J Dent Res 1997;76:1587–1595.

22. Reynolds EC, Cai F, Shen P, Walker GD. Retention in plaque and remineralization of enamel lesions by various forms of calcium in a mouthrinse or sugar-free chewing gum. J Dent Res 2003;82:206–211.

23. Sales-Peres SH, Pessan JP, Buzalaf MA. Effect of an iron mouthrinse on enamel and dentine erosion subjected or not to abrasion: an *in situ/ex vivo* study. Arch Oral Biol 2007;52:128–132.

24. Shen P, Cai F, Nowicki A, Vincent J, Reynolds EC. Remineralization of enamel subsurface lesions by sugar-free chewing gum containing casein phosphopeptide-amorphous calcium phosphate. J Dent Res 2001;80:2066–2070.

25. Venables MC, Shaw L, Jeukendrup AE, Roedig-Penman A, Finke M, Newcombe RG, Parry J, Smith AJ. Erosive effect of a new sports drink on dental enamel during exercise. Med Sci Sports Exerc 2005;37:39–44.

26. Wefel JS. NovaMin: likely clinical success. Adv Dent Res 2009;21:40–43.

27. Willershausen B, Schulz-Dobrick B, Azrak B, Gleissner C. In-vitro-Studie zur Überprüfung einer möglichen Remineralisation durch caseinphosphopeptidhaltige, amorphe Calciumphosphatkomplexe (CPP-ACP). DZZ 2008;63:134–139.

7 Antibacterial agents for the prevention of caries

Svante Twetman and Klaus Neuhaus

▪ Introduction

Caries is the result of acids produced by bacteria that dissolve the dental hard tissues and these bacteria are generally members of commensal microflora. Therefore, an antibacterial approach to prevent and control caries simply by removing bacteria would be logical. However, caries is a multi-factorial disease and a common clinical experience is that antibacterial action is not always followed by a subsequent reduction or arrest of lesion development. When evaluating research, it is consequently important to distinguish between results obtained with clinical or microbial outcomes. The latter are called intermediate or surrogate outcomes since they, at best, may be indicative from an evidence-based point of view. The aim of this section is to review the efficacy of antibacterial agents in preventing and controlling caries and to discuss the possible reasons for the often rather mediocre outcome.

▪ Antibacterial approaches

There are several principle home-based and professional strategies to combat oral microorganisms:

- Exclusion or reduction of fermentable carbohydrates from diet
- Mechanical removal of plaque
- Topical application of antiseptic agents
- Interference with bacterial acquisition and initial oral colonization

Although tooth cleaning is probably the most common way of eliminating bacteria, this aspect will not be further addressed here. Likewise, diet control and possible antibacterial effects of fluoride is beyond the scope of this section. The focus below is on topical applications of chemotherapeutic agents and measures taken to interfere with the initial colonization of caries-associated pathogens in the oral biofilm.

▪ Topical application of antibacterial agents

The most commonly suggested antiseptic agents to prevent and manage caries are chlorhexidine (CHX), povidine iodine (PI), triclosan, and silver diamine fluoride (SDF).

Chlorhexidine

Among the antibacterial agents used in the oral cavity, CHX is considered the gold standard. CHX is available in the form of rinsing solutions, gels, or dental varnishes in various concentrations (0.1–40%, Fig 7-1). CHX rinses are the treatment of choice for plaque control, after surgery, and for temporary support of oral hygiene in medically compromised and disabled patients. After a 0.2% CHX rinse, the bacterial population in plaque and saliva is reduced by approximately 80%.

The drug has a strong affinity for oral structures and interferes with cell wall transportation and the metabolic pathways of susceptible bacteria (Fig 7-2). Chlorhexidine has a general and broad effect on Gram-positive bacteria and mutans streptococci are particularly sensitive. Gram-negative bacteria and lactobacilli are less susceptible and many oral strains are in fact unaffected by CHX.

Long-term use of CHX mouth rinse do not seem to confer any significant changes in bacterial resistance, overgrowth of potentially opportunistic organisms, or other adverse changes in the oral microbial ecosystem. It is however important to stress that the number of bacteria in plaque always returns to baseline within weeks or months after the discontinuation of therapy. Continued use of products containing chlorhexidine for long periods can cause stained teeth, especially on silicate and resin restorations, and a prolonged use can also alter taste sensation.

> The long-term use of CHX products may lead to tooth discoloration, discoloration of composite resin restorations, and impaired sensation of taste.

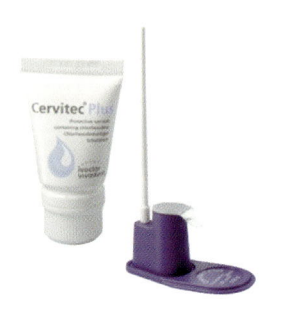

Fig 7-1 A dental varnish containing chlorhexidine for professional topical application.

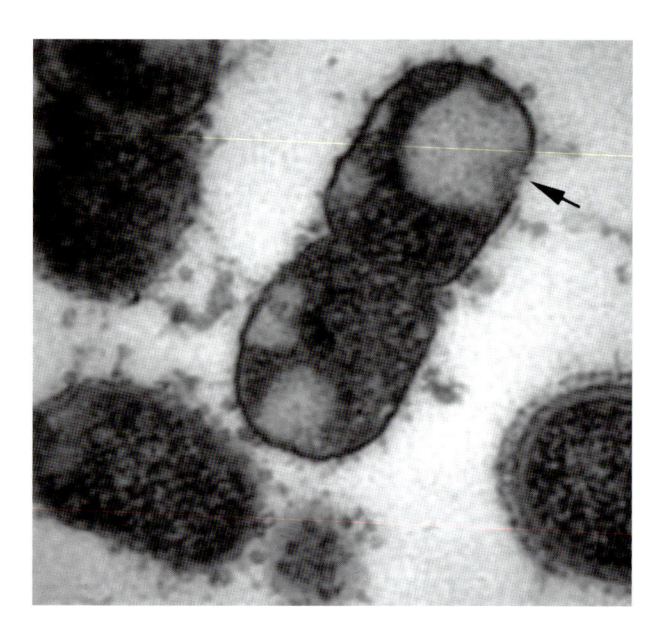

Fig 7-2 Bacterial wall breakdown after 5 min chlorhexidine exposure.

CHX treatments are normally carried out professionally in the dental office but can be self-applied depending on patient motivation and cooperation. The indication is increased caries risk or proven caries activity. The best mode of professional treatment seems to be an intensive regimen with gel in custom-made soft trays, 3 times for 5 minutes for 2 consecutive days. For home-care use, a 5-minute application once a day for 14 days is preferred. Varnishes exert a local slow-release but must be re-applied with regular intervals. Detergents in toothpaste can inactivate CHX and tooth brushing should therefore be separated from the agent by at least 2 hours.

The role of chlorhexidine in caries prevention is controversial.[1] A meta-analysis of the pioneering investigations carried out with CHX-gel applications in custom trays revealed a prevented proportion of 46%, but this figure was likely affected by publication bias since positive and novel findings are more likely to be published than negative. Later reviews on the use of chlorhexidine-containing dental varnishes have resulted in more cautious conclusions indicating a moderate caries-preventive effect, especially in occlusal fissures.[24,30] Based on the available reviews, it can be stated that chlorhexidine rinses, gels, and varnishes, or combinations of these items with fluoride, have variable effects. Due to the current lack of evidence on long-term clinical outcomes and reported side effects, chlorhexidine rinse should not be recommended for caries prevention.[1] The evidence for gels and varnishes are mixed and inconclusive, and further research is therefore warranted.

In long-term clinical trials, the application of CHX does not lead to less caries than the use of fluoride. Based on the data currently available and in view of the known side effects, it should not be advocated as a single measure for caries prevention but may be used on short term basis as an adjunct to fluoride in high-risk individuals. CHX gels or varnishes may be used for root caries, but the published studies on this usage are not conclusive.

Povidone iodine

PI is known to be a powerful broad-spectrum germicidal agent effective against a wide range of bacteria, viruses, fungi, protozoa, and spores. In medicine, PI is commonly used as a skin disinfectant and for the treatment of wounds. A 10% solution can be used for topical oral applications in which the iodine is carried in a complexed form and the concentration of free iodine is very low. PI has primarily been used to combat early childhood caries, but studies have produced contrasting findings. A moderate effect in reducing and suppressing the levels of mutans streptococci in plaque and saliva is evident. While Lopez et al[14,15] reported favorable results in Puerto Rican infants, other researchers have been unable to confirm an additional effect as an adjunct to fluoride and extensive restorative procedures.[26,29] Thus, no firm conclusions on the efficacy of PI in preventing caries can be drawn and its use should therefore be questioned. Restricted use is further justified by the fact that PI may cause skin irritation and severe allergic reactions.

Application of povidone iodine for caries prevention should be avoided due to a lack of evidence of efficacy and because of its known potential side effects.

Triclosan

Another antimicrobial agent that is used against oral bacteria is triclosan (2,4,4'-trichloro-2'-hydroxydiphenyl ether). It is a synthetic broad-spectrum agent with antibacterial and partially antiviral and fungicidal properties, which is used in numerous cosmetics. Triclosan blocks the active center of the enzyme enoyl-acyl carrier protein reductase (ENR), which is essential for bacterial fatty acid synthesis but is not produced by humans. As a result of this enzyme inactivation, triclosan prevents the bacterial synthesis of cell wall membranes. Even small doses of triclosan are enough to block ENR.[19] Recently there have been objections to triclosan as a ubiquitous additive in dentifrice because it was thought to promote antibiotic resistance.[27] In a few Scandinavian countries, the use of triclosan as an additive in cosmetics is prohibited. The evidence that resistance or cross-resistance of clinically relevant microorganisms is in any way due to the use of triclosan cannot be regarded as substantiated. For instance, the Scientific Committee on Consumer Products of the European Union stated that, based on the available information, the use of triclosan in cosmetic products can be regarded as safe and there is currently no evidence of clinical resistance or cross-resistance.[20]

Triclosan/copolymer as an active ingredient in dentifrices has been shown to reduce supragingival plaque and gingivitis in clinical tests.[8] In adult patients, randomized controlled trials using fluoridated dentifrice containing triclosan/copolymer have been performed with the caries increment rate as the outcome. Compared with dentifrice containing 1,100 ppm fluoride[6] and 1,500 ppm fluoride,[16] the addition of triclosan/copolymer did not have an additional anticaries effect, but it also did not diminish the effect of fluoride. However, in a controlled 2-year clinical trial comparing a 2,430 ppm fluoridated dentifrice with and one without triclosan/copolymer, a significantly greater anticaries effect was reported for the triclosan group, which led to a reduction of the caries increment by 12.2 % in the first year and 16.6 % in the second year.[17] After 3 years, 1,357 patients were still included in this study. Analysis showed that there was a significantly smaller caries increment for both root and coronal caries in the group receiving triclosan/copolymer.[25] However, as the published study results cannot be regarded as unbiased, it cannot be proven at present that using dentifrice with triclosan/copolymer causes a decrease in the caries increment rate over and above the result achievable with fluoride.

Triclosan is an antibacterial active substance that is used in dentifrice. An effect exceeding that of fluoride is not proven beyond a doubt.

Silver diamine fluoride

The antimicrobial use of silver compounds has a long history within dentistry and has traditionally been used to halt rampant caries in young children (Howe's solution). The rationale is that Ag^+ can effectively kill bacteria and inhibit biofilm formation at concentrations exceeding 50 ppm. Silver salts are also associated with stimulation of calcified dentin formation. The application of silver salts is simple and inexpensive, but the silver fluoride makes caries lesions stain black, which is an esthetic drawback. A recent systematic review by Rosenblatt et al[18] has examined the clinical evidence for SDF. They identified two studies that met the inclusion criteria and reported a proportion for caries arrest and caries prevention of 96% and 70%, respectively. The staining was troublesome for 7% of the patients and a few experienced transient tissue irritations. The research on SDF is limited to children and there are still many open questions as to whether or not this "historical" therapy to prevent and arrest caries will have a place in future practice.

Silver diamine fluoride may be used in pediatric dentistry. It causes pronounced and irreversible black discoloration of treated teeth.

■ Measures to combat vertical transmission of cariogenic bacteria

The concept of treating parents for the benefit of their offspring' is termed "primary-primary prevention." This has been evaluated in pediatric dentistry with the purpose of combating or delaying the initial acquisition of mutans streptococci. The intervention is most often directed to pregnant women and/or mothers of newborn babies with high counts of salivary mutans streptococci assessed by a pre-study screening. The findings from the major clinical trials are summarized in Table 7-1. Some of the studies were carried out with antiseptic measures as part of a comprehensive program that was compared with untreated controls (no intervention). Some reported only the offspring's mutans streptococci colonization as an intermediate outcome while others focused on caries increment in the primary dentition. Therefore, mixed results were reported; none of the investigations with PI proved to be successful while four of six trials with CHX reported beneficial findings on either bacterial suppression or caries development.

There were two investigations with xylitol that were perhaps the most interesting.[12,23] They tested the hypothesis that the vertical transmission of mutans streptococci could be delayed or hampered by maternal use of xylitol-containing chewing gum during the period of primary tooth eruption. Caries prevalence was scored when the children were 5 and 4 years of age, respectively, and a prevented proportion of 72% was displayed in both projects. The tentative explanation for the beneficial outcome was that the trans-

Table 7-1 Clinical trials on influencing the mother-to-child transmission of caries-associated mutans streptococci (MS)

First author, year published	Intervention group	Control group	Intervention, months	MS (child)	Caries (child)	Age, years
Tenovuo et al (1992)[22]	CHX + F gel	none	12–48	ns	–	4
Dasanyake et al (1993)[3]	povidone iodine	placebo	6	ns	ns	3
Köhler and Andréen (1994)[13]	prev. prog. + CHX	none	3–36	↓	↓	7
Brambilla et al (1998)[2]	F + CHX rinse	F	prenatal	↓	–	2
Isokangas et al (2000)[12]	xylitol gum	CHX/F varnish	3–24	–	↓	5
Söderling et al (2001)[21]	xylitol gum	CHX/F varnish	3–24	↓	–	6
Dasanyake et al (2002)[4]	CHX varnish	placebo	6–36	ns	ns	4
Gripp and Schlagenhauf (2002)[10]	CHX varnish	none	1–24	↓	–	2
Zanata et al (2003)[28]	prev. prog. + iodine	none	prenatal–12	–	ns	2
Thorild (2006)[23]	xylitol gum	CHX/F, gum	6–18	ns	↓	4
Ercan et al (2007)[5]	restoration + CHX/xyl	none	2–36	↓	↓	4
Fontana et al (2009)[7]	xylitol gum	sorbitol/no gus	0–5	ns	–	ns

↓ = statistically significant reduction; ns = statistically not significant

mission of mutans streptococci was decreased by a xylitol-induced shift from "sticky" to less adhesive strains of the caries-associated bacterium. A 10-year follow-up of the pioneering Finnish project has recently been performed. A cost-benefit analysis indicated an average net gain of 3.2 "caries-free years" in the xylitol gum group compared to the controls.

The findings from the Nordic countries were however recently challenged by Fontana et al[7] in which xylitol failed to affect the mother-child transmission of mutans streptococci. This demonstrates that the mother-child approach may not be effective or even applicable everywhere and illustrates the importance of repeating studies in various cultural and socioeconomic settings. At present, the body of evidence of primary-primary prevention of caries is limited, but parents would likely benefit from information on the common routes of transmission and advice on safe handling of pacifiers and baby bottles.

■ Limitations of the antibacterial approach to prevent caries

What is the reason for the limited outcome of the antibacterial measures taken for caries prevention and control? A simple answer would be that neither fluoride nor chemotherapeutics can fully counteract or compensate the carbohydrate (sucrose) challenge that is one key factor in caries etiology. Caries is not a "classic" infectious disease that can be cured with 1 week of antibiotic treatment. It is well known that even extensive efforts to control the disease can fail and, in addition, genetic differences with respect to caries susceptibility may be overlooked.

A more complex answer may be found in recent insights concerning the functions of the oral biofilm. Antibacterial agents, such as CHX and PI, are extremely efficient for skin disinfection and there is no doubt that caries-associated bacteria are also sensitive to these agents, especially in plantonic monocultures using traditional culturing techniques. However, the complex and diverse biofilm in the oral cavity, consisting of over 700 different species, is characterized by an increased tolerance to antibacterial agents,[9] and the effect *in vivo* may, at best, be short term and transient. The reasons for this impaired efficacy in biofilms are not fully known but factors such as inhibition of diffusion, adaption, bacterial cross-talk, reactions to stress, and up-regulation of protein production are likely to play an important role. Another key question is whether or not it is advisable, or even realistic, to try to eradicate certain pathogenic strains from the biofilm. The ecological plaque hypothesis suggests that no single species, not even *Streptococcus mutans*, mediates the initiation or progression of dental caries. It is well established that various bacteria may act "friendly" or "hostile" and oral health is associated with a diverse and balanced microbial community (microbial homeostasis) that is protective against invasions of pathogens. The ecological long-term strategy to combat oral diseases would therefore be to restore the microbial balance rather than removing or killing selective pathogens, especially since the "kill" approach may create sites that are susceptible to a rapid repopulation by the pathogens.[11] Thus, novel antibacterial approaches to modify the oral biofilm diversity beneficially are currently emerging as an alternative to selective killing. Examples are replacement therapy, probiotics, and plant-derived agents and peptides regulating bacterial metabolism. Even if some of these methods will prove promising, the safety and efficacy must of course be established in well-conducted randomized controlled trials.

Caries is a multifactorial disease. The nonspecific killing of bacteria in the mouth cannot be the therapeutic objective. Approaches that influence the ecological balance in the oral cavity, so that a less cariogenic flora can become permanently established, are more promising.

Conclusions

There is insufficient evidence to support and recommend topical applications of antibacterial agents, such as chlorhexidine and povidone iodine, in order to prevent or arrest caries lesions. Although the evidence for various antibacterial measures to combat the vertical transmission of mutans streptococci from mothers to their offspring is still limited, parents of infants and toddlers should be encouraged to reduce behaviors that promote the early transmission of mutans streptococci. It is also clear that any antibacterial treatment should be combined with a fluoride program.

References

1. Autio-Gold J. The role of chlorhexidine in caries prevention. Oper Dent 2008;33:710–716.
2. Brambilla E, Felloni A, Gagliani M, Malerba A, García-Godoy F, Strohmenger L. Caries prevention during pregnancy: results of a 30-month study. J Am Dent Assoc 1998 Jul;129:871–877.
3. Dasanayake AP, Caufield PW, Cutter GR, Stiles HM. Transmission of mutans streptococci to infants following short term application of an iodine-NaF solution to mothers' dentition. Community Dent Oral Epidemiol 1993 Jun;21:136–142.
4. Dasanayake AP, Wiener HW, Li Y, Vermund SV, Caufield PW. Lack of effect of chlorhexidine varnish on Streptococcus mutans transmission and caries in mothers and children. Caries Res 2002 Jul-Aug;36:288–293.
5. Ercan E, Dülgergil CT, Yildirim I, Dalli M. Prevention of maternal bacterial transmission on children's dental-caries-development: 4-year results of a pilot study in a rural-child population. Arch Oral Biol. 2007 Aug;52(8):748–752.
6. Feller RP, Kiger RD, Triol CW, Sintes JL, Garcia L, Petrone ME, Volpe AR, Proskin HM. Comparison of the clinical anticaries efficacy of an 1100 NaF silica-based dentifrice containing triclosan and a copolymer to an 1100 NaF silica-based dentifrice without those additional agents: a study on adults in California. J Clin Dent 1996;7:85–89.
7. Fontana M, Catt D, Eckert GJ, Ofner S, Toro M, Gregory RL, Zandona AF, Eggertsson H, Jackson R, Chin J, Zero D, Sissons CH. Xylitol: effects on the acquisition of cariogenic species in infants. Pediatr Dent 2009;31:257–266.
8. Gaffar A, Afflitto J, Nabi N. Chemical agents for the control of plaque and plaque microflora: an overview. Eur J Oral Sci 1997;105:502–507.
9. Gilbert P, Das J, Foley I. Biofilm susceptibility to antimicrobials. Adv Dent Res 1997;11:160–167.
10. Gripp VC, Schlagenhauf U. Prevention of early mutans streptococci transmission in infants by professional tooth cleaning and chlorhexidine varnish treatment of the mother. Caries Res 2002 Sep-Oct;36:366–372.
11. He X, Lux R, Kuramitsu HK, Anderson MH, Shi W. Achieving probiotic effects via modulating oral microbial ecology. Adv Dent Res 2009;21:53–56.
12. Isokangas P, Söderling E, Pienihäkkinen K, Alanen P. Occurrence of dental decay in children after maternal consumption of xylitol chewing gum, a follow-up from 0 to 5 years of age. J Dent Res 2000;79:1885–1889.
13. Köhler B, Andréen I. Influence of caries-preventive measures in mothers on cariogenic bacteria and caries experience in their children. Arch Oral Biol 1994 Oct;39:907–911.
14. Lopez L, Berkowitz R, Spiekerman C, Weinstein P. Topical antimicrobial therapy in the prevention of early childhood caries: a follow-up report. Pediatr Dent 2002;24:204–206.
15. Lopez L, Berkowitz R, Zlotnik H, Moss M, Weinstein P. Topical antimicrobial therapy in the prevention of early childhood caries. Pediatr Dent 1999;21:9–11.
16. Mann J, Karniel C, Triol CW, Sintes JL, Garcia L, Petrone ME, Volpe AR, Proskin HM. Comparison of the clinical anticaries efficacy of a 1500 NaF silica-based dentifrice containing triclosan and a copolymer to a 1500 NaF silica-based dentifrice without those additional agents: a study on adults in Israel. J Clin Dent 1996;7:90–95.
17. Mann J, Vered Y, Babayof I, Sintes J, Petrone ME, Volpe AR, Stewart B, De Vizio W, McCool JJ, Proskin HM. The comparative anticaries efficacy of a dentifrice containing 0.3 % triclosan and 2.0 % copolymer in a 0.243 % sodium fluoride/silica base and a dentifrice containing 0.243 % sodium fluoride/silica base: a two-year coronal caries clinical trial on adults in Israel. J Clin Dent 2001;12:71–76.

18. Rosenblatt A, Stamford TC, Niederman R. Silver diamine fluoride: a caries "silver-fluoride bullet". J Dent Res 2009;88:116–125.
19. Russell AD. Whither triclosan? J Antimicrob Chemother 2004;53:693–695.
20. Scientific Committee on Consumer Products, SCCP. Opinion on TRICLOSAN. In: European Commission, ed. Brussels: Directorate C - Public Health and Risk Assessment, 2006:1–9.
21. Söderling E, Isokangas P, Pienihäkkinen K, Tenovuo J, Alanen P. Influence of maternal xylitol consumption on mother-child transmission of mutans streptococci: 6-year follow-up. Caries Res 2001 May-Jun;35:173–177.
22. Tenovuo J, Häkkinen P, Paunio P, Emilson CG. Effects of chlorhexidine-fluoride gel treatments in mothers on the establishment of mutans streptococci in primary teeth and the development of dental caries in children. Caries Res 1992;26:275–280.
23. Thorild I, Lindau B, Twetman S. Caries in 4-year-old children after maternal chewing of gums containing combinations of xylitol, sorbitol, chlorhexidine and fluoride. Eur Arch Paediatr Dent 2006;7:241–245.
24. Twetman S. Antimicrobials in future caries control? A review with special reference to chlorhexidine treatment. Caries Res 2004;38:223–229.
25. Vered Y, Zini A, Mann J, DeVizio W, Stewart B, Zhang YP, Garcia L. Comparison of a dentifrice containing 0.243 % sodium fluoride, 0.3 % triclosan, and 2.0 % copolymer in a silica base, and a dentifrice containing 0.243 % sodium fluoride in a silica base: a three-year clinical trial of root caries and dental crowns among adults. J Clin Dent 2009;20:62–65.
26. Xu X, Li JY, Zhou XD, Xie Q, Zhan L, Featherstone JD. Randomized controlled clinical trial on the evaluation of bacteriostatic and cariostatic effects of a novel povidone-iodine/fluoride foam in children with high caries risk. Quintessence Int 2009;40:215–223.
27. Yazdankhah SP, Scheie AA, Hoiby EA, Lunestad BT, Heir E, Fotland TO, Naterstad K, Kruse H. Triclosan and antimicrobial resistance in bacteria: an overview. Microb Drug Resist 2006;12:83–90.
28. Zanata RL, Navarro MF, Pereira JC, Franco EB, Lauris JR, Barbosa SH. Effect of caries preventive measures directed to expectant mothers on caries experience in their children. Braz Dent J. 2003;14:75–81.
29. Zhan L, Featherstone JD, Gansky SA, Hoover CI, Fujino T, Berkowitz RJ, Den Besten PK. Antibacterial treatment needed for severe early childhood caries. J Public Health Dent 2006;66:174–179.
30. Zhang Q, van Palenstein Helderman WH, van't Hof MA, Truin GJ. Chlorhexidine varnish for preventing dental caries in children, adolescents and young adults: a systematic review. Eur J Oral Sci 2006;114:449–455.

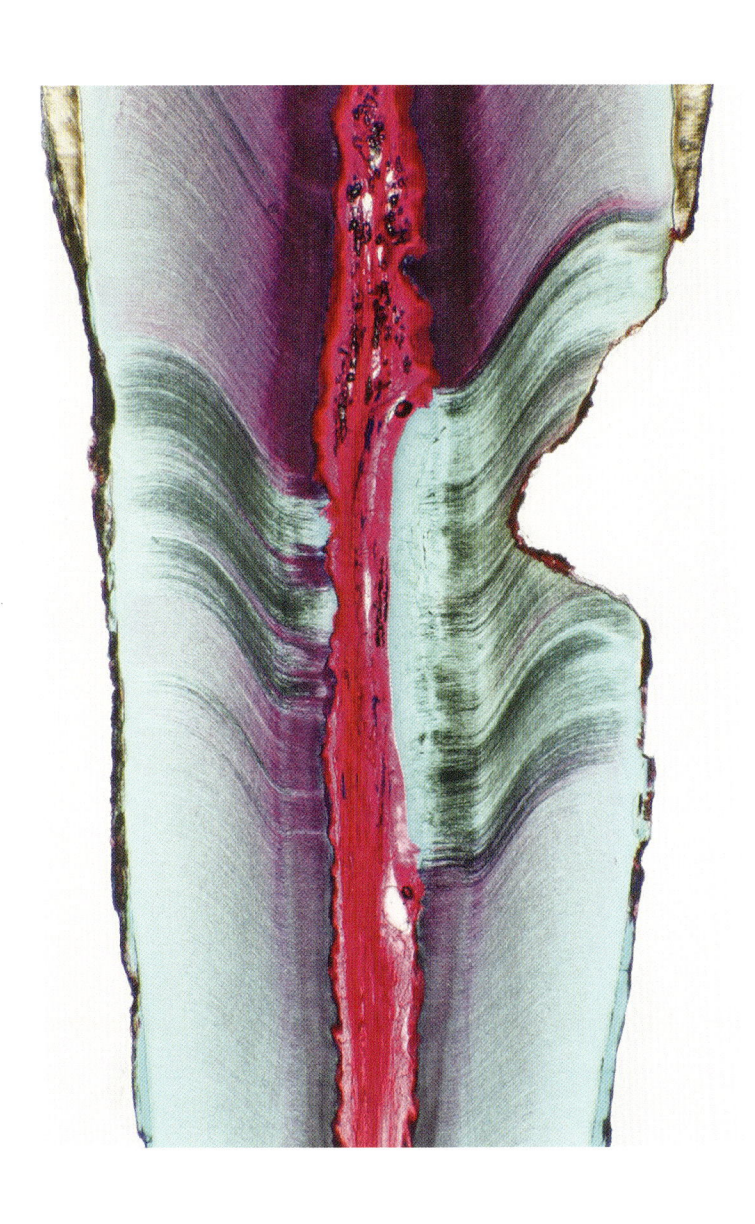

Caries

III

8 Diagnosing caries and caries activity

Adrian Lussi, Markus Schaffner, Jonas Rodrigues, and Klaus Neuhaus

■ Introduction

If a dentition is caries-free or the caries is stable, balance is maintained by mineral loss and mineral gain. If mineral loss predominates, active caries with progression exists, whereas remission is the consequence of a net mineral gain (see chapter 1, Fig 1-26). Caries starts with demineralization of the affected enamel or dentin/cementum surfaces, which is only visible under the microscope. As caries progresses further, chalky changes arise in the enamel, sometimes involving the dentin and finally resulting in breakdown of the surface. It is difficult to diagnose lesions with macroscopically intact surfaces. This chapter explores the problems of diagnosing caries on the various surfaces.

■ Smooth surface caries

Smooth surface caries is rare nowadays in Europe. If oral hygiene is good, it progresses slowly, remains constant, or disappears, as shown in the classic study by Backer-Dirks[1]: with good oral hygiene, over half of the initial lesions (white spots) altered so much after a 7-year observation period that they were classified as healthy in the second examination. As well as remineralization, remission of the decalcification caused by abrasive processes will probably occur. A healthy band of enamel between white spot and gingiva and a shiny and glossy lesion indicate a lengthy inactive phase. Active smooth surface caries borders the gingiva and appears matt and rough (Figs 8-1 to 8-3).

Smooth surface lesions with an intact surface or only localized and small breakdown of the surface are treated by optimized preventive measures, including the application of fluoride. Restoration is only necessary if surface breakdown has occurred.

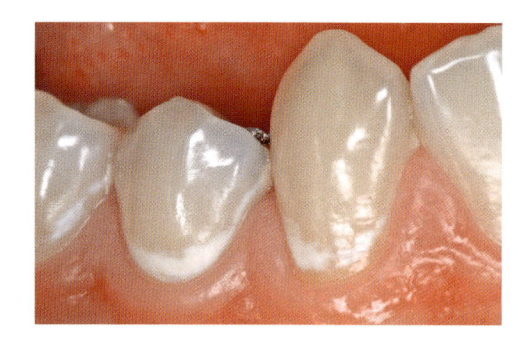

Fig 8-1 Smooth surface caries with intact surface.

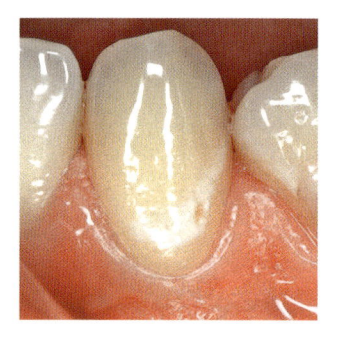

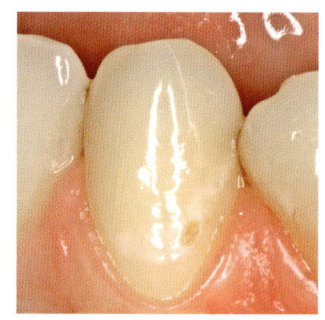

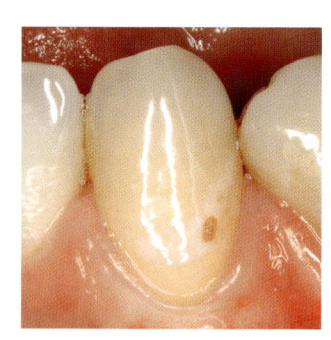

Fig 8-2 Smooth surface caries with local surface breakdown. Left: initial finding. Centre: after 10 years. Right: after 20 years.

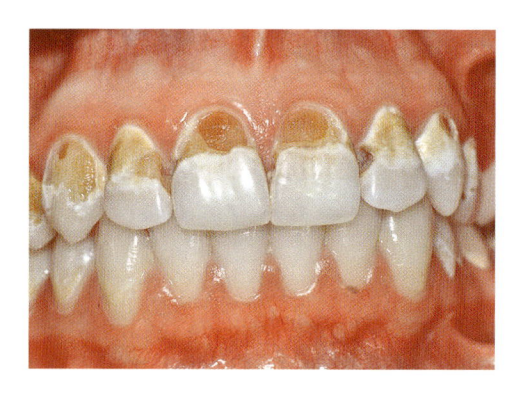

Fig 8-3 Smooth surface caries with pronounced breakdown of surfaces.

■ Pit and fissure caries

Studies have shown that the occlusal surfaces of the permanent molars in children and adolescents are most commonly affected by caries. The proportion of pit and fissure caries in children with minimal caries is between 75% and 92% depending on age. Thus pit and fissure caries is bound to be a common diagnosis. There are various possible reasons for the high caries prevalence in fissures:

- Until final occlusion-finding, an increased accumulation of plaque can be seen in the fissures.
- The enamel is prone to caries in the first few years following eruption. Maturation of enamel involves remineralization and demineralization cycles. The reduced susceptibility of mature enamel to caries is not fissure-specific, but makes a greater impact there.
- The unfavorable fissure morphology prevents adequate cleaning of the fissure base and impedes saliva access (Figs 8-4 to 8-7).

Diagnosing caries and caries activity

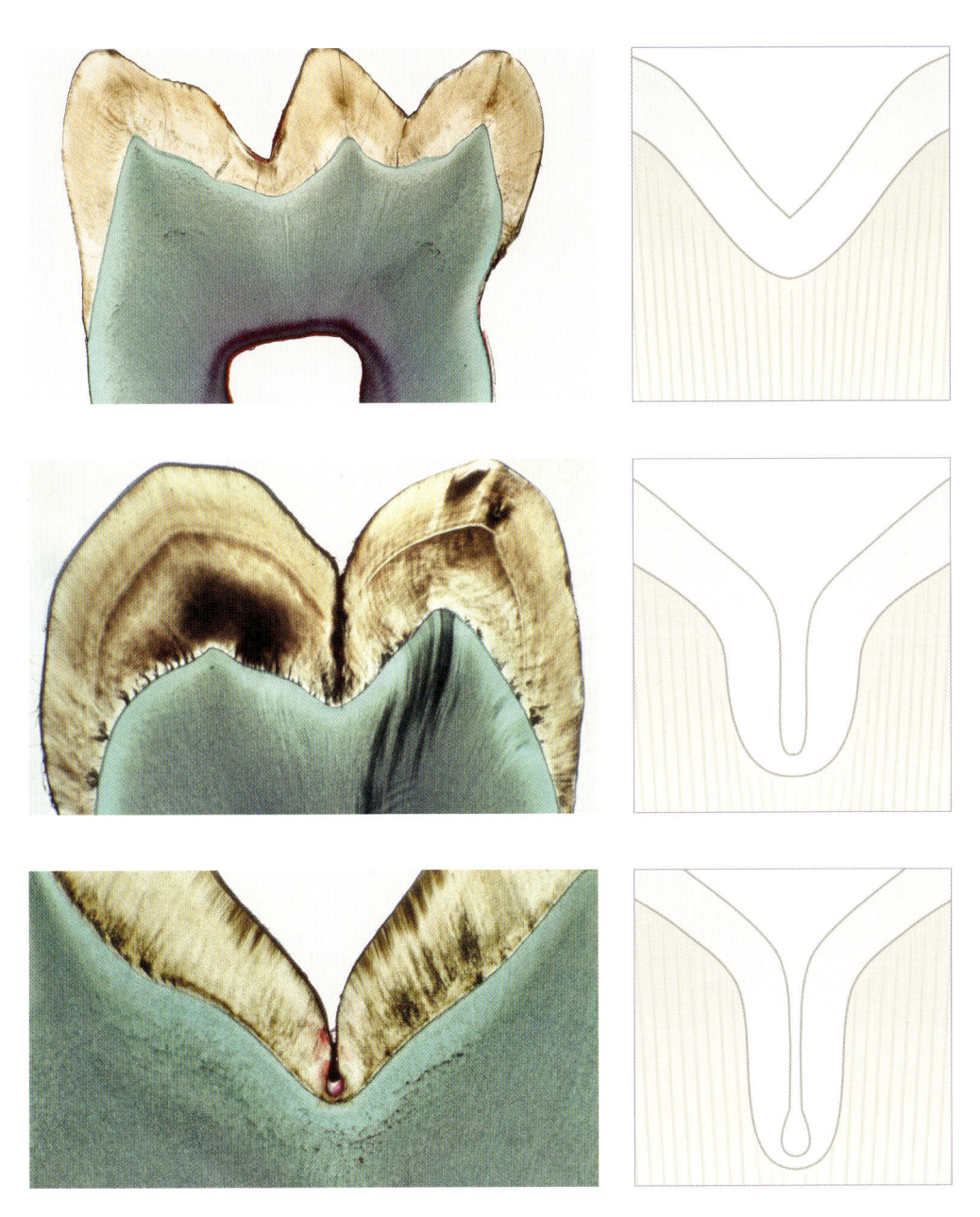

Fig 8-4 to 8-6 Different types of fissure morphology.

It is important for the teeth to be cleaned before diagnosis so that white spots at the fissure entrance can be identified (Fig 8-8). If a white spot is already visible before drying, it is reasonable to assume that the caries is more advanced than in a white spot which needs to be dried before it can be detected. This long-known fact was recently systematized with the ICDAS system, one of the aims being to publicize comparable diagnostic criteria in all countries.[5]

Diagnosis is difficult because dentin caries can exist underneath an apparently intact surface. In most cases, however, drying and close inspection will reveal an area of decalcification at the fissure entrance. The frequency of the so called "hidden caries" in molars varies between 10% and 50%. It appears to be a direct consequence of suboptimal technique in clinical diagnostics.

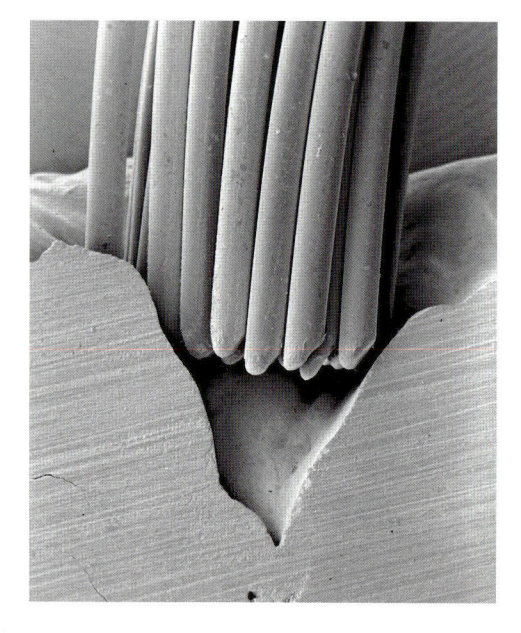

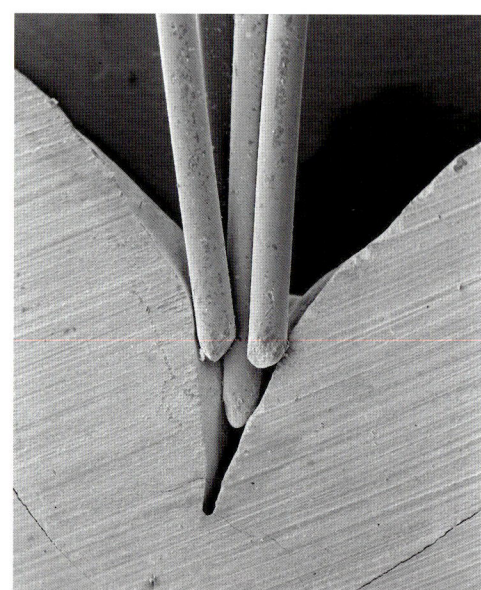

Fig 8-7 *It is not possible to clean the base of the fissure with a toothbrush and individual bristles.*

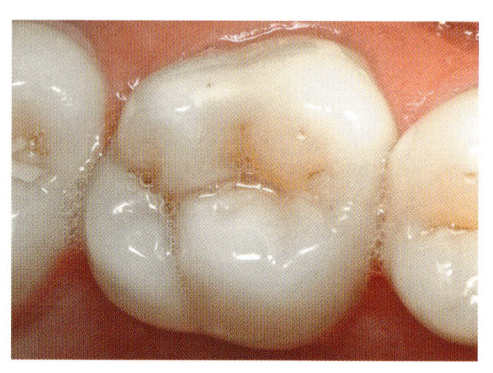

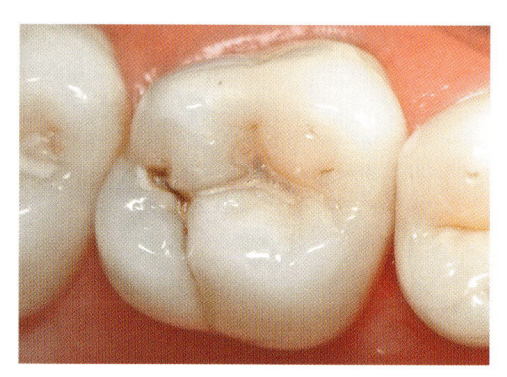

Fig 8-8 *White spots before and after drying of the fissure.*

> The use of a probe does not improve the diagnostic investigation of pit and fissure caries. Furthermore, a disadvantage of probing with pressure is that enamel areas decalcified at the surface are destroyed and this can accelerate the progression of caries. Drying the surface will reveal an area of decalcification that is a definite sign of caries.

Occlusal caries that has penetrated into the dentin can be diagnosed by bitewing radiographs. Dentin caries that is visible on a radiograph but which has an intact surface is generally treated by minimally invasive treatment and restoration (Figs 8-9 and 8-10).

■ Fluorescence measurement

Tools enabling caries to be detected early, even when the surface is apparently intact, have been sought for a number of years. The systems now available on the market and suitable for daily use take advantage of the fluorescence of dental hard substance that has been altered by caries.

Diagnosing caries and caries activity

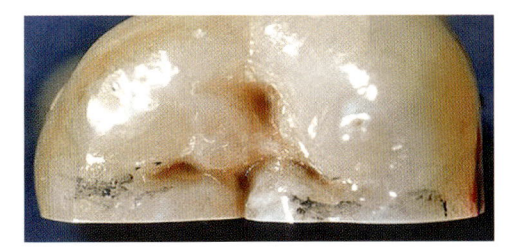

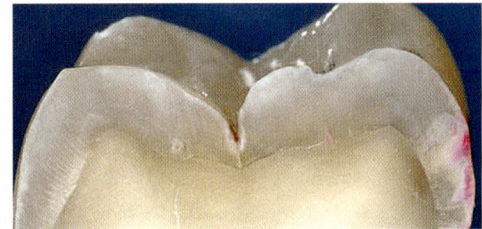

Fig 8-9 Left: intact fissure surface with discoloration. Right: no caries despite pronounced fissure discoloration.

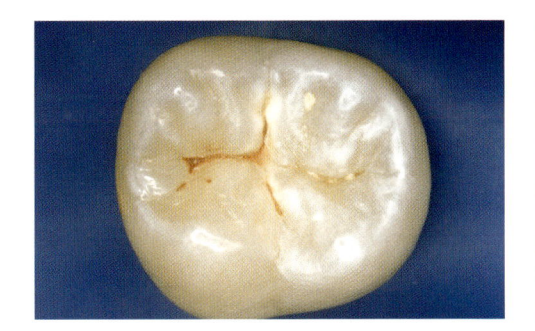

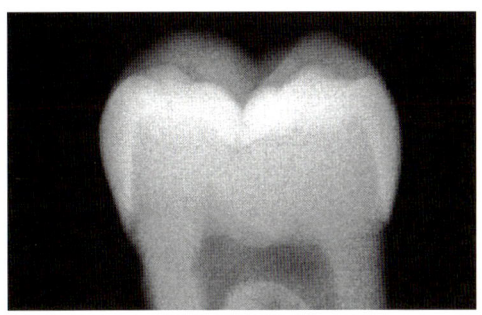

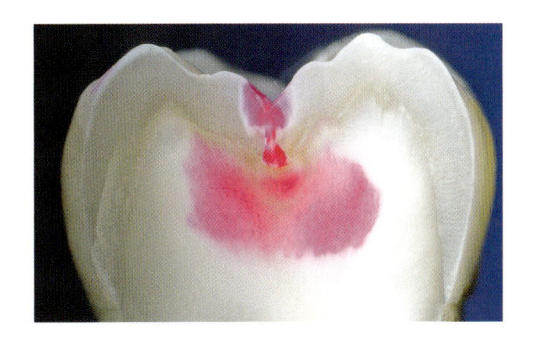

Fig 8-10 Top left: intact fissure surface. Top right: seemingly, the radiograph shows early radiolucency in the dentin. Bottom: pronounced enamel and dentin caries.

When radiant energy is applied to a tooth it causes a temporary transition of certain molecules into an excited state. That energy is then released as the molecules return to their initial state; part of the energy is released into the surrounding tissue as heat, while another part is lost as an emission of light, namely fluorescent radiation. The fluorescent light emitted has a longer wavelength (> 680 nm) than the light causing the excitation (655 nm).

This principle was developed into a practical device for caries detection in the form of the DIAGNOdent® (DD) and DIAGNOdent® pen (DD pen) (KaVo, Biberach) (Fig 8-11). Unwanted light is retained by a filter system. An acoustic signal that changes in pitch as the tip of the device is rotated enables the operator to locate the point of highest fluorescence at a specific site without having to look at the display on the device (Fig 8-12). The maximum value is read off after the measuring process. Existing studies prove that the DIAGNOdent based on laser fluorescence has good sensitivity for detecting dentin caries. As previously mentioned, clinical inspection achieves good specificity levels. Therefore, the advantages of the higher specificity and speed of clinical diagnostic examination can usefully be combined with the advantages of this device.

Light with a wavelength of 488 nm is another possible way to excite fluorescence. Autofluorescence alters in the presence of demineralization, therefore a decrease in fluorescence, which is evident as a dark appearance, indicates a carious lesion. This effect can even indicate initial caries. Quantitative laser fluorescence (QLF) is particularly suitable for smooth surfaces and the occlusal plane, where it enables even small changes to be detected.

Findings, diagnosis, and proposed treatment for pit and fissure caries are summarized in Tables 8-1 and 8-2.

It is advisable to perform a clinical examination of the patient first and, if drying raises doubts about the health of a particular site, to use the laser device for a "second opinion".

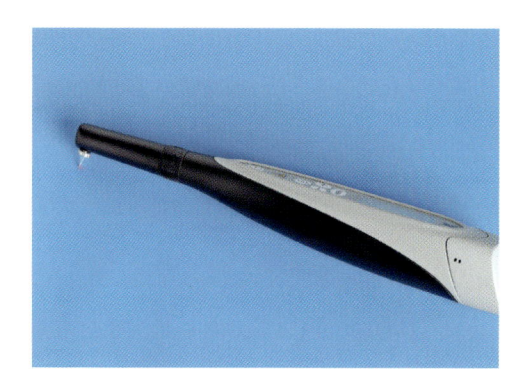

Fig 8-11 DIAGNOdent® pen.

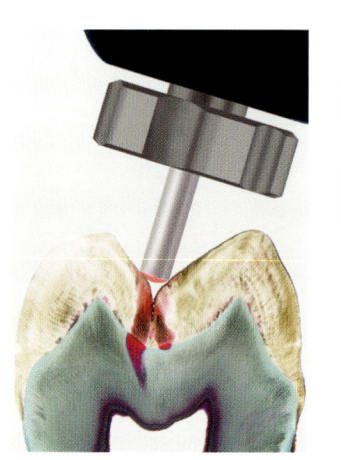

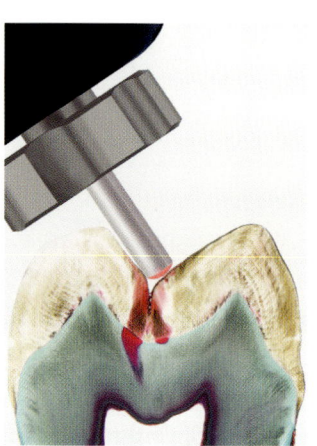

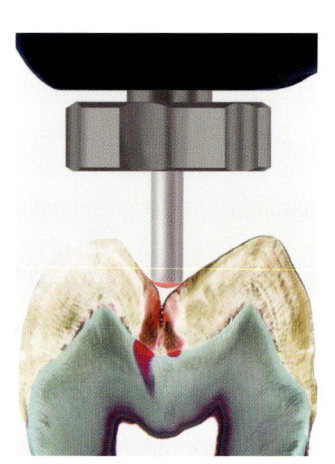

Fig 8-12 Rotation of the tip makes it possible to locate the strongest fluorescence.

Table 8-1 Recommended treatment on the occlusal surface depending on the DIAGNOdent (DD) display values

Display value	Diagnosis	Treatment
0–20	D_0–D_2	Prophylaxis
21 – ~30:		Intensified prophylaxis or restoration Indication is dependent on: • Caries activity • Recall interval, etc • Caries risk
≥ ~30	D_3, D	Restoration and intensified prophylaxis

Table 8-2 Findings, diagnosis, and recommended treatment for pit and fissure caries

Findings	Diagnosis	Treatment
Deep, retentive fissure, no change to the surface	D_0	• Prophylaxis • Pit and fissure sealing
• Fissure with white discoloration (dry!) (Brown discolorations are not a definite sign of caries in permanent teeth!!) • Radiograph: no dental lesion • Second opinion DD, DD pen	D_1, D_2	• Second opinion: DIAGNOdent (DD) • DD values < ~30: intensified prophylaxis • DD values > ~30: extended sealing
• Fissure with chalky white discoloration and/or visible surface defect • Radiograph: radiolucency in dentin	D_3, D_4	• Extended pit and fissure sealing or minimally invasive restoration • Reduction of caries risk

■ Approximal caries

Clinical examination, bitewing radiography, measurement of laser fluorescence, and fiber-optic transillumination (FOTI) can be used for diagnosing approximal (interproximal) caries. Bitewing radiographs are still the method of choice today for diagnosing approximal caries; around three-quarters of dentin caries is detected by this method. Most examinations reveal surface breakdown in the case of dentin lesions, such that remineralization is impossible. New, more sensitive x-ray films or digital systems seem to be equivalent to earlier methods in terms of diagnosing caries, but their use should be preferred because they significantly reduce the radiation exposure.

It is particularly difficult to detect whether the surface has broken down. However, it is important to detect surface breakdown so that a decision can be made about whether more-intensive prevention or more-invasive therapy is necessary. Only if the surface is intact can intensified prophylaxis be expected to halt the progression of surface breakdown or possibly bring about remineralization. A direct method for detecting approximal surface cavitation involves using an orthodontic separator which is left in place for 2 days prior to diagnosis. This method has been used to record the relationship between extension in the bitewing radiograph and cavitation. It was shown that around 10% of the approximal surfaces of permanent teeth with radiolucency on the bitewing radiograph extending as far as the dentoenamel junction had surface breakdown (Figs 8-13 and 8-14).

Teeth with a radiolucency confined to the enamel (hence without surface breakdown) are generally not treated operatively. Preventive measures and periodic check radiographs are indicated.

Given good oral hygiene, it can take more than 5 years before caries penetrates the enamel of mature permanent molars. This means it is possible to refrain from invasive therapy initially and simply to observe the progression or regression of the caries (Table 8-3). The penetration speed can be assessed with the aid of newly taken, standardized radiographs, which are then

Fig 8-13 Approximal caries: radiograph, D3 – there is distinct surface breakdown.

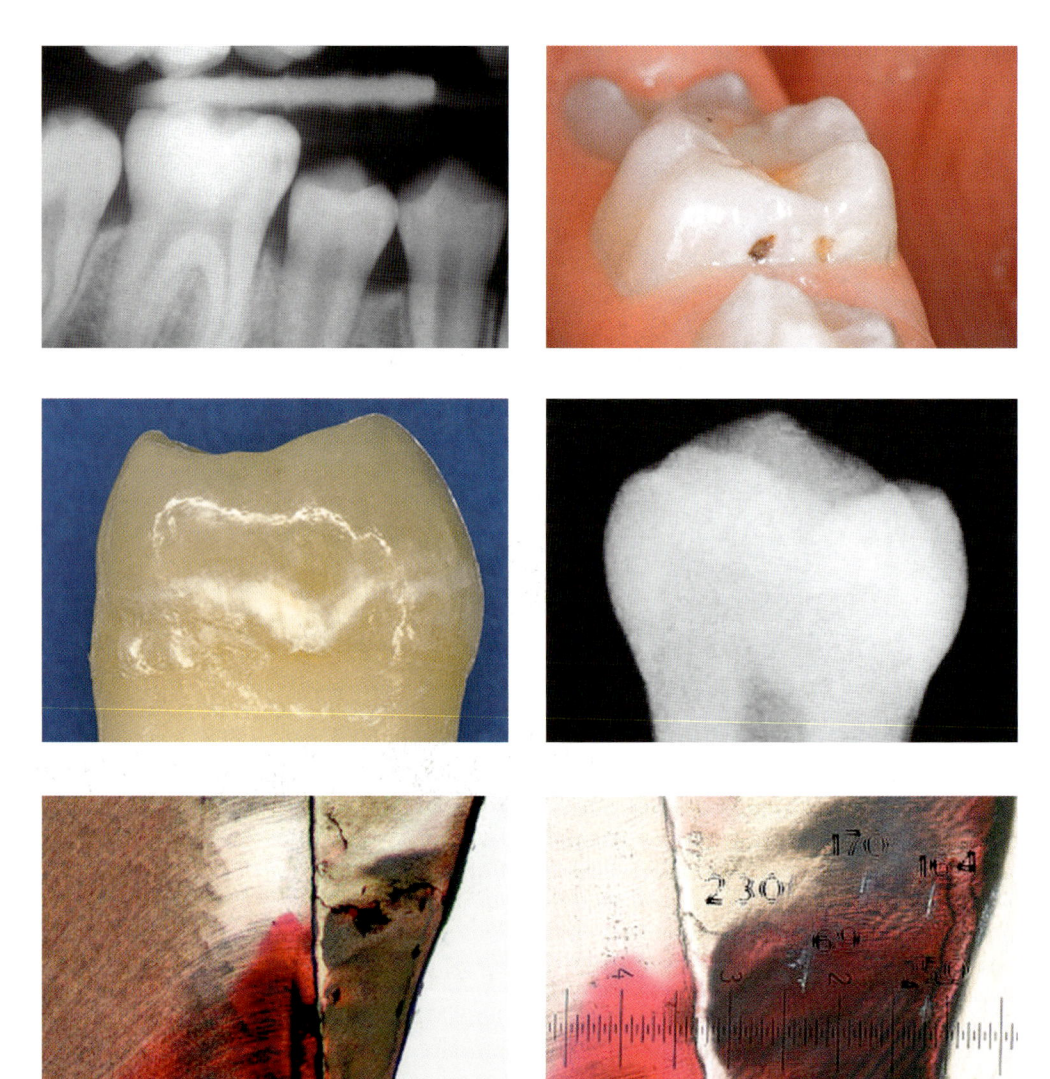

Fig 8-14 Approximal caries: Top: radiograph, D1 – the surface is intact. Bottom: However, enamel and dentin caries are histologically detectable.

compared with the existing radiographs. It should be noted that the penetration time of teeth is significantly shorter following eruption than it is in mature teeth, a fact which must be taken into consideration when planning the recall interval.

A film holder is recommended in order to reduce overlaps in the approximal area. Horizontal deviations of the x-ray tube by only a few degrees of angle can substantially impair correct diagnosis (Fig 8-15, left). Projection of enamel caries into the dentin area arises, which can lead to a false positive diagnosis. The radiographs should be examined under magnification and isolated from effects of light from the sides (Table 8-4).

FOTI can be used as an additional tool alongside bitewing radiographs if interproximally there is no interference from adjacent non-tooth-colored restorations. More than 70 % of the dentin lesion can be detected in anterior teeth by means of FOTI (Fig 8-16). However, it is difficult to distinguish enamel lesions in the posterior region.

The DIAGNOdent pen can be used for both occlusal and approximal surfaces.[3,4] Table 8-5 provides an overview of values based on a two-center study (Munich – Berne).[2]

Table 8-3 Time intervals for radiographs

No fixed time intervals (eg, a bitewing radiograph every year)
The interval varies between 6 months and 2 years and depends on various factors: • Caries risk, caries activity, expected progression • Age • Performance of other methods in detecting caries

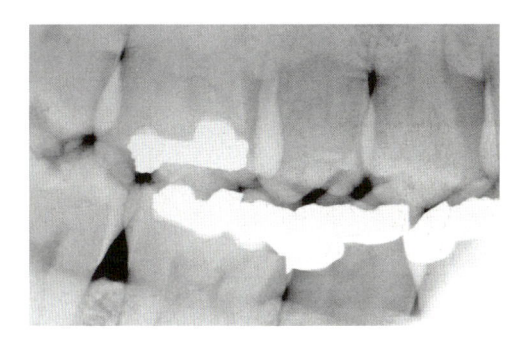

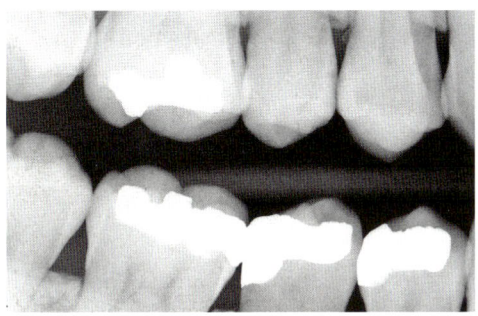

Fig 8-15 Overlaps in radiographic image due to faulty technique (left).

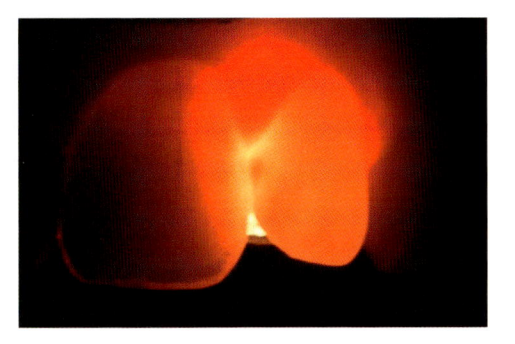

Fig 8-16 Approximal caries in the anterior region becomes visible with FOTI (image: P. Hotz).

Table 8-4 Findings, diagnosis and proposed treatment for approximal caries

Findings	Diagnosis	Treatment
Radiograph: lesion grade 1 and 2 (radiolucency in enamel) (comparisons with earlier radiographs; second opinion: DD pen)	D_1, D_2	Prophylaxis (interdental cleaning, fluoride)
Radiograph: lesion grade 2 (- > 3) (radiolucency in enamel which starts to extend into dentin) (comparisons with earlier radiographs; second opinion: DD pen)	D_3	Prophylaxis for low caries risk Restoration for high caries risk Reduction of caries risk!
Radiograph lesion grade 3 and 4 (radiolucency in dentin, surface breakdown) (comparisons with earlier radiographs; second opinion: DD pen)	D_3, D_4	Restoration

Table 8-5 DIAGNOdent pen – Prophylaxis when? (approximal caries)[2]

Measurement	Recommended treatment/further diagnostic investigations
0 – ~7	Standard prophylactic measures
~8 – ~15	Intensified prophylaxis with recall interval, dependent on caries risk
≥ ~16	Take a bitewing radiograph as a "second opinion", then decide on future action If radiography contraindicated (phobia, pregnancy): the sensitivity of DD pen is 84%

■ Root caries

With advancing age, most people have gingival recession affecting one or more teeth. As a result, parts of the root surfaces are exposed and, in keeping with the characteristic structures and chemical composition of cementum and dentin, these parts are more prone to mechanical trauma and caries than enamel surfaces. The labial/buccal surfaces are most commonly affected, followed by the approximal and palatal surfaces.

Primary root caries only occurs when the root surfaces are exposed to the oral environment and plaque attack. In this context it is important to bear in mind that the critical pH for root caries is about 6.3, whereas the critical pH is markedly lower in enamel at about 5.5. Root caries is hence a disease that appears in dentate individuals more frequently with advancing age.

Once again diagnosis is extremely important because, even if mineral loss is up to 50%, the dentin structure will remain sufficiently intact for remineralization to be possible. Root caries often appears as soft, discolored destruction of the dentin that is not very deep.

Interdental diagnosis, in particular, is not easy. Although root caries is associated with loss of attachment, direct inspection can be rendered impossible by periodontal pockets. The progression of such dentin defects, which are not accessible to cleaning, is faster than

Diagnosing caries and caries activity 8

in coronal caries. The lesion is often so far advanced that the endodontium is affected and root canal treatment becomes essential. A radiograph for areas that cannot be viewed and cautious use of the probe for accessible sites have proved effective diagnostic methods (Figs 8-17 to 8-19).

Diagnostically it is important to differentiate active from inactive lesions. Root caries with a soft surface harbors significantly more mutans streptococci and lactobacilli than lesions with a hard surface. All carious defects display discolorations from light brown to dark brown and black. Significantly more mutans streptococci and lactobacilli have been found in black lesions than in dark brown ones. Thus the color of root caries is not a criterion of caries activity.

Inactive root caries is characterized by a relatively hard surface, while active lesions – regardless of the discoloration of dental tissue – are characterized by softened dental substance and often border the gingival margin.

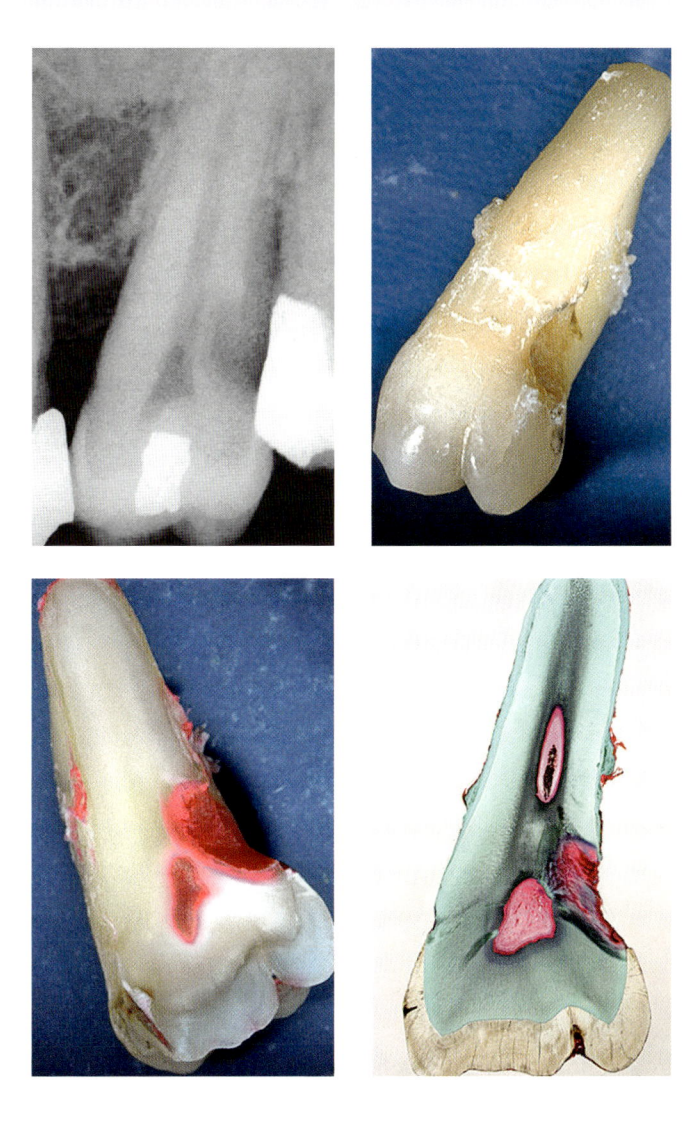

Fig 8-17 Root caries in a molar.

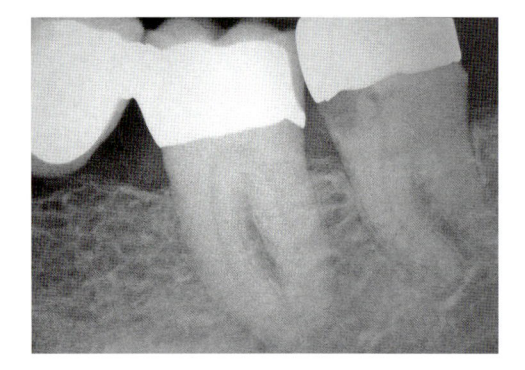

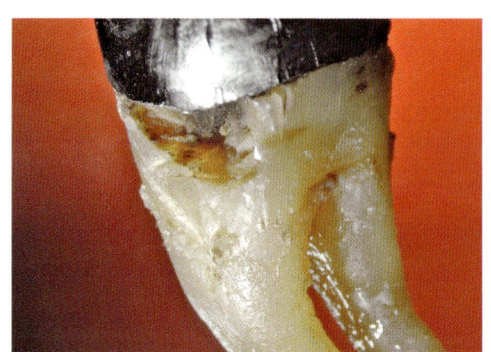

Fig 8-18 Root caries under a crown.

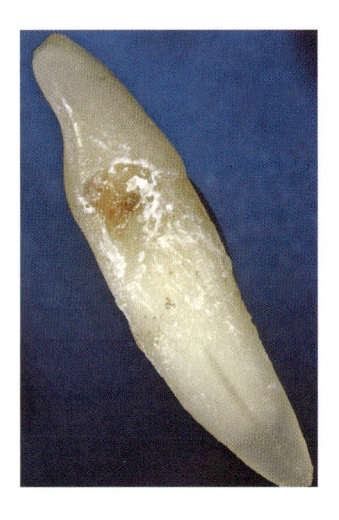

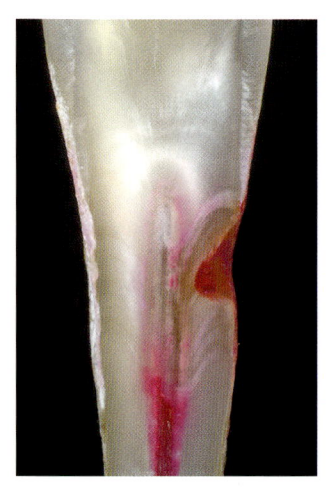

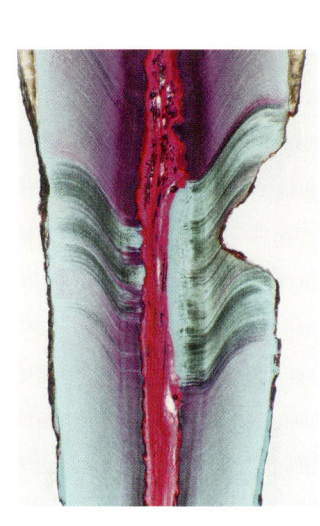

Fig 8-19 Root caries in an anterior tooth: the pulp reacted to the carious attack with substantial tertiary dentin formation.

Inactive lesions do not require any restorative treatment but can be kept under control by suitable preventive measures (Table 8-6). However, appreciably higher fluoride concentrations are required in dentin caries than enamel caries in order to achieve the same effect (see chapter 3).

Provided the defect has not advanced to a depth that endangers the pulp, active lesions are polished smooth. They are also managed by preventive measures. Active root caries can be converted into an inactive stage, especially on buccal or labial surfaces, by means of suitable oral hygiene measures and adequate fluoride application.

■ Caries activity and caries risk

As mentioned above, on the smooth surface in question a healthy band of enamel between a lesion and the gingiva is indicative of a lengthy inactive phase. Furthermore the surface of an inactive lesion appears smooth and glossy; unlike active lesions, which border the gingiva and have a matt surface. In the approximal area, however, it can be difficult to tell whether inactive or active caries is present. Bleeding on probing in healthy periodontal conditions, where a lesion is visible on radiograph or on clinical examination, indicates active caries. Other variables are used to estimate the current risk of caries. Oral hygiene and dietary habits, the number of caries pathogens in the interproximal space, the flow

Table 8-6 Findings, diagnosis and proposed treatment for root caries

Findings	Diagnosis	Treatment
Surface hard	Inactive caries	Prophylaxis (oral hygiene, fluoridation, dietary advice)
Surface leathery	Active caries	Polishing with (abrasive) fluoride paste (removal of softened substance), prophylaxis, fluoride varnishes and/or dentifrice with increased F- content
Surface soft	See active caries	as above
Surface soft, larger defect	See active caries	Restoration: composite resin or compomer with dentin adhesion; glass ionomer cement, light-curing for high risk of secondary caries

rate and buffer capacity of oral fluid, fluoride intake, and previous caries attacks are important factors.

In addition to appropriate care, patients with active (initial) caries require understandable information about the etiology, preventive measures, and possible consequences. In particular, knowing about the possiblility of stagnation or remineralization of the initial lesion can motivate the patient to continue cooperating, but it may still be necessary to alter dietary habits, improve oral hygiene, and introduce or optimize fluoridation measures.

Caries-pathogenic microorganisms on a specific approximal surface or in the whole mouth can be detected in the dental practice with the aid of kits. These test kits also make it possible to monitor bacterial colonization of the oral cavity and can be used to motivate patients. Where patients have active caries and a high number of caries-pathogenic bacteria, it may additionally be desirable to reduce the bacterial burden using chlorhexidine gel applied in a thermoformed splint or by means of chlorhexidine varnish.

The risk of caries can easily be estimated by assigning risk points to different factors. The risk assessment is based on published experience and does not require a great deal of time (Table 8-7). It can also be performed simply for infants, using just a few variables (Table 8-8).

Table 8-7 Caries risk assessment (CRA)

Risk factor	Points
Drugs that affect dental health	5
Reduced saliva flow (clinically assessed)	5
Oral hygiene less than twice daily	5
Oral hygiene without fluoride toothpaste	10
No interdental cleaning	5
Sugar urges more than 5 times a day	5
Bleeding on probing 30 %	5
New caries in the past 2 years	10
Existing white spots	5
Exposed necks of teeth	5
Fixed orthodontic appliances	5
Total risk points	

0–5 points: low caries risk; 10–20 points: moderate caries risk; > 20 points: high caries risk

Table 8-8 Estimate of caries risk in infants

Visible plaque on the upper anterior teeth
Sugary drinks several times a day, or use of baby's bottle containing sugary drinks during the night

■ Summary

The early, correct diagnosis of a carious lesion is important as it will ensure that the right preventive and therapeutic measures can be taken. Depending on the location of the carious change to the dental hard substance (approximal, smooth surface, fissure, or root caries) different tools are used for diagnostic and monitoring purposes.

The bitewing radiograph is suitable for diagnosing approximal caries, visual inspection for pit and fissure as well as smooth surface caries, and careful probing combined with radiography for root caries. Devices can be used to provide a "second opinion" in the decision-making process. When diagnosing caries progression, it is important to bear in mind that a patient's risk of caries is not a constant value but can change.

■ References

1. Backer-Dirks O. Posteruptive changes in dental enamel. J Dent Res 1966;45: 503–511.
2. Huth KC, Neuhaus KW, Gygax M et al. Clinical performance of a new laser fluorescence device for detection of occlusal caries lesions in permanent molars. J Dent 2008;36:1033–1040.
3. Lussi A, Hack A, Hug I, Heckenberger H, Megert B, Stich H. Detection of approximal caries with a new laser fluorescence device. Caries Res 2006;40:97–103.
4. Lussi A, Hellwig E. Performance of a new laser fluorescence device for detection of occlusal caries *in vitro*. J Dentistry 2006;34:467–471.
5. Pitts NB. 'ICDAS' – an international system for caries detection and assessment being developed to facilitate caries epidemiology, research and appropriate clinical management. Community Dent Health 2004;21:193–198.

9 Sealing and infiltration of caries – is this the future?

Brigitte Zimmerli and Simon Flury

■ Introduction

Fissure sealants have been used with great success for 50 years in the prevention of pit and fissure caries. If the caries risk is correctly assessed, dental sealant treatments are a simple and cost-effective individual preventive measure. As far as possible, premature, "preventive" opening of surface lesions should be avoided. In cases of regular recall, delaying invasive therapy and opening the lesion only when the caries has progressed further does not lead to any greater loss of tooth substance.[6]

As well as preventing loss of dental substance due to caries, sealing of teeth based on a correct diagnosis can also serve as a form of treatment. The idea underlying this therapeutic approach – namely to inhibit the supply of substrate to the bacteria, with the sealant acting as a diffusion barrier and thereby preventing any progression of the caries – has already existed for some time. For instance, there are studies from as early as 1976 assessing the possibility of bacterial survival underneath sealants.[7] Despite this, only a few articles concerning the sealing of carious lesions have been published so far, and this subject is a matter of extremely heated debate. More recent studies show, however, that the spectrum of bacteria alters if they are cut off from the supply of substrate by sealants or restorations: after a while, both bacterial count and genotype diversity are markedly reduced.[15] The sealing of carious lesions effects a 100 to 1,000-fold decrease in the bacterial count and reduces by 50 % the probability of culturable bacteria on sealed surfaces.[14]

It was shown in a 10-year study that, in the presence of composite resin and amalgam restorations, residual caries does not progress any further after additional sealing.[10] Preventing caries progression by separating bacteria from the substrate supply was described by Oliveira and coworkers.[13] Where a coronal radiolucency approaching the vicinity of the pulp was seen on radiographs of permanent posterior teeth but no clinical symptoms were observed, the caries was only partially removed and tightly sealed after application of calcium hydroxide. Over an observation period of 14 to 18 months, no statistical differences in caries progression were recorded in comparison with the fully excavated control group.

In view of these observations, studies were performed on the treatment of initial carious lesions with sealants. In the case of approximal lesions it was shown that sealing the surface led to significantly less progression of lesions than in the nonsealed control group.[9]

Furthermore the approximal sealing was more successful than the application of fluoride varnish.[3] In a review analysis it was established that 19.4% of sealed carious lesions per year were subject to progression, whereas the caries continued to progress in 59.3% of nonsealed lesions.[5]

■ Noninvasive treatment techniques for initial lesions

The following three noninvasive therapeutic approaches for preventing caries progression from initial lesions are currently under discussion: conventional sealing, the infiltration technique, and application of a resin patch.

Conventional sealing

Procedure
- Tooth cleaning
- Creation of a dry operating field (rubber dam)
- Application of phosphoric acid for 60 seconds; move the gel!
- Application of the sealant or adhesive system, penetration time at least 20 seconds, light curing
- Polishing
- Fluoridation

Access to the diseased site on a tooth is difficult with approximal lesions. This is why the interdental space must be opened slightly with wedges, or preferably with orthodontic separators, prior to treatment, which adds to the treatment time involved.[4] Phosphoric acid etching is not successful with initial lesions because the outermost enamel layer cannot be adequately conditioned. Therefore, methods for removing this surface layer prior to sealing by means of polishing discs or strips have also been described. This treatment step is difficult to control, especially in the approximal area. The penetration depth of conventional adhesives to the underlying, porous lesion body is limited. Lengthening the penetration time from 15 to 30 seconds before the sealant or adhesive sets will increase the penetration depth for most products.[11] The protection against further progression of caries provided by sealing is primarily achieved by its acting as a diffusion barrier on the initial lesion and not by penetration of the sealing material into the lesion.[16,17]

Infiltration technique

Procedure
- Tooth cleaning
- Creation of a dry operating field (rubber dam)
- Application of hydrochloric acid (2 minutes), rinse
- Application of ethanol solution (30 seconds), dry
- First application of the infiltrant, penetration time 3 minutes, light curing

Sealing and infiltration of caries – is this the future?

- Second application of the infiltrant, penetration time 1 minute, light curing
- Check for excess material, polishing
- Fluoridation

A further development of the sealing technique is intended to penetrate the entire carious lesion with a methacrylate-based infiltrant. Unlike conventional sealing, the purpose here is to create a diffusion barrier within the lesion. Hydrochloric acid removes the outermost, fluoride-rich and caries-resistant enamel layer of the initial lesion and exposes the underlying porous lesion body. It has been shown that the application of hydrochloric acid markedly improves penetration by the infiltrant.[12] The lesion is then dried with ethanol. This ensures the necessary drying of the porous lesion body, which has an increased water content. A low-viscosity, light-curing resin infiltrant is applied and light-cured after a few minutes' penetration time. A second application should be carried out to ensure complete infiltration.

Various types of methacrylate and different ethanol concentrations have been researched in order to achieve ideal wetting and infiltration of the lesion and also good polymerization properties of the material.[16] The infiltration technique can mask the esthetically detrimental white spots better than conventional sealing because the lesion body is almost completely infiltrated (Fig 9-1). Clinical trials are currently under way, but there are still no long-term data regarding the methodology. A material set for the infiltration of carious lesions recently came onto the market (Icon®, DMG, Hamburg). Special applicators for the infiltration technique in the approximal area are an interesting feature of this set (Fig 9-2). The advantage is that the teeth only need to be separated briefly using wedges.

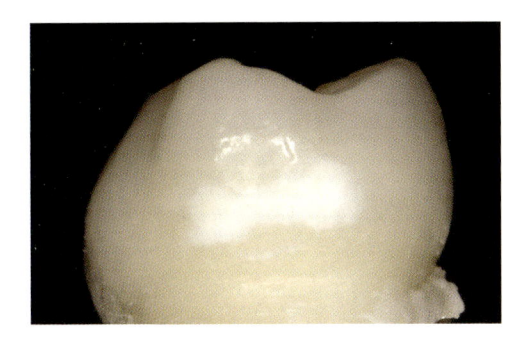

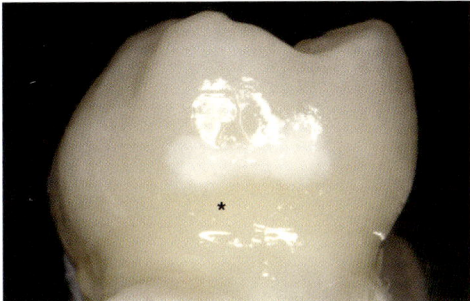

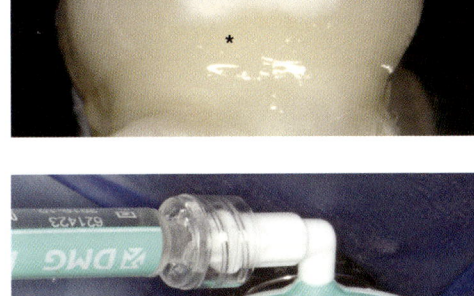

Fig 9-1a White opaque initial lesion without surface breakdown.

Fig 9-1b Initial lesion after infiltration technique. The masking is more effective with discrete opacities (*).

Fig 9-2 Approximal applicator for the infiltration technique (Icon®). The thin plastic film is perforated on one side so that only the desired approximal surface is treated.

Resin patch

Procedure
- Tooth cleaning
- Creation of a dry operating field (rubber dam)
- Application of phosphoric acid (60 seconds)
- Application of the adhesive system
- Application of the resin patch, light curing
- Check for excess material, polishing
- Fluoridation

This form of treatment involves covering the carious lesion with a resin patch (Poly-Strip). This technique cannot be used occlusally. The teeth have to be separated (with separators) for application in the approximal space.

The enamel surface concerned is etched with phosphoric acid. The patch, which is made of polyurethane dimethacrylate, is fixed onto the enamel surface with a conventional adhesive system and light cured. The aim of this type of sealing is to create a diffusion barrier on the site of the lesion. Under laboratory conditions, the patch seems to protect efficiently against further demineralization.[19] In addition, the patch can be used for marginal sealing of Class II restorations or as a caries-inhibiting layer in the case of brackets, the bracket being affixed to the preapplied patch.[20,21] For the most part, there is a lack of clinical data on use of the patch,[1] but the existing data are promising. The product is not available on the market and the company rules out any sale at the present time (development by Ivoclar Vivadent AG, Schaan, Liechtenstein) (Fig 9-3).

■ Discussion

In summary, new approaches have been developed on the basis of knowledge gained from conventional fissure sealing. As well as the occlusal area of application, expansion into other locations can be seen, and noninvasive treatment techniques have been developed from primarily preventive ideas and efforts (Table 9-1).

Nevertheless, all the described therapeutic approaches and most of the materials for approximal sealing (except the conventional etching/adhesive or sealing systems) are still in the trial and development phase. Sealing of lesions involving surface breakdown must still be rejected as an option. While fissures and occlusal surfaces are relatively easy to view, it is not simple to make a clinical diagnosis of an intact surface in the case of approximal lesions because of their interdental location. Radiologically, approximal lesions should not exceed a D_2 stage (lesion extending as far as the dentoenamel junction) or, at the very most, an early D_3 stage (parts of the caries in dentin areas that are close to the dentoenamel junction). Furthermore, regular check radiographs and radiographic documentation are required with all types of sealing to ensure early detection of any progression of the lesion. It is also possible to measure fluorescence through transparent sealants using DIAGNOdent® without any significant change of signal.[2,8]

Sealing and infiltration of caries – is this the future?

Table 9-1 Possible applications of the different noninvasive techniques for the treatment of carious lesions

Technique	Material	Application: occlusal surfaces	Application: smooth surfaces	Products
Sealing	Sealant	Possible	Possible, approximal separation necessary	Established products from various manufacturers
Infiltration	Infiltration system (hydrochloric acid, ethanol, infiltrant)	Possible (not investigated)	Possible, with special applicator; approximally often no appreciable separation required	System new, available on the market (Icon®, DMG)
Resin patch	Adhesive system, patch (Poly-Strip)	Not possible	Possible, approximal separation necessary	In development phase, not commercially available (Ivoclar Vivadent AG)

Clinical trials are needed to obtain more precise information about the use of the new sealing methods and materials in daily dental practice. At present, clinical data on the use of the infiltration technique and the resin patch are almost nonexistent. Application technique, penetration depth, closure, and tightness of the sealing are important variables in terms of long-term clinical success.

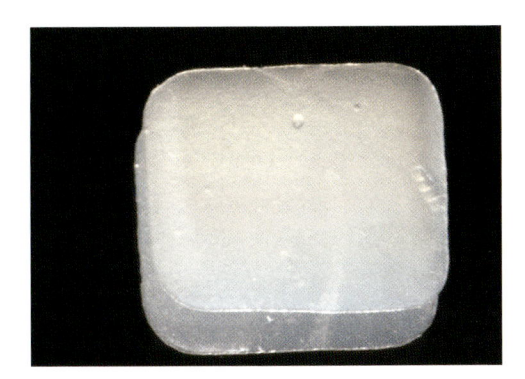

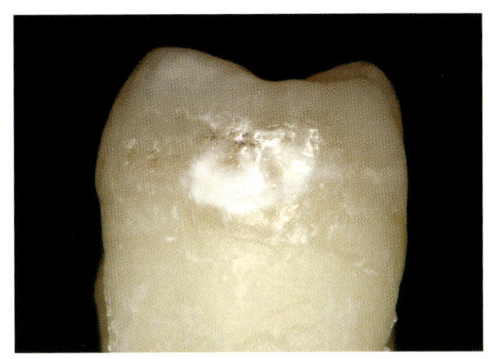

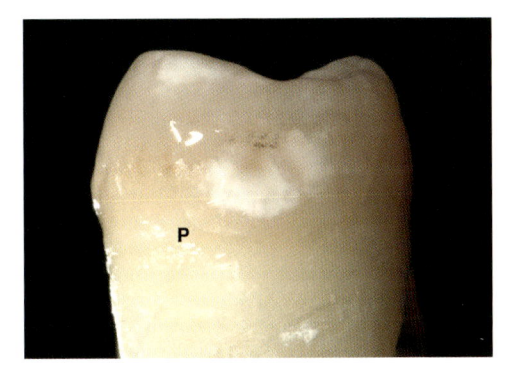

Fig 9-3
Top left: resin patch (Poly-Strip). Top right: initial situation: initial approximal lesion without breakdown. Bottom right: resin patch after being cut to lesion size and applied using adhesive system. Owing to the thickness of the patch, the marginal areas have to be finished (P: marginal area of the patch).

References

1. Alkilzy M, Berndt C, Meller C, Schidlowski M, Splieth C. Sealing of proximal surfaces with polyurethane tape: a two-year clinical and radiographic feasibility study. J Adhes Dent 2009;11:91–94.
2. Diniz MB, Rodrigues JA, Hug I, Cordeiro RCL, Lussi A. The influence of pit and fissure sealants on infrared fluorescence measurements. Caries Res 2008;42:328–333.
3. Gomez SS, Basili CP, Emilson CG. A 2-year clinical evaluation of sealed noncavitated approximal posterior carious lesions in adolescents. Clin Oral Investig 2005;9:239–243.
4. Gomez SS, Onetto JE, Uribe SA, Emilson CG. Therapeutic seal of approximal incipient noncavitated carious lesions: technique and case reports. Quintessence Int 2007;38:e99–105.
5. Griffin SO, Oong E, Kohn W, Vidakowitch B, Gooch BF, CDC Dental Sealant Systematic Review Work Group, Bader J, Clarkson, Fontana MR, Meyer DM, Rozier RG, Weintraub JA, Zero DT. The effectiveness of sealants in managing caries lesions. J Dent Res 2008;87:169–174.
6. Hamilton JC, Dennison JB, Stoffers KW, Gregory WA, Welch KB. Early treatment of incipient carious lesions: a two-year clinical evaluation. J Am Dent Assoc 2002;133:1643–1651.
7. Handelman SL, Mashburn F, Wopperer P. Two year report of sealant effect on bacteria in dental caries. JADA 1976;93:967–970.
8. Krause F, Braun A, Frentzen M, Jepsen S. Effects of composite fissure sealants on IR laser fluorescence measurements. Lasers Med Sci 2008;23:133–139.
9. Martignon S, Ekstrand KR, Ellwood R. Efficacy of sealing proximal early active lesions: an 18-month clinical study evaluated by conventional and subtraction radiography. Caries Res 2006;40:382–388.
10. Mertz-Fairhurst EJ, Curtis JW jr, Ergle JW, Rueggeberg FA, Adair SM. Ultraconservative and cariostatic sealed restorations: results at year 10. Am Dent Assoc 1998;129:55–66.
11. Meyer-Lueckel H, Paris S, Mueller J, Cölfen H, Kielbassa AM. Influence of the application time on the penetration of different dental adhesives and a fissure sealant into artificial subsurface lesions in bovine enamel. Dent Mater 2006;22:22–28.
12. Meyer-Lueckel H, Paris S, Kielbassa AM. Surface layer erosion of natural caries lesions with phosphoric and hydrochloric acid gels in preparation for resin infiltration. Caries Res 2007;41:223–230.
13. Oliveira EF, Carminatti G, Fontanella V, Maltz M. The monitoring of deep caries lesions after incomplete dentin caries removal: results after 14-18 months. Clin Oral Investig 2006;10:134–139.
14. Oong EM, Griffin SO, Kohn WG, Gooch BF, Caufield PW. The effect of dental sealants on bacteria levels in caries lesions: a review of the evidence. J Am Dent Assoc 2008;139:271–178.
15. Paddick JS, Brailsford SR, Kidd EAM, Beighton D. Phenotypic and genotypic selection of microbiota surviving under dental restorations. Appl Environ Microbiol 2005;71:467–472.
16. Paris S, Meyer-Lueckel H, Mueller J, Hummel M, Kielbassa AM. Progression of sealed initial bovine enamel lesions under demineralizing conditions *in vitro*. Caries Res 2006;40:124–129.
17. Paris S, Meyer-Lueckel H, Kielbassa AM. Resin infiltration of natural caries lesions. J Dent Res 2007;86:662–666.
18. Paris S, Meyer-Lueckel H, Cölfen H, Kielbassa AM. Penetration coefficients of commercially available and experimental composites intended to infiltrate enamel carious lesions. Dent Mater 2007;23:742–748.
19. Schmidlin PR, Zehnder M, Zimmermann MA, Zimmermann J, Roos M, Roulet JF. Sealing smooth enamel surfaces with a newly devised adhesive patch: a radiochemical *in vitro* analysis. Dent Mater 2005;21:545–550.
20. Schmidlin PR, Seemann R, Filli T, Attin T, Imfeld T. Sealing of minimally invasive class II fillings (slot) using an adhsive patch: sealant margin extension for prevention. Oper Dent 2007;32:482–287.
21. Schmidlin PR, Schätzle M, Fischer J, Attin T. Bonding of brackets using a caries-protective adhesive patch. J Dent 2008;36:125–129.

Magnification aids in restorative dentistry

IV

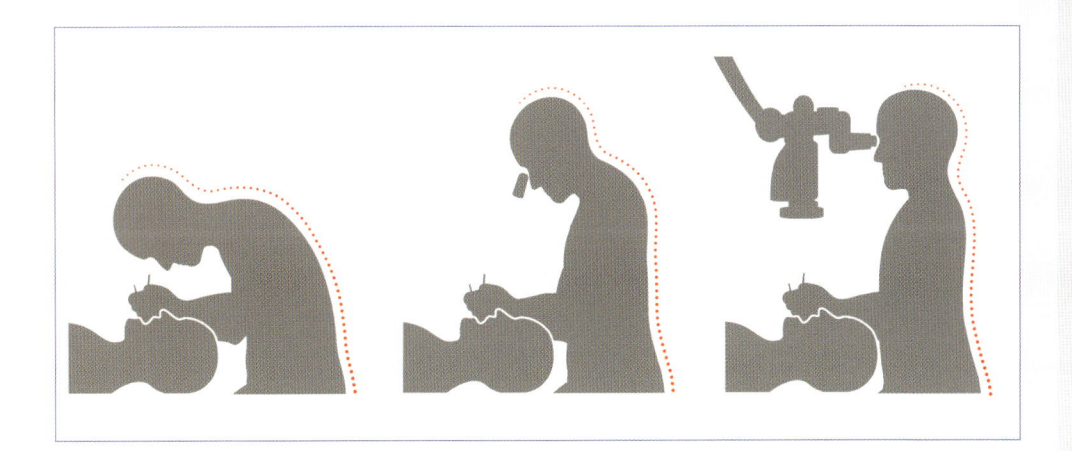

10 Utility and futility of magnification aids in restorative dentistry

Martina Eichenberger, Philippe Perrin, Daniel Jacky, and Adrian Lussi

■ Introduction

The precision of any manual activity is limited not by the hands but by vision – a fact that has long been known by watchmakers. The maxim "You can do what you can see," which has been true in microsurgery specialisms of general medicine for decades, explains the use of optical magnification aids by surgeons. It is therefore obvious that optical magnification aids also offer advantages in dentistry given the small spatial dimensions encountered.[1]

This is particularly true for restorative dentistry, where thanks to intensive caries prevention, new preparation instruments, and adhesive, flowable restoration materials, the trend is towards minimally invasive and defect-specific cavity shaping. The only limiting factor is visual checkability. In practice, magnification aids and adequate light are found to be essential for such minimally invasive restorations.[8]

A wide range of visualization instruments are available, but loupes and operating microscopes have proved especially practical. These will be explored in more detail in this chapter.

■ Discrepancy between subjective perception and scientific evidence

Nearly all users of loupes and microscopes are subjectively convinced that these instruments bring advantages and improve both the quality of their work and their ergonomic conditions. However, there is a noticeable discrepancy between this subjective conviction and the scientific evidence. This is mainly related to the complexity of the visual system. There are not only wide differences in natural visual acuity,[4] but also age-dependent variables, such as accommodation capacity (which can act as a natural magnification system) and contrast sensitivity.[3] Added to this is the influence of the light and variables within the optical systems (focal distance, light loss, quality of the lenses).

There are obviously other variables that impact on the key question of how optical instruments affect the quality of dentistry work. This is why most publications on the subject of visual acuity and quality of work are confined to case studies, review articles, or expert opinions. There are only a few scientific studies and these mainly originate from the areas of endosurgery (where innovative instruments also play a role) and endodontology, where most studies concern the identification of accessory root canals. Here, optical magnification aids have had a proven positive effect.[2,5,9–11] By contrast, a study on the subject of loupes and damage to adjacent teeth during approximal preparation revealed no improvement in quality, although this might have been due to the above-mentioned variables.[6]

> The positive subjective perception when using magnification aids is not yet scientifically confirmed in all areas of dentistry.

■ Loupes

The simplest and most affordable form of loupe is the single lens clip but, for physical reasons, there are some limitations to this magnification aid. At 2× magnification the working distance is so small that ergonomic problems will arise. However, this closeness does afford an amazingly precise view.[4]

With *Galilean* loupes, the user is free to choose the working distance, which can be adjusted to suit ergonomic requirements. Magnification is limited to 2.5× by the lenses, but it can be augmented to as much as 3.5× with some compromises (restricted visual field, blurry periphery). Galilean loupes are recognizable by their conical design.

Prismatic or *Kepler* loupes offer a choice of working distance and magnification factor. For dental work, 3× to 7× magnification seems reasonable because the depth of field becomes too small at higher magnifications; even small head movements can cause interference. Prismatic loupes are optically superior and produce a high-quality image; however, their complex optics mean that these loupes are bigger and heavier than Galilean loupes. Prismatic loupes are recognizable by their cylindrical shape.

The magnified image achieved with loupes affords a good view at a greater working distance. For the best possible adjustment, users can vary the different parameters (working distance, loupe inclination, convergence angle) to suit their needs. This allows the practitioner to adopt a more comfortable posture and maintain a reasonable practitioner-patient distance, to protect the privacy of patient and dentist.[12] Nevertheless, some curvature of the cervical spine and a static posture are unavoidable, which is why the extolled ergonomic advantages of a loupe are a matter of controversy among experts.[7]

Advantages of loupes	Disadvantages of loupes
• Magnification	• Magnification limited
• Increased working distance	(depth of field, head movements)
• Relief to the back area	• Strain on the neck area
(musculature and spine)	• Limited overview

Operating microscope

Operating microscopes enable the required magnification to be selected by means of a manual magnification changer or a continuously adjustable electric zoom. The working distance should be adjusted to the user's height; it can be altered using exchangeable lenses of different focal lengths or, depending on the model, by an electric zoom. The microscope is usually fixed above the dental unit or to the dental chair by means of a swivel supporting arm; this type of mounting is preferable to a mobile stand.[7]

Unlike loupes, there is no controversy over the ergonomic advantages of operating microscopes. An upright, more relaxed working posture and suitable working distance from the patient can be achieved using an operating microscope (Fig 10-1). In addition, the variable magnification and centered light guarantee an excellent view at all times.

There is also no doubt that microscope use can sometimes result in a steep learning curve. However, attending suitable courses can make this learning curve far easier to manage.[7]

Advantages of the microscope
- Free choice of magnification
- Excellent view
- Ergonomics
- Focusing on a very small operating field

Disadvantages of the microscope
- Acquisition costs
- Learning curve
- Limited overview

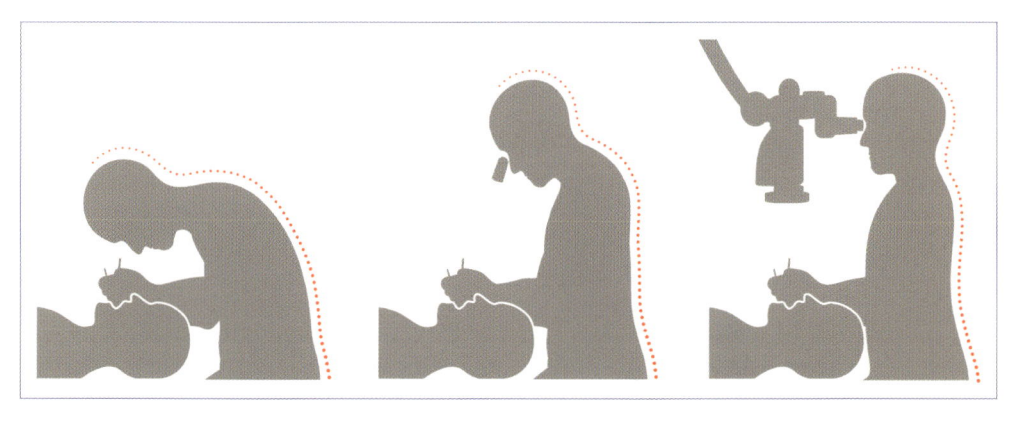

Fig 10-1 Position/back strain without magnifying aid (left), with loupe (center), when using a microscope (right).[7]

Minimally invasive restorations

Thanks to the latest preparation instruments and restorative techniques, restorations in shapes and locations that were previously thought impossible can now be achieved, with minimally invasive techniques predominating (Figs 10-2 to 10-16).[8] However, visual control with the naked eye places limits on this minimally invasive caries therapy. As previously mentioned, this limit varies widely from one individual to another. Nevertheless, visual acuity can be improved in all individuals by the use of loupes and microscopes.[4]

Case 1: Minimally invasive treatment of primary caries (Figs 10-2 to 10-9)

Fig 10-2 The caries at the distolingual cementoenamel border on the right mandibular first molar is clearly visible in the radiograph.

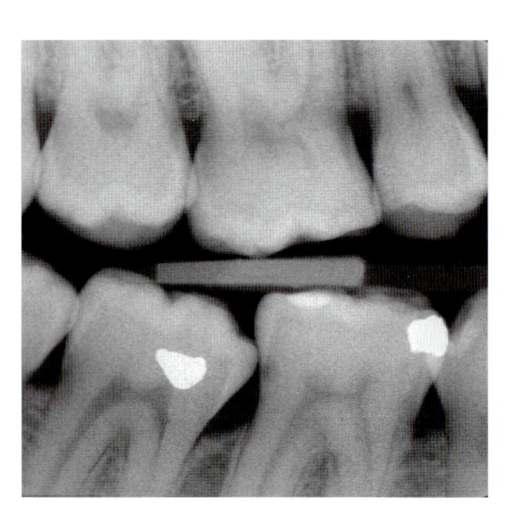

Fig 10-3 Same situation clinically: without rubber dam and at a low magnification, the caries cannot be detected.

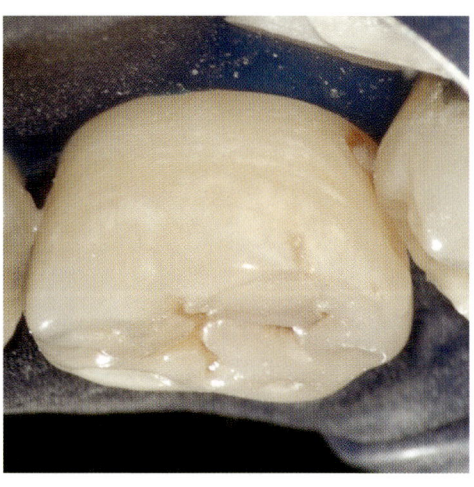

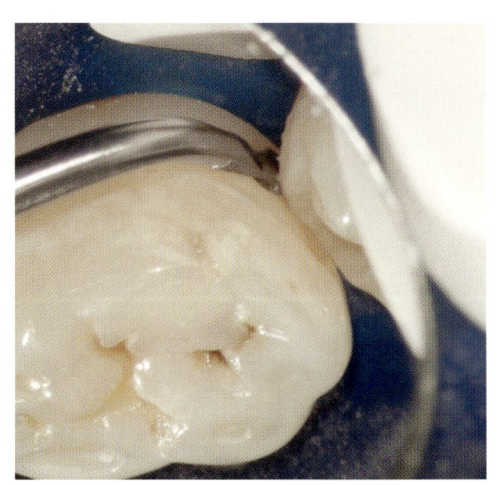

Fig 10-4 After placement of the rubber dam, the caries can be visually located using the microscope.

Fig 10-5 Preparation with ultrasound (KaVo Sonicsys).

Utility and futility of magnification aids in restorative dentistry

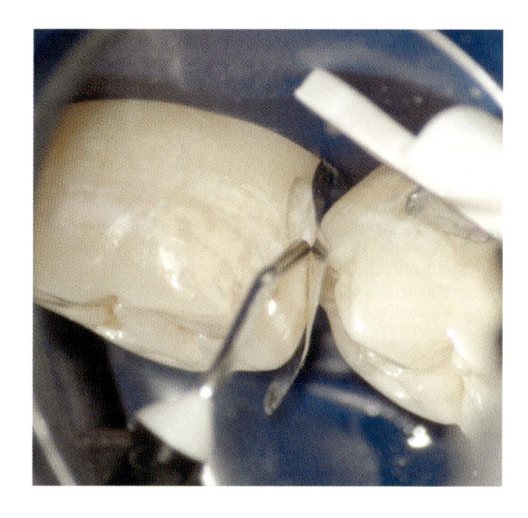

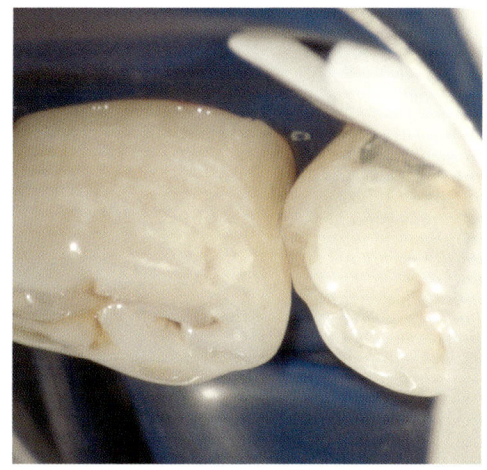

Fig 10-6 Drying the prepared cavity with a fine air jet (Stropko attachment).

Fig 10-7 Fully finished composite resin restoration; the rubber dam is slightly damaged.

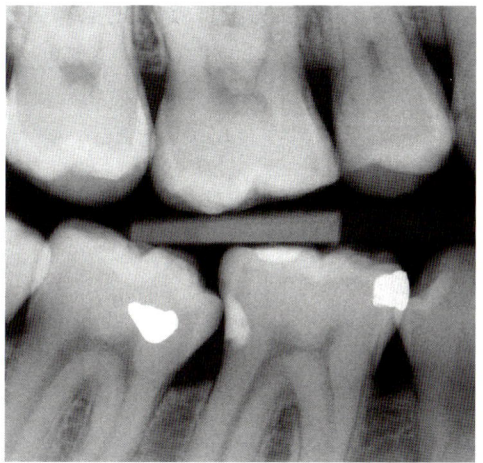

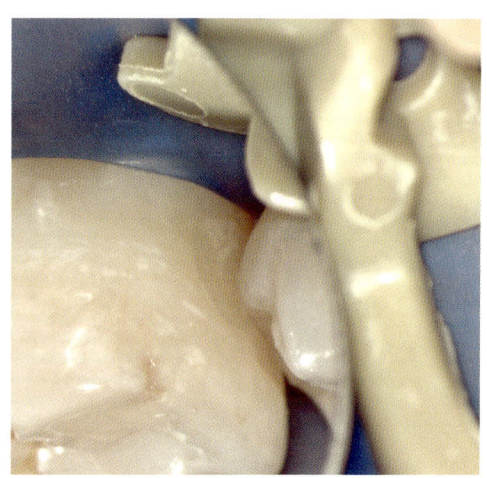

Fig 10-8 The restoration at the check-up after 18 months. Although the small air bubble inside the composite resin is not clinically relevant, it does illustrate how difficult it is to achieve bubble-free restoration of small cavities.

Fig 10-9 After 10 years the restoration is intact.

Case 2: Minimally invasive treatment of secondary caries (Figs 10-10 to 10-16)

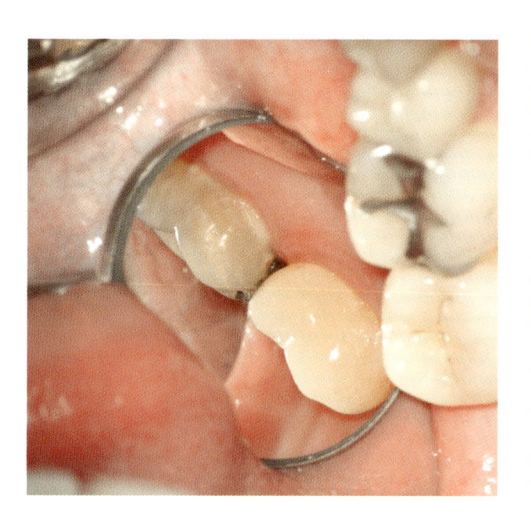

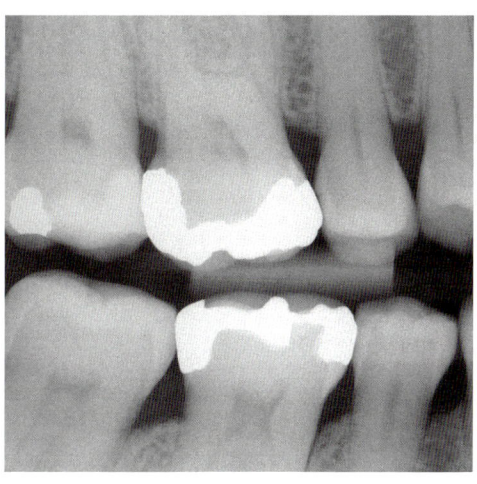

Fig 10-10 Localized secondary caries distolingual to the mandibular right first molar; amalgam restoration otherwise intact. It should be noted that the situation is visually unclear despite the 2.5× magnification.

Fig 10-11 The clinically detected secondary caries distal to the first molar cannot be detected on the bitewing radiograph.

Fig 10-12 After placement of the rubber dam and under stronger magnification, the caries can clearly be assessed.

Fig 10-13 Finished preparation, the transition between enamel and amalgam is entirely caries-free.

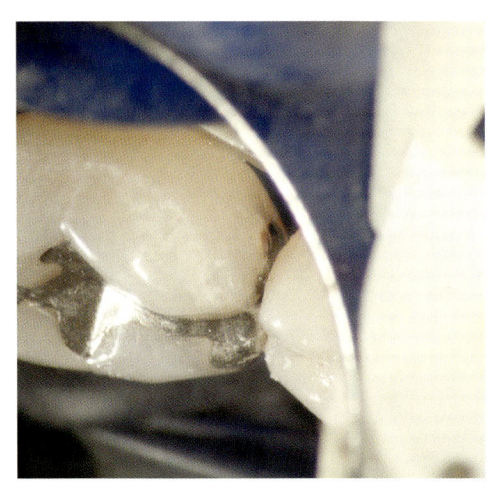

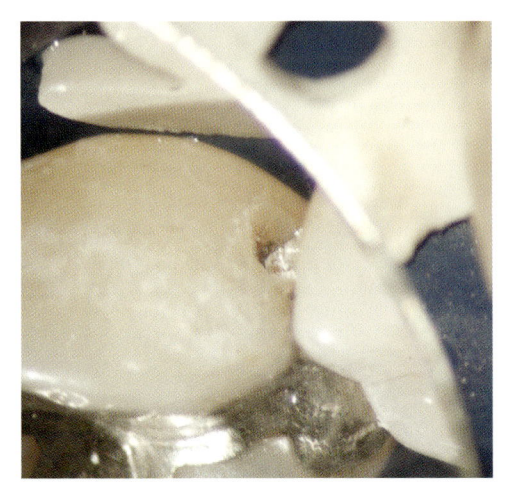

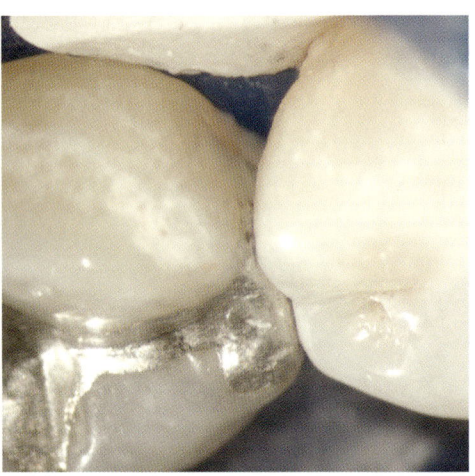

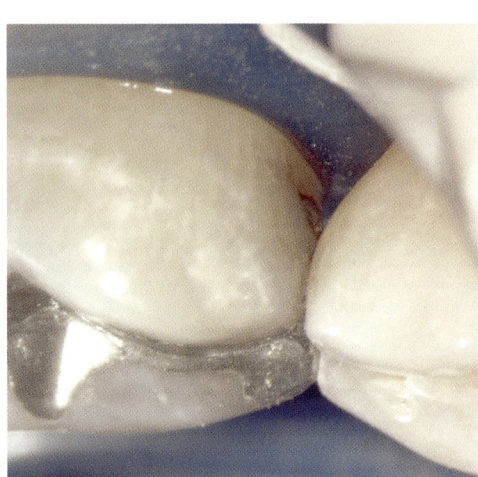

Fig 10-14 Finished composite resin restoration.

Fig 10-15 Clinical image nearly 10 years later.

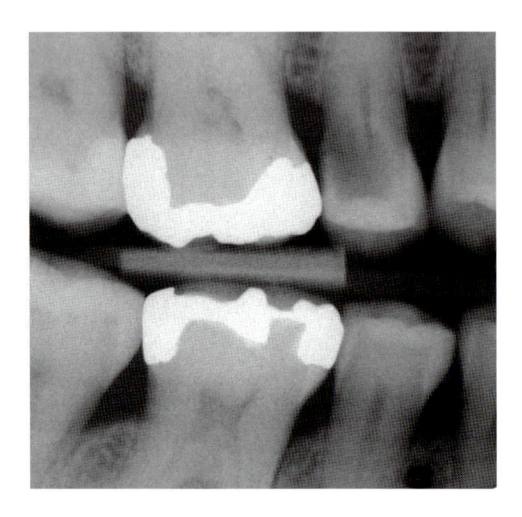

Fig 10-16 Bitewing radiograph also 10 years later. The restoration is intact and there is no caries. Deep caries affecting the maxillary second premolar, which developed within 2 years because of medication-induced xerostomia, should be noted.

References

1. Arens DE. Introduction to magnification in endodontics. J Esthet Restor Dent 2003;15:426–439.

2. Buhrley LJ, Barrows MJ, BeGole EA, Wenckus CS. Effect of magnification on locating the MB2 canal in maxillary molars. J Endod 2002;28:324–327.

3. Burton JF, Bridgeman GF. Presbyopia and the dentist: the effect of age on clinical vision. Int Dent J 1990;40: 303–312.

4. Eichenberger M, Perrin P, Neuhaus KW, Bringolf U, Lussi A. Influence of loupes and microscopes on the near visual acuity of practicing dentists. J Biomed Opt 2011;16(3):035003.

5. Görduysus Ö, Görduysus M, Friedman S. Operating microscope improves negotiation of second mesiobuccal canals in maxillary molars. J Endod 2001; 27:683–686.

6. Lussi A, Kronenberg O, Megert B. The effect of magnification on the iatrogenic damage to adjacent tooth surfaces during class II preparation. J Dent 2003;31:291–296.

7. Perrin P, Jacky D, Hotz P. Das Operationsmikroskop in der zahnärztlichen Allgemeinpraxis. Schweiz Monatsschr Zahnmed 2000;110:947–954.

8. Perrin P, Jacky D, Hotz P. Das Operationsmikroskop in der zahnärztlichen Praxis: minimalinvasive Füllungen. Schweiz Monatsschr Zahnmed 2002;112:723–729.

9. Schwarze T, Baethge C, Stecher T, Geurtsen W. Identification of second canals in the mesiobuccal root of maxillary first and second molars using magnifying loupes or an operating microscope. Aust Endod J 2002;28:57–60.

10. Velvart P. Das Operationsmikroskop in der Wurzelspitzenresektion. Teil II: Die retrograde Versorgung. Schweiz Monatsschr Zahnmed 1997;107:507–521.

11. Velvart P. Das Operationsmikroskop in der Wurzelspitzenresektion. Teil I: Die Resektion. Schweiz Monatsschr Zahnmed 1997;107:969–978.

12. Zitzmann NU, Danzkay Chen M, Zenhäusern R. Häufigkeit und Auswirkungn von Rückenbeschwerden im zahnärztlichen Beruf. Schweiz Monatsschr Zahnmed 2008;108:610–618.

Damage to adjacent teeth and minimally invasive preparation

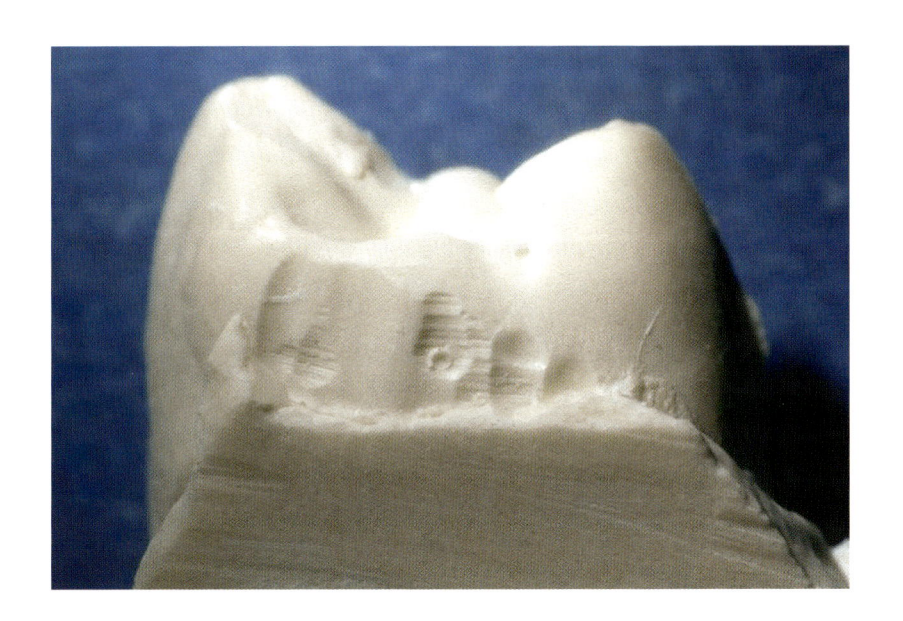

11 Damage to adjacent teeth and minimally invasive preparation

Martina Eichenberger, Philippe Perrin, and Adrian Lussi

■ Introduction

For nearly a whole century, Black's principle of *"extension for prevention"* predominated in restorative dentistry. Preparation guidelines based on this principle are now obsolete and have been superseded by a more sophisticated, minimally invasive approach. Thus *"prevention of extension"* has taken the place of *"extension for prevention"*.[14]

This development has been made possible by a better understanding of carious processes and by the availability of adhesive materials. If lesions are detected early, further progression can be halted in the initial stage by suitable preventive measures. If invasive therapy in indicated, the affected teeth are treated using the smallest possible defect-specific restorations.

Intensive preventive measures and minimally invasive therapy are a major focus of modern dentistry.

The pursuit of minimally invasive therapy also requires preparation of the smallest possible approximal cavities, which, using conventional instruments, is difficult to do without damaging the adjacent teeth.[6,10,12] This damage to adjacent teeth, which is contrary to the principal aim of substance preservation, often remains undetected. This chapter therefore examines the problem of damage to adjacent teeth and how to prevent it through the use of various aids.

■ The origin and consequences of damage to adjacent teeth

Studies have shown that minimally invasive approximal cavity preparation is not the only cause of damage to adjacent teeth. Iatrogenic grinding marks are left on adjacent teeth in 69 % of conventional Class II preparations[15] and at least 73 % of cases of crown preparations[3] (Table 11-1). These marks are frequently overlooked because they are often inconspicuous in the enamel and because attention is focused on the cavity. Cervical damage is more com-

Damage to adjacent teeth and minimally invasive preparation

Table 11-1 Adjacent tooth damage in crown and Class II preparations

Preparation	Adjacent tooth damage	Practitioner	Study
Crown preparation	73%	Dentists, private practice	Moopnar and Faulkner (1991)[13]
	94%	Students	Moopnar and Faulkner (1991)[13]
	90%	Dentists, private practice	Strübig and Opitz (2000)[17]
Class II preparation	69%	Dentists, advanced training courses	Qvist et al (1992)[15]
	100%	Dentists, private practice	Lussi and Gygax (1998)[8]
	64%	Dentists, university	Medeiros et al (2000)[12]
	100%	Dentists, laboratory study	Hahn et al (2000)[2]

mon than coronal damage, primarily due to the preparation technique. In the case of traditional Class II preparatory work, the initial access is from the occlusal direction, leaving a thin approximal enamel ridge that is subsequently removed. The cavity usually has to be widened slightly in the apical area because the carious defect has been underestimated. This widening leads to the above-mentioned damage to adjacent teeth (Fig 11-1).[10]

Surface damage does not inevitably lead to the formation of caries but it does increase the risk of caries: check-ups over a period of up to 7 years showed that tooth surfaces with iatrogenic damage had to be restored with a significantly higher frequency than undamaged tooth surfaces.[15] This is due to the fact that the affected surfaces accumulate more plaque and lie in an area that is difficult to access for hygiene purposes.[3,4] In addition, the damage exposes deeper enamel layers which are more easily demineralized.

> Iatrogenic grinding marks favor the formation of caries and result in more restorations to the tooth surfaces concerned.

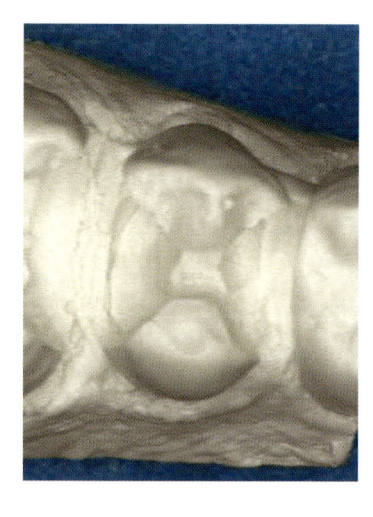

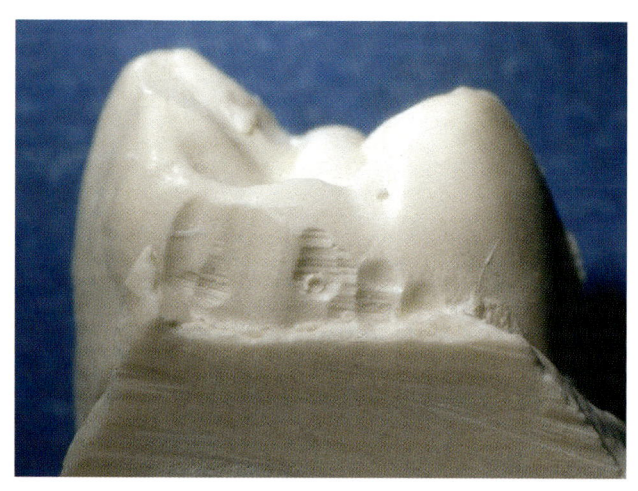

Fig 11-1 Left: from the occlusal view no damage to the adjacent tooth can be seen. Right: from the distal view, distinct iatrogenic grinding marks can be seen, which are particularly pronounced in the cervical third.

Damage to adjacent teeth and minimally invasive preparation

■ Aids to prevent adjacent tooth damage

Metal matrices

The adjacent tooth can be protected by the insertion of a metal matrix, but there are certain limitations (Fig 11-2). Matrices make accessibility and viewing difficult during preparation and matrices that are particularly thin offer only minimal mechanical protection because they are destroyed relatively quickly.[8] Placement of a metal matrix, however, increases the attention paid to the adjacent tooth surface and facilitates diagnosis of any damage.

Oscillating instruments

Oscillating instruments can be divided into low-frequency oscillating (eg, Prepcontrol) and high-frequency oscillating (eg, SONICflex) preparation systems. In studies, both systems showed a significant reduction of adjacent tooth damage, especially when they were used in combination with countersink drilling using a front-end cutting diamond bur with a recessed cutting face (Fig 11-3).[6,8]

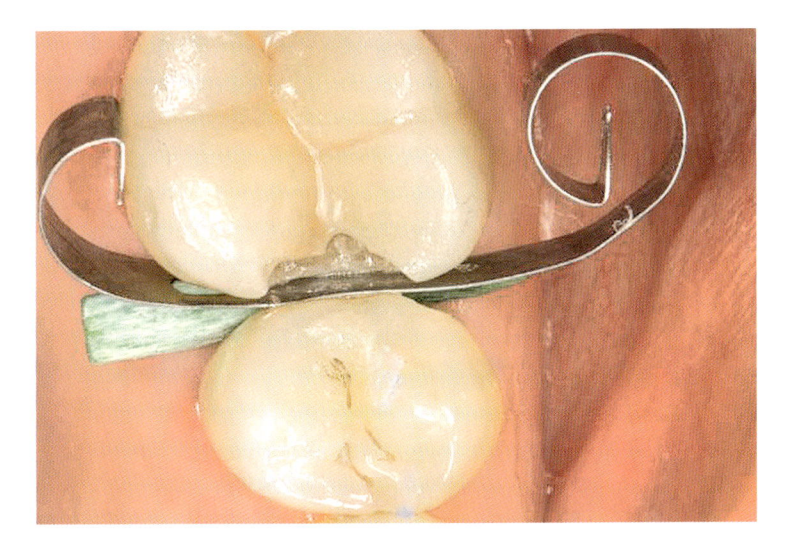

Fig 11-2 Metal matrix inserted to protect the adjacent tooth.

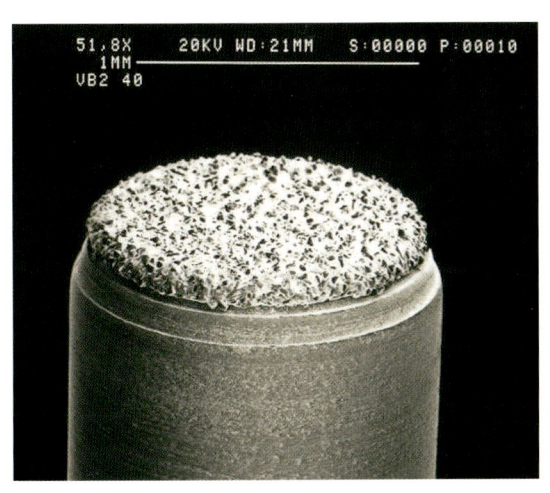

Fig 11-3 Front-end cutting diamond bur with recessed cutting face (Intensiv tcb-diamond).

Damage to adjacent teeth and minimally invasive preparation

The Prepcontrol system (KaVo) is based on the familiar EVA system and comprises an oscillating contra-angle handpiece with lockable file positions and 0.8 mm stroke height (Fig 11-4). After basic preparation with rotary instruments, the approximal enamel lamella created is broken away with a vertical drill or with hand instruments and the cavity floor is deepened and finished as required. To avoid damage to adjacent teeth, only the above-mentioned countersink drills should be used. Lateral walls and the side wall of the box can be finished using the Cavishape file. The Bevelshape file, which produces good edge quality quickly and easily, is suitable for edge beveling (Figs 11-5 and 11-6).[3,4,9] The newly developed Intensiv Margin Shaper is even more efficient for edge beveling; it can be used to prepare and bevel the lateral walls and the cervical shoulder in a single step.[16] Bevelshape files and the Intensiv Margin Shaper can also be used for finishing the chamfer in crown or veneer preparations (Figs 11-7 and 11-8). The Proxoshape file is employed for removing excess material after placement of the restoration (Fig 11-9).

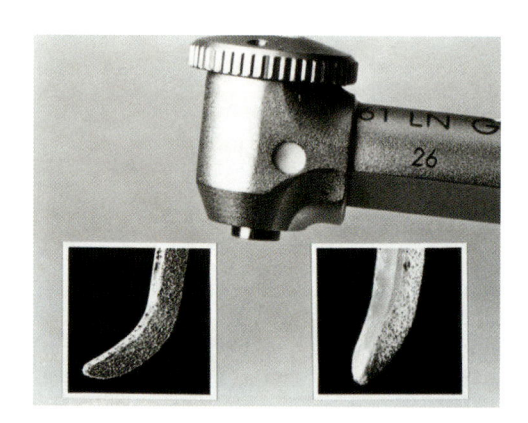

Fig 11-4 Prepcontrol with original Cavishape file (left) and Bevelshape file.

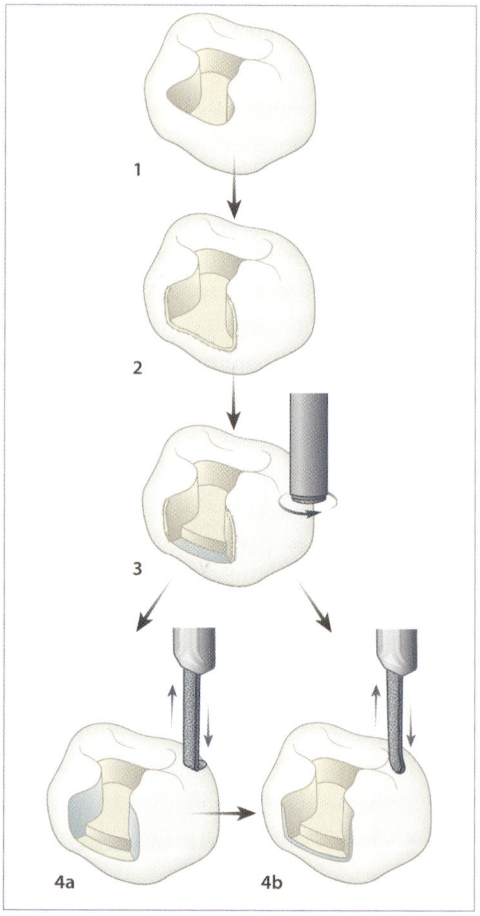

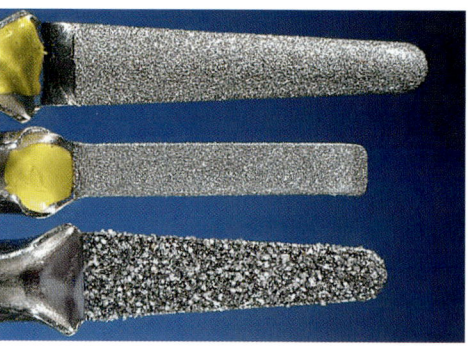

Fig 11-6 Bevelshape file (top), Cavishape file (center), and Proxoshape file (bottom).

Fig 11-5 Preparation and finishing of the cavity floor using Intensiv tcb-diamond (3), finishing of the side walls of the box using Cavishape file (4a), beveling of the lateral walls and the cervical shoulder using Bevelshape file (4b).

Damage to adjacent teeth and minimally invasive preparation

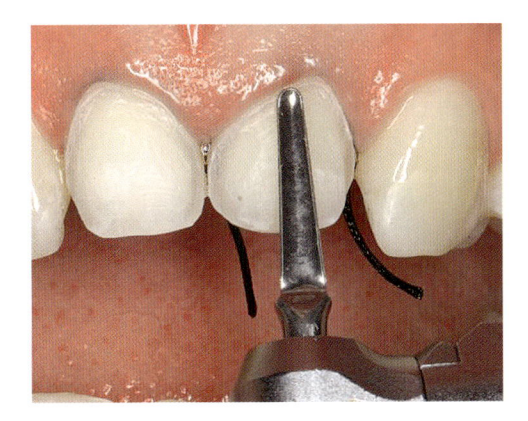

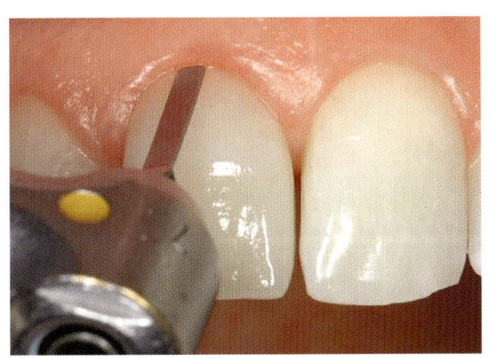

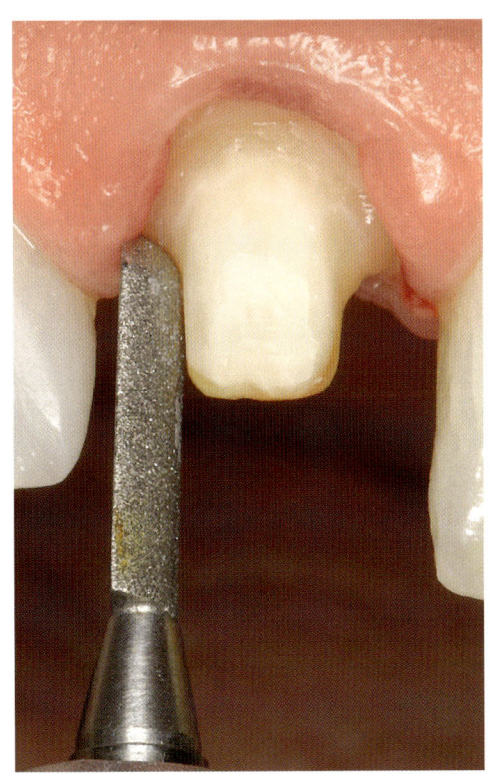

Fig 11-7 (Top left) Finishing of veneer preparation with the Bevelshape file.

Fig 11-8 (Right) Finishing a crown preparation with the Intensiv Margin Shaper.

Fig 11-9 (Bottom left) Removal of excess after adhesive cementing of the veneer.

The Prepcontrol system, with its different file shapes, has a diversity of uses and protects not only the adjacent tooth surfaces, but also the gingiva. It is suitable primarily for cavity preparation. The former disadvantages of poor abrasive efficiency and unpleasant sensations experienced by patients have largely been eliminated by the development of a damped EVA head with an altered stroke (0.8 mm instead of 0.4 mm).[3,4,9]

One example of a high-frequency oscillating system is the SONICflex Airscaler (KaVo), which oscillates in the sonic range (< 6.5 kHz). Owing to the sonic drive, a transverse movement component of the working tip is achieved in addition to the longitudinal oscillation.[3,4] The special micropreparation instrumentation with fine hemispherical tips that are diamond-coated on one side enables the smallest cavities to be prepared, even in poorly accessible areas (Fig 11-10). The tips display good abrasive efficiency, especially in enamel, and therefore allow primary opening of the defect, while the side without a diamond coating faces the adjacent tooth surface. In addition to the micropreparation tips, box-shaped SONICsys approx tips, which flare slightly in the occlusal direction and have a circular contact angle of 45 degrees, are available in a range of sizes (Fig 11-11). Their abrasive efficiency compared with rotary instruments and with the finer tips is rather low, which is why they are mainly suitable for the final shaping and finishing.[3,4]

Simple and precise preparation of suitable cavity shapes can be achieved using high-frequency oscillating systems. However, a disadvantage of these systems is the fixed position of the attachment in the handpiece.

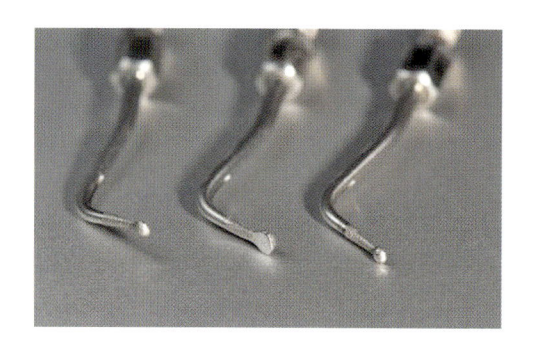

Fig 11-10 SONICflex tips diamond-coated on one side only for minimally invasive preparations.

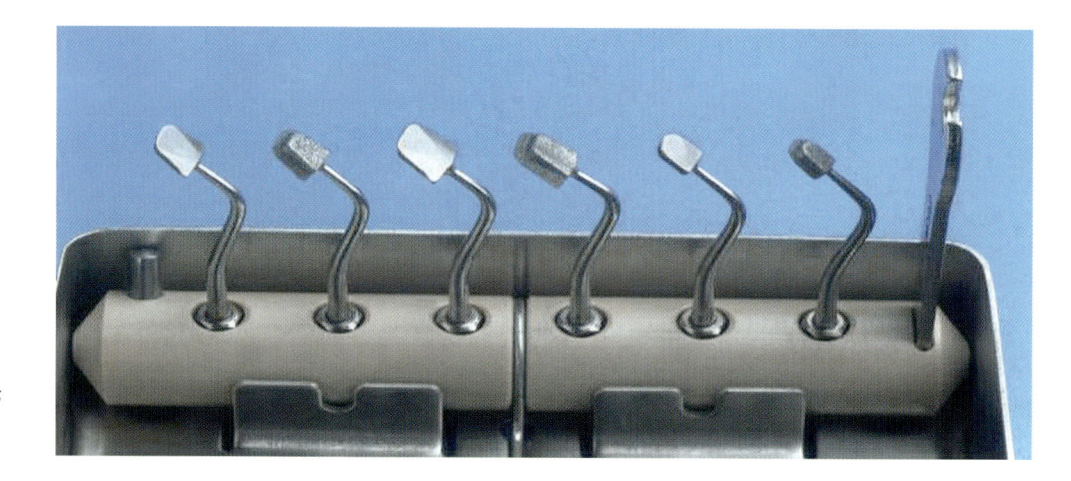

Fig 11-11 Box-shaped SONICsys approx tips in different sizes for both mesial and distal surfaces.

> Oscillating instruments are mainly used for minimally invasive cavity preparation and finishing in the marginal area. Damage to adjacent teeth can largely be prevented.

Hand instruments

Hand instruments for edge shaping of approximal cavities cause very little damage to adjacent teeth. However, their abrasive efficiency, especially in enamel, is very low and so the quality of the finished edges is usually poor. Hand instruments cannot, therefore, be recommended for the finishing of cavities.

Magnification

Studies have shown that magnifying aids offer advantages when removing restorations[1] and diagnosing caries.[5,7] However, whether magnifying aids are useful during preparation, especially in respect of adjacent tooth damage, is a matter of intense debate. For instance, a study by Lussi et al[11] showed no significant differences in terms of damage to adjacent teeth between preparations prepared with and without loupe glasses. How the complex visual system and the quality of dental work are influenced by magnifying aids has not been fully resolved; chapter 10 of this book explores the relevant issues.

Conclusions

Damage to adjacent teeth has an adverse effect on the prognosis of the affected teeth. Such damage is common with both conventional and minimally invasive preparations if nonspecific techniques and instruments are used. The refinement and improvement of these instruments is therefore particularly important for modern minimally invasive dentistry.

References

1. Forgie AH, Pine CM, Pitts NB. Restoration removal with and without the aid of magnification. J Oral Rehabil 2001;28:209–313.
2. Hahn P, Günther F, Hellwig E. Einfluss verschiedener Präparationstechniken auf die Verletzung von Nachbarzähnen und die Qualität der Schmelzabschrägung. Dtsch Zahnärztl Z 2000;55:118–123.
3. Hugo B. Oszillierende Verfahren in der Präparationstechnik (Teil I). Schweiz Monatsschr Zahnmed 1999a;109:140–153.
4. Hugo B. Oszillierende Verfahren in der Präparationstechnik (Teil II). Schweiz Monatsschr Zahnmed 1999b;109:269–280.
5. Lussi A. Comparison of different methods for the diagnosis of fissure caries without cavitation. Caries Res 1993;27:409–416.
6. Lussi A. Verletzung der Nachbarzähne bei der Präparation approximaler Kavitäten. Schweiz Monatsschr Zahnmed 1995;105:1259–1264.
7. Lussi A. Impact of including or excluding cavitated lesions when evaluating the performance of occlusal caries diagnostic methods. Caries Res 1996;30:389–393.
8. Lussi A, Gygax M. Präparationstechnik zur signifikanten Minimierung von Nachbarzahnverletzungen. Eine In-vivo-Studie. Acta Med Dent Helv 1996;1:3–6.
9. Lussi A, Jaeggi T, Gygax M. Einfluss des Hubes und der Kraftdämpfung beim Gebrauch des EVA-Systems. Acta Med Dent Helv 1997;2:273–276.
10. Lussi A, Gygax M. Iatrogenic damage to adjacent teeth during classical approximal box preparation. J Dentistry 1998;26:435–441.
11. Lussi A, Kronenberg O, Megert B. The effect of magnification on the iatrogenic damage to adjacent tooth surfaces during class II preparation. J Dentistry 2003;31:291–296.
12. Medeiros VAF. Iatrogenic damage to approximal surfaces in contact with Class II restorations. J Dentistry 2000;28:103–110.
13. Moopnar M, Faulkner KD. Accidental damage to teeth adjacent to crown-prepared abutment teeth. Aust Dent J 1991;36:136–140.
14. Peters MC, McLean ME. Minimally invasive operative care. II Contemporary techniques and materials: an overview. J Adhesive Dent 2001;3:17–31.
15. Qvist V, Johannessen L, Bruun M. Progression of approximal caries in relation to iatrogenic preparation damage. J Dent Res 1992;71:1370–1373.
16. Schmidlin PR, Wolleb K, Imfeld T, Gygax M, Lussi A. Influence of beveling and ultrasound application on marginal adaptation of box-only Class II (slot) resin composite restorations. Oper Dent 2007;32:291–297.
17. Strübig W, Opitz J. Präparationsdefekte an Nachbarzähnen bei Inlay- und Kronenversorgungen. Dtsch Zahnärztl Z 2000;55:101–103.

12 Novel preparation and excavation methods

Klaus Neuhaus, Franziska Jeger, Philip Ciucchi, and Adrian Lussi

■ Introduction

Preparation of diseased hard dental substance is usually performed at high speed with rotary diamond burs or with tungsten carbide rotary burs. In contrast, excavation of dentin softened by caries is done at slow to medium speed using round burs. These methods, used in conjunction with water cooling, offer the advantages of speed and the possibility of sterilizing used abrasives and burs and using them several times. Another advantage is the tactile feedback created by the working ends being in contact with the tooth. The noise, the discomfort caused by vibration, and the relative inaccuracy during preparation can be seen as disadvantages of these methods. Healthy hard dental substance often has to be sacrificed in order to gain access to the lesion body. This is why other preparation and excavation methods are being investigated; methods which are likely to embrace the principles of minimally invasive dentistry.

■ Kinetic preparation using air abrasion

Air abrasion was introduced into dentistry by *Black* in the 1950s,[5] but was then abandoned in favor of high-speed turbines. In recent years, however, it has been used increasingly as an alternative to conventional preparation with diamond abrasives. It has been shown that patients' acceptance of air abrasion devices is high. Younger patients, in particular, appreciate the lower noise level and the reduced pain and vibration compared with micromotor-driven abrasive instruments. Occlusal discolorations and primary caries can both be removed efficiently and delicately by this method.[7] Furthermore it has been shown that the process of diagnosing occlusal caries is improved after air abrasion.[10] In a recently published *in vitro* study, air abrasion with aluminum oxide powder resulted in markedly better diagnostic information in relation to primary molars for both laser fluorescence measurements and visual inspection.[21]

The principle of air abrasion technology involves blasting the tooth surface with abrasive particles using high pressure air (around 5 bar). The most commonly used powder for blasting away hard dental substance is aluminum oxide (Al_2O_3) with an average particle size of 27.5 μm. These particles blast small quantities of hard dental substance out of the biological matrix, as a result of the kinetic energy released, and leave small craters on the tooth surface. The surface thus treated appears rough under the microscope and is therefore ideal for subsequent restoration using the adhesive technique (Fig 12-1).[2] One disadvantage of this technique is that, during treatment, a potentially harmful powder-and-water aerosol is produced, especially when nonsoluble aluminum oxide is used. It has been shown, however, that the quantity of powder particles produced in the aerosol is too small to pose a health risk to patient or dental practitioner.[23] The resulting aerosol can be effectively controlled by the use of efficient water cooling (always use maximum water feed) and powerful suction. Nevertheless, the lack of tactile feedback and generally low specificity seem to be an obstacle to more widespread use of this technology.[16]

Air abrasion is currently used mainly for cleaning fissures, to aid caries detection and to make probing wholly superfluous. This is because forced probing of a questionable lesion can sometimes induce progression of that lesion.[15] However, it is advised that the method is applied conservatively and with caution when used for diagnostic purposes as the aluminum powder can cause damage to healthy fissures or arrested initial lesions.[20] An alternative is the air-polishing technique, in which sodium bicarbonate ($NaHCO_3$) is used instead of aluminum oxide to remove plaque and occlusal discolorations and thus allow more accurate visual diagnosis.

Preparation of delicate cavities is possible with air abrasion because, unlike round burs or rotary diamond abrasives, it is end-cutting.[22] Therefore, this method is ideally suited to extended pit and fissure sealing (Fig 12-2).

By contrast, the poor selectivity between healthy and demineralized dental hard substance and between enamel and dentin is problematic.[12] This characteristic of nonspecific preparation, combined with a lack of tactile feedback, carries a risk of overpreparation; ie, causing injury to healthy dental hard substance. Thus air abrasion is less well suited to the preparation of larger and deeper lesions. This is why efforts are being made to develop new powders with selective preparation characteristics so that only carious enamel or only carious dentin, for instance, is removed. Bioactive glass might be such a powder: it can be used to clean and polish tooth surfaces selectively and, after debonding of orthodontic brackets, it results in a cleaner surface than preparation with tungsten carbide finishers.[4] However, bioactive glass – like aluminum oxide – is not resorbable and is therefore potentially harmful.

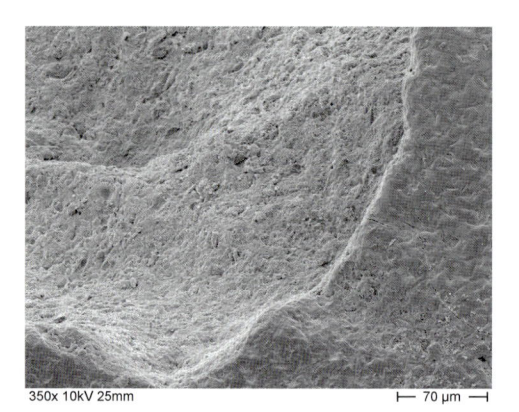

Fig 12-1 Air abrasion with aluminum oxide leads to a rough enamel surface which is ideally suited to adhesive restorations.

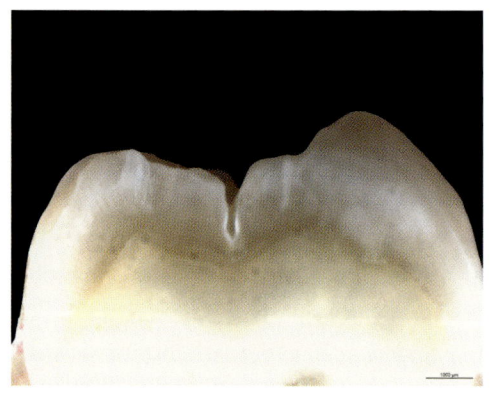

Fig 12-2 Widened fissure after kinetic preparation with aluminum oxide.

Novel preparation and excavation methods

Air abrasion with aluminum oxide powder is a suitable method for preparation of delicate cavities. However, the preparation of larger and deeper defects is problematic because of its low specificity. The technique has high patient acceptance because there is less noise and less pain than with rotary preparation.

■ Laser preparation

Laser (acronym for *"light amplification by stimulated emission of radiation"*) has been used in more and more areas of medicine over recent years. In dentistry, too, laser therapy is interesting from the viewpoint of both dental practitioner and patient. Acceptance among patients seems to be considerable.[13] In dentistry, four types of laser are particularly valuable:

- Diode laser $\lambda =$ 610 nm
- Er,Cr:YSGG $\lambda =$ 2,790 nm
- Er:YAG laser $\lambda =$ 2,940 nm
- CO_2 laser $\lambda =$ 10,600 nm

Laser treatments operate on the principle of absorption of electromagnetic energy in body tissue. The various types of laser differ in terms of the media that they excite. The energy difference between the excited and the unexcited states of the medium is equivalent to the energy of the emitted photons.

Different lasers produce different wavelengths (λ), and the wavelength is inversely proportional to the energy. Therefore, the amount of energy emitted is specific to the type of laser. Unlike the wavelength, a laser's frequency is directly proportional to the energy. A laser with a higher frequency is therefore more energy-rich.

A distinction is often made between soft and hard lasers. The difference is that a soft laser is characterized by much lower power at a lower energy density than a hard laser. Soft lasers can also be used for biostimulation.

The process underlying the laser removal of tissues is the absorption of electromagnetic radiation by substances in the tissue, which causes the substance being worked to vaporize explosively (Table 12-1).

The CO_2 laser was introduced by *Patel* as early as the 1960s.[17] This type of laser is excellent for surgical procedures on soft tissues because of the high absorption in water. However, preparation of dental hard substance is poor with this type of laser. Diode and Nd:YAG lasers are also unsuitable for the preparation of dental hard substance because of their poor absorption in hydroxyapatite.

By contrast, enamel and dentin, and also cementum, bone, and even composite resin, can be abraded with the Er:YAG laser. Only amalgam cannot be prepared with this laser. The

Table 12-1 Overview of different types of laser

Wavelength	< 750 nm	750–2,500 nm	> 2,500 nm	> 10,000 nm
Laser type	Diode laser (soft laser)	Nd:YAG laser, Ho:YAG laser	Er:YAG laser, Er,Cr:YSGG laser	CO_2 laser
Absorption	Hemoglobin, pigments	Hemoglobin, hydroxyapatite	Water, hydroxyapatite	Water (high absorption)
Principal use	Periodontology, surgery, endodontology	Coagulation	Enamel and dentin preparation	Soft tissue surgery

Er,Cr:YSGG laser, which has a similar wavelength to the Er:YAG laser, can similarly be used for hard tissue preparation. From the patient's point of view, the greatest advantage of dental treatment by laser is undoubtedly that anesthesia can often be dispensed with.[8] With different settings of the Er:YAG laser, more or less specific cutting of enamel or dentin can rapidly be performed.

After cavity preparation, the entire preparation should be finished with a low energy density because loose enamel and dentin chips (Fig 12-3) otherwise reduce adhesive bond strength. Another advantage is that the prepared tooth surface, deemed sterile after finishing obviously, does not have to be selectively etched and the bonding system can be directly applied (Figs 12-4 and 12-5).[3] Which bonding systems are especially suitable has not yet been adequately investigated. Some research studies show that repairs to existing composite resin restorations can also be carried out more simply. Working the composite resin surface with the Er:YAG laser is likely to render silanization unnecessary.[6]

Irrespective of the above advantages, it is important to be aware that preparation using laser demands a great deal of adjustment and familiarization on the part of the practitioner. The depth of the cavity is difficult to assess as it is constantly filled with cooling water, and the practitioner lacks any tactile control because of the 2 to 3 mm working distance between the laser and the cavity. Furthermore, the practitioner needs to be able to estimate the correct laser parameters for optimum cutting of the particular dental hard substance, which is an added difficulty.

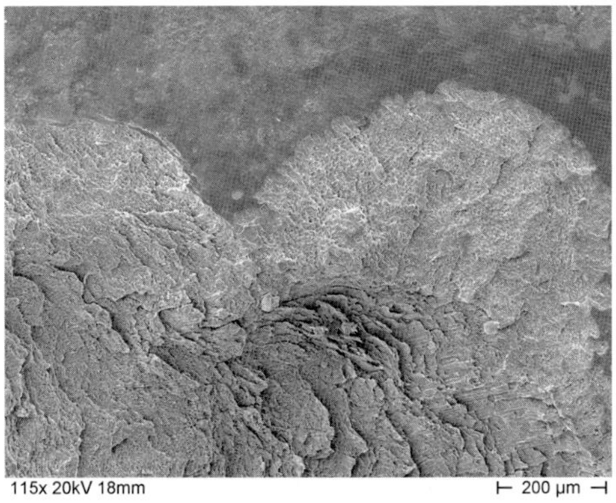

Fig 12-3 Er:YAG laser preparation in enamel (bottom: 300 mJ/25 Hz; middle of picture: after finishing the preparation with 100mJ/35 Hz).

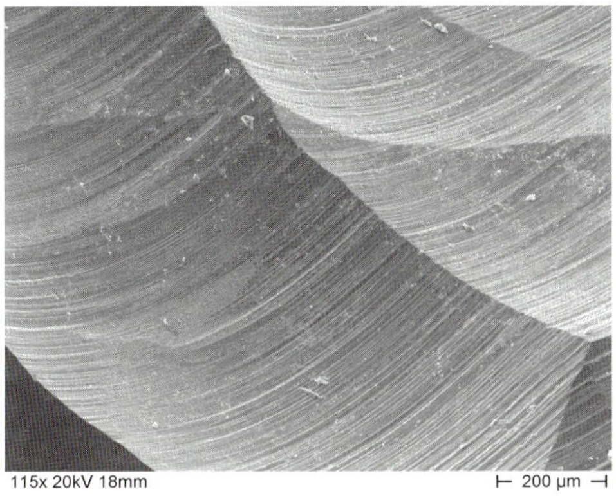

Fig 12-4 Enamel preparation with finishing diamond.

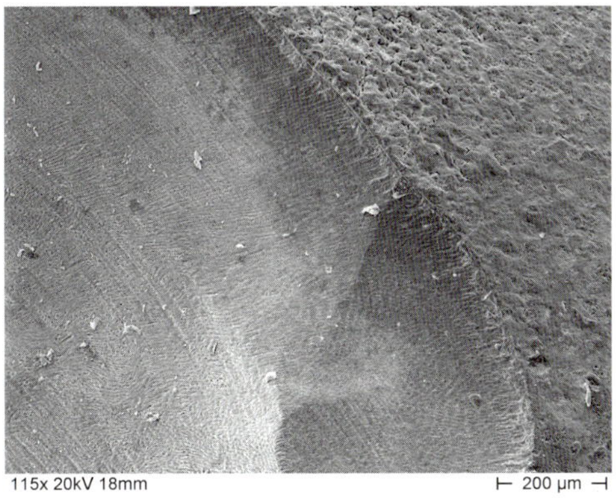

Fig 12-5 Enamel preparation with finishing diamond plus etching with 37 % phosphoric acid for 30 seconds.

The preparation of dental hard substance with the Er:YAG laser offers advantages for both the patient and the practitioner. However, the fact that the user needs to develop specific skills must not be underestimated. Further research studies, particularly clinical trials, are necessary to investigate the durability of adhesive restorations after laser preparation.

■ Selective removal of dentin caries

The question of how much dentin has to be excavated before placement of a restoration is a matter of some debate. Removal of infected and soft dentin is generally required, but dentin that is hard on probing, which has in fact been altered by the carious process and harbors around 1,000 times fewer viable bacteria, should be excluded from excavation.[14] "Soft" dentin characteristically displays denaturation of collagen fibers, while "hard" dentin may be demineralized but has remineralization potential. Testing residual dentin hardness using a probe often leads to overextension of the cavity into healthy dentin. The use of caries-detecting solutions is also not without its problems because they are subject to variability and wide interpretation.[9,24]

Conversely, it has been shown that self-limiting dentin excavation methods might be able to preserve healthy dentin substance. Specific enzymes are involved in these self-limiting excavation methods, for example, the digestive enzymes trypsin and pepsin, which appear to have no effect on healthy dentin.[1] In a caries model with artificial dentin caries, it was shown that the use of enzymes for self-limiting excavation of dentin caries can produce promising results because only denatured collagen is removed while remineralizable dentin is preserved.[1]

Another method for self-limiting caries excavation is chemomechanical excavation with Carisolv™, a gel containing 10 % sodium hypochlorite.[11] The gel is placed in the cavity and becomes cloudy as a result of the reaction with denatured dentin. A layer of dentin softened by caries is then removed using hand excavators. This step is repeated until the gel is no longer cloudy. The long treatment time must be regarded as a downside, which can be up to eight times longer than traditional excavation with round burs. In a clinical trial involving 50 children, more than 40% of lesions were still not caries-free after 15 minutes, so that the remaining dentin had to be removed with a round bur.[19] Nevertheless, chemomechanical excavation with Carisolv in pediatric dentistry may be regarded as advantageous because it causes less pain than traditional excavation but enables clinically equivalent restorations to be achieved.[18]

> Self-limiting methods for dentin excavation are a promising addition to the conservative treatment arsenal. Chemomechanical excavation using Carisolv™ offers advantages in pediatric dentistry or in the treatment of anxious patients, but it takes much longer than conventional methods. The latest excavation methods using proteolytic enzymes still need to have their practicality demonstrated in clinical trials.

■ References

1. Ahmed AA, García-Godoy F, Kunzelmann KH. Self-limiting caries therapy with proteolytic agents. Am J Dent 2008;21:303–312.
2. Antunes LA, Vieira AS, Alves Dos Santos MP, Maia LC. Influence of kinetic cavity preparation devices on dental topography: an *in vitro* study. J Contemp Dent Pract 2008;9:146–154.
3. Bader C, Krejci I. Marginal quality in enamel and dentin after preparation and finishing with Er:YAG laser. Am J Dent 2006;19:337–342.
4. Banerjee A, Paolinelis G, Socker M, McDonald F, Watson TF. An *in vitro* investigation of the effectiveness of bioactive glass air-abrasion in the 'selective' removal of orthodontic resin adhesive. Eur J Oral Sci 2008;116:488–492.
5. Black GV. Airabrasive: some fundamentals. J Am Dent Assoc 1950;41:701–710.
6. Burnett LH Jr, Shinkai RS, Eduardo CDE P. Tensile bond strength of a one-bottle adhesive system to indirect composites treated with Er:YAG laser, air-abrasion, or fluoridric acid. Photomed Laser Surg 2004;22:351–356.
7. Christensen GJ. Air-abrasion tooth cutting: state of the art 1998. J Am Dent Assoc 1998;129:484–485.
8. Delmé K, Meire M, De Bruyne M, Nammour S, De Moor R. Cavity preparation using an Er:YAG laser in the adult dentition. Rev Belge Med Dent 2009;64:71–80.
9. Fusayama T. Clinical guide for removing caries using a caries-detecting solution. Quintessence Int 1988;19:397–401.
10. Goldstein RE, Parkins FM. Using air-abrasive technology to diagnose and restore pit and fissure caries. J Am Dent Assoc 1995;126:761–766.
11. Hannig M. Effect of Carisolv™ Solution on sound, demineralized and denatured dentin. An ultrastructural investigation. Clin Oral Invest 1999;3:155–159.
12. Horiguchi S, Yamada T, Inokoshi S, Tagami J. Selective caries removal with air-abrasion. Oper Dent 1998;23:236–243.
13. Keller U, Hibst R, Geurtsen W, Schilke R, Heidemann D, Klaiber B, Raab WH. Erbium:YAG laser application in caries therapy. Evaluation of patient perception and acceptance. J Dent 1998;26:649–656.
14. Kidd EAM. How "clean" must a cavity be before restoration? Caries Res 2004;38:305–313.
15. Neuhaus KW, Ellwood R, Lussi A, Pitts NB. Traditional Lesion Detection Aids. Monogr Oral Sci 2009;21:42–51.
16. Paolinelis G, Watson TF, Banerjee A. Microhardness as a predictor of sound and carious dentine removal using alumina air-abrasion. Caries Res 2006;40:292–295.
17. Patel CKN. Interpretation of CO_2 - optical maser experiments. Phys Rev Lett 1964;12:588–590.
18. Peric T, Markovic D, Petrovic B. Clinical evaluation of a chemomechanical method for caries removal in children and adolescents. Acta Odontol Scand 2009;18(5):1–7.

19. Peters MC, Flamenbaum MH, Eboda NN, Feigal RJ, Inglehart MR. Chemomechanical caries removal in children: efficacy and efficiency. J Am Dent Assoc 2007;137:1658–1666.
20. Ricketts DN, Pitts NB. Novel operative treatment options. Monogr Oral Sci 2009;21:174–187.
21. Rodrigues JDE A, de Vita TM, Cordeiro RDE C. *In vitro* evaluation of the influence of air-abrasion on detection of occlusal caries lesions in primary teeth. Pediatr Dent 2008;30:15–18.
22. Santos-Pinto L, Peruchi C, Marker VA, Cordeiro R. Effect of handpiece tip design on the cutting efficiency of an air-abrasion system. Am J Dent 2001;14:397–401.
23. Wright GZ, Hatibovic-Kofman S, Millenaar DW, Braverman I. The safety and efficacy of treatment with air-abrasion technology. Int J Paediatr Dent 1999;9:133–140.
24. Yip HK, Stevenson AG, Beeley JA. The specificity of caries detector dyes in cavity preparation. Br Dent J 1994;176:417–421.

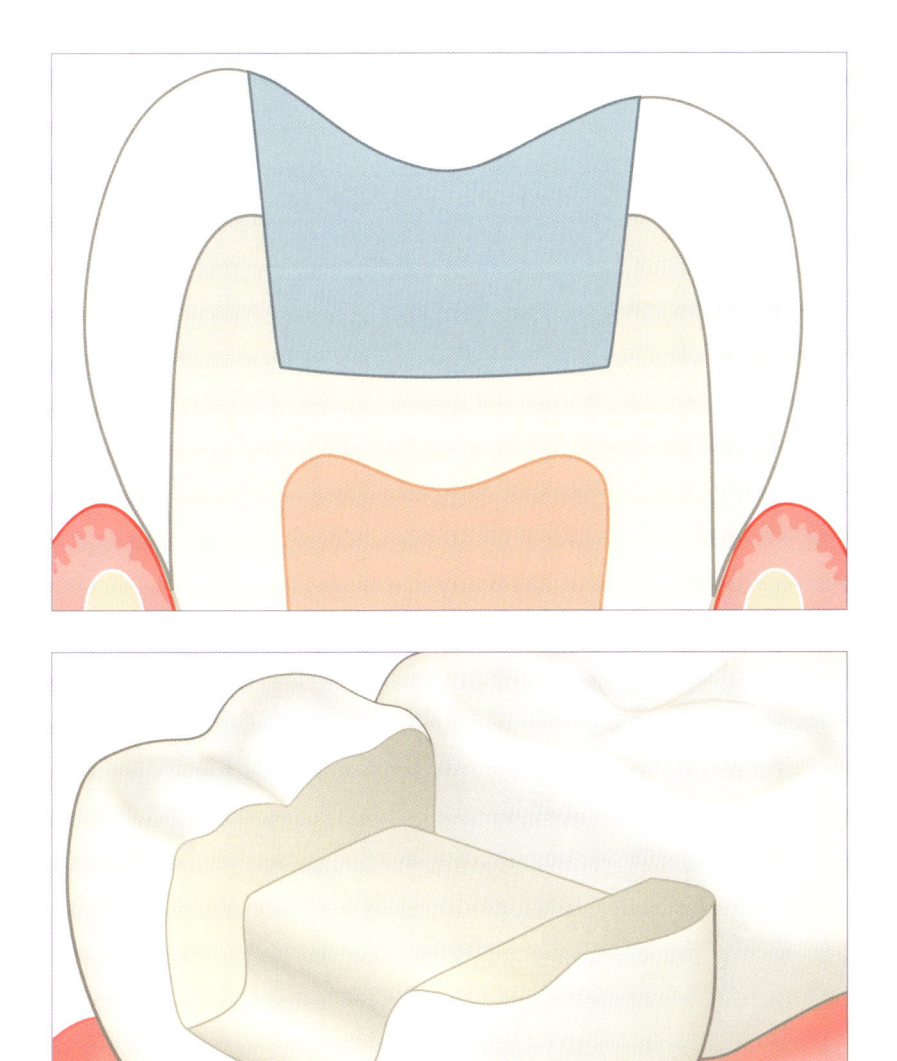

Yesterday retention – today adhesion?

VI

13 Adhesive techniques for dental restorations

Brigitte Zimmerli and Matthias Strub

▪ Introduction

The change from the "extension for prevention" preparation principle to minimally invasive restorations is based on the development of adhesive techniques. With its introduction, the preparation of undercuts or retention grooves became obsolete, which means that the preparation of tooth substance is less invasive. A reliable adhesive system is crucial to the long-term success of adhesively bonded restorations. It forms the interface between the restorative material (hydrophobic) and dental hard tissues (hydrophilic). The bonding agent has to form a strong interlocking with the two surfaces to resist the polymerization shrinkage and also to prevent gaps between tooth and restorative material. While the bond to the restorative material is primarily due to the C=C double bonds that remain in the surface layer of the adhesive due to oxygen inhibition, the bond to the tooth surface is more complex. Not least the tooth structure itself plays a decisive role because enamel and dentin display different properties.

Every adhesive system aims to achieve a sufficient bond between composite resin and the tooth surface. This is basically achieved in four steps:

1. Conditioning of the enamel surface with acid → etching pattern allows micromechanical interlocking.
2. Conditioning of the dentin surface with acid → (partial) dissolution of the smear layer, demineralization of the surface and the entrances to tubules, exposure of the collagen network.
3. Hydrophilic primer → diffusion into the collagen network and into opened tubules.
4. Adhesive → penetration and stabilization of the collagen network to form a hybrid layer in dentin → penetration into the etched enamel surface and bind to the composite resin.

▪ Classification of adhesive systems

The classification of adhesive systems into generations, based on the timing of market launch, is difficult to remember. It is far simpler and more intuitive to classify bonding agents according to their basic properties with regard to tooth conditioning and the number of individual components in the system.[13] A differentiation is made between "etch-and-rinse" systems (bonding agents where an acid is applied to the surface and then sprayed off with water) and the "self-etch" adhesive systems (where the etching is done by acidic monomers that do not have to be sprayed off). Depending on the number of individual components or steps, the range of systems extends from "one-step" adhesives (one-bottle systems) through to "four-step" adhesives (four-bottle systems) (Table 13-1).

> In etch-and-rinse systems, conditioning is performed by applying an acid that has to be sprayed off again. Self-etch systems condition using acidic monomers that do not have to be sprayed off.

The manufacturers' instructions must be carefully followed when using adhesive systems to obtain optimal bond strength. The individual components require enough time to penetrate into the tooth structure. Most hypersensitivities in the area of composite resin restorations after restoration placement can be attributed to inadequate application of the adhesive system. The individual components of a system must not be combined with those from another system. It is unacceptable to combine the primer from adhesive system A with the adhesive from system B. Conversely, an adhesive system from manufacturer X can be used in combination with a restorative material from manufacturer Y. There are only a few exceptions. For instance, it is imperative to use the restorative material Filtek Silorane® with its specific adhesive (Filtek Silorane System Adhesive®). Furthermore there are incompatibilities between self-curing composite resin materials and certain self-etch bonding agents (AdheSE one, Admira Bond, Adper Prompt L-Pop, Adper Scotchbond SE, Clearfil Protect Bond, Clearfil SE Bond, iBond self etch, Solobond M, Xeno). The acidic ingredients of these adhesives might neutralize the tertiary amine that is responsible for the polymerization of the self-curing materials.

Table 13-1 Overview of different adhesive systems (simplified representation)

Technique	Components	Conditioning	Primer	Adhesive	Product example
Etch-and-rinse	4-step				Syntac classic®[1]
	3-step				Optibond FL®
	2-step				ExciTE® One Coat Bond® Prime&Bond NT® XP Bond®
Self-etch	2-step				AdheSE® Clearfil SE Bond® One Coat SE Bond®
	1-step				Adper Prompt L-Pop®[2] Xeno III®[2] und V® AdheSE One® G-Bond®

[1] With this system, conditioning is subdivided into enamel and dentin conditioning. Syntac Primer® is thus applied for dentin conditioning, Syntac Adhesive® for the "primer step", and the product Heliobond® as an adhesive.

[2] With these systems two components have to be mixed together before application.

According to the data currently available, the etch-and-rinse adhesive systems Syntac classic® and Optibond FL® can continue to be regarded as the gold standards. Their bond strengths are reliable and both systems show promising long-term results. However, there are considerable differences between the self-etch systems. While the bond strength of Clearfil SE Bond® does not differ greatly from those of the gold standards, other systems have markedly lower bond strength. The one-step self-etch adhesive systems are still inferior to the multiple-step systems, according to most studies. The chemical stability of these products is limited and, at most, a minimal time saving is achieved, as one-bottle systems often have to be applied several times. With the one-bottle systems there is a pronounced decrease in bond strength observed over time, especially after a prolonged period *in situ*.

■ Adhesion to prepared enamel

The etching technique of enamel was developed in 1955.[2] Etching the enamel results in a microretentive surface with high surface energy, which makes wetting easier for the adhesive system.

Various analyses have revealed that the etching effect is better in vertically cut enamel prisms than in ones that run laterally. This is the main reason why beveling of the cavity is advantageous in the approximal area. Aprismatic enamel can only be etched poorly; in this situation the etching time needs to be lengthened from 30 to 60 seconds. It has been shown that orthophosphoric acid at a concentration of 30% to 40% by weight achieves the best etching effect. The efficiency of the etching performance of phosphoric acid gel and liquid is identical. However, selective etching of enamel can only be done with a gel. As a result of enamel etching, the prisms and the interprismatic enamel are dissolved to a variable extent (see Fig 1-6). This results in a microretentive surface texture. The etching process alters the enamel surface down to a depth of 30 to 50 μm. To ensure there are no precipitates left on the surface which might weaken the bond, after the application time the etching gel must be rinsed off with water spray for about 10 seconds. A white, matt-opaque surface color after drying is a clinical sign that the enamel has been sufficiently etched.

Although the bond strength on the enamel surface is generally lower when using self-etch systems than when using etch-and-rinse systems,[14] thoroughly satisfactory bonding strengths can be achieved with some multiple-step self-etch adhesives. Markedly lower strengths are achieved by one-step systems.[6] Instead of phosphoric acid, self-etch adhesives contain acidic monomers that partially dissolve the smear layer and demineralize the enamel layer. The resulting etching pattern is less pronounced than after conditioning with phosphoric acid. The bond strength of self-etch adhesive systems may be improved, however, by conditioning the enamel surface with phosphoric acid before application of the bonding agent.[12]

After the acid conditioning, bonding onto enamel can be achieved directly using the adhesive system. Application of a primer does not improve the bonding strength, but does not worsen it either. The adhesive system should have only low viscosity in order to permit adequate wetting of the enamel surface. In addition, the system requires a certain amount of time to be able to flow into the microretentions. A penetration time of around 20 seconds must therefore be allowed prior to light curing.

> On an enamel surface, the best adhesion can be achieved after phosphoric acid etching (30% to 40% by weight) with an etching time of approximately 15 to 30 seconds.

■ Adhesion to dentin

A perfect bonding of the adhesive system to the dentin surface is the key to a long-lasting composite resin restoration. Furthermore, it minimizes the postoperative hypersensitivity. The outer surface of dentin must be demineralized to achieve a micromechanical interlocking with the restorative material. For this purpose, inorganic fractions are dissolved by acid and collagen is exposed. The primer then penetrates the exposed collagen network. Ideally this is then penetrated and stabilized by the adhesive as far as the demineralization front. The dentin layer infiltrated by the adhesive is called the *hybrid layer*.

Demineralization of dentin is a highly sensitive process. Hydroxyapatite has a high surface energy, while that of collagen is low. This means that wetting of demineralized dentin with an adhesive system is more difficult than for enamel. However, the wettability of dentin can be markedly improved by prior application of a primer.

If working with an etch-and-rinse system, it is essential to ensure that the phosphoric acid does not remain on the surface for longer than 15 seconds. The bond strength diminishes if the etching time is too long. An additional etching step prior to application of a self-etch adhesive also reduces the bonding strengths on dentin.[12] In both cases, because there is too much demineralization, the adhesive is not able to penetrate the collagen network completely and therefore the hybrid layer will be prone to degradation processes.

> The formation of a stable hybrid layer on a dentin surface is crucial for a long-term bonding of the restoration. The maximum etching time with phosphoric acid is 15 seconds for permanent teeth dentin.

The adhesive system penetrates not only the exposed collagen network, but also the dentinal tubules and their branches. The resulting tags provide further anchorage of the adhesive system to the tooth surface. However, stable formation of the hybrid layer is more important for bond strength. In the etch-and-rinse systems, the entire smear layer on the tooth surface is removed. After the acid has been sprayed off the dentin surface, the dentin should not be overdried because this will cause the collagen network of the conditioned dentin surface to collapse, preventing the adhesive system from penetrating. One approach, especially when using primers containing acetone, is to adopt wet-bonding; ie, the application of primer to the dentin while it still has a wet surface. The problem of overdrying can be reduced if the primer contains water. The etching process and subsequent application of primer are therefore highly technique-sensitive. Self-etch systems promise a decrease in the number of working steps and are time saving because the etching process can be omitted. These systems do not fully remove the smear layer on the dentin surface but modify it.

Primers contain amphiphilic monomers, ie, both hydrophilic and hydrophobic constituents, and are thus able to build a bridge between dentin and the adhesive or restorative material. To achieve this, the primer has to replace the water of the spaces between the individual collagen fibers, which means a sufficient exposure time ($\geq$ 20 seconds) has to be observed. Primers very often contain HEMA (hydroxyethyl methacrylate) because, as a very small molecule, it is able to penetrate the collagen network well and it has good wetting properties. However, HEMA has an allergenic potential and, due to its small molecular size, can even penetrate gloves. It is essential to take care when working with this substance – as with all dental materials – and to avoid contact with skin or gloves when the material is not polymerized.

Penetration by the adhesive into the pretreated dentin surface leads to formation of the hybrid layer. Before polymerization, the material again needs enough time to penetrate into the microstructure. When direct restorations are applied, the adhesive system is polymerized before application of the restorative material. With indirect restorations, on the other hand, the adhesive is polymerized together with the luting composite, or it has to be applied in a very thin layer and cured so that the restoration can be luted without any marginal gaps.

■ Adhesive technique for primary teeth

The adhesive technique for primary teeth does not differ fundamentally from that used with permanent teeth. The enamel of primary teeth has a higher aprismatic content, which makes a regular etching pattern difficult to achieve. The dentin contains a small proportion of inorganic components and is characterized by larger dentinal tubules than permanent teeth. The choice of system and the correct application of the technique are also key to a successful restoration in primary teeth. A complicating factor when restoring primary teeth is often poor compliance or noncompliance by the young patients.

Enamel etching with phosphoric acid for 30 seconds also seems to be sufficient for the aprismatic enamel of primary teeth. In dentin, on the other hand, the etching time should not exceed 10 seconds because of the lower mineral content. If etching times are longer, the adhesive system no longer succeeds in coating the exposed collagen fibers.

The trend in adhesive systems for primary teeth is clearly towards two-step self-etch adhesives. This is for several reasons: approximately only a small amount of enamel is often available at the bottom of the box for efficient bonding and hence phosphoric acid etching can be omitted; two-step systems achieve a better adhesive bond to dentin than one-bottle adhesives; and as no water spray is needed for elimination of the phosphoric acid, children's compliance is better.

For primary teeth the enamel should be etched for 30 seconds, while the etching time for dentin is 8 to 10 seconds. Self-etch adhesives offer advantages because they allow optimum bonding to dentin and approximately there is often no enamel available at the bottom of the box.

Classification of adhesive luting agents

Demand for adhesive cementing materials increased with the introduction of all-ceramic inlays. Unlike conventional cements for fixation of metal frameworks, adhesive luting agents have to form an adhesive bond to both the tooth structure and the restorative material in order to guarantee the long-term success of the restoration. Such a bond is important as it has been demonstrated that adhesive luting agents also increase the flexural strength of ceramic inlays.[1] In addition, adhesive luting agents are able to optimize the color match of a restoration. Another indication for adhesive luting agents emerged through the technology of fiber posts.

The functioning of adhesive luting agents is based on that of composite resin restoration materials, except that viscosity is reduced by a lower filler content in order to simplify cementation. Most cements are dual-cure; meaning they polymerize with or without light activation. Purely light-curing adhesive luting agents have a limited indication and should only be used for ceramic restorations not exceeding 2 mm thickness and which are sufficiently translucent (eg, veneers).

In a similar way to adhesive systems, adhesive luting agents are classified according to the type of tooth conditioning. A distinction is made between luting agents that use an etch-and-rinse adhesive (eg, Variolink II® with Syntac Classic), those that use self-etching primer (eg, Panavia F®) and self-adhesive luting agents (eg, RelyX Unicem®) (Table 13-2).

Etch-and-rinse luting agents result in the best bonding strength to enamel, followed by self-etch luting agents. The bonding of self-etch and self-adhesive luting agents to enamel can be improved by pre-etching of the enamel surface with phosphoric acid. Self-etch luting agents and etch-and-rinse luting agents are today equivalent in terms of dentin bonding. By contrast, the bond strengths that can be achieved with self-adhesive luting agents are usually markedly lower.

Table 13-2 Classification of adhesive luting agents (list not complete)

Type of adhesive luting agent	Product	Manufacturer
Etch-and-rinse luting agent	Calibra®/XP Bond™	Dentsply DeTrey, Konstanz, Germany
	Nexus/Optibond FL®	Kerr, Orange, USA
	Variolink II®/Syntac classic	Ivoclar Vivadent, Schaan, Liechtenstein
Self-etch luting agent	Multilink® Automix	Ivoclar Vivadent, Schaan, Liechtenstein
	Panavia™ F	Kuraray, Tokyo, Japan
Self-adhesive luting agent	BisCem®	Bisco, Schaumburg, USA
	GCem	GC, Tokyo, Japan
	MaxCem™	Kerr, Orange, USA
	RelyX™ Unicem	3M Espe, St. Paul, USA
	SpeedCEM	Ivoclar Vivadent, Schaan, Liechtenstein

The development of self-adhesive luting agents in 2002 marked a simplification in the bonding of materials. Unfortunately, only a few long-term data are currently available. The stability of these luting agents during storage is subject to limitations and they often have to be stored in a refrigerator. However, their bonding strengths are better at room temperature. This means that the luting agent needs to be taken out of the refrigerator prior to the cementation.[3] While dentin bonding more or less works, there are greater problems with enamel bonding.[10] This is why it is advisable to etch the enamel margin selectively with phosphoric acid. Self-adhesive cements should still be used with caution. While crown fixation does not seem to be problematic, there are increased risks with more complex forms of restoration, such as inlays or onlays, as the majority of the restoration margin with these restorations lies in the enamel. According to an *in vitro* study, luting agents being used in combination with an adhesive system performed better than self-adhesive luting agents with regard to marginal integrity.[5] These results have since been clinically confirmed.[11]

Luting agents that are advertised as being dual-cure should always be light polymerized. The material properties are improved by the light polymerization.[8,9]

Another way of classifying adhesive luting agents is according to their viscosity. Above a filler content of around 76% by weight, sonic activation during cementation is recommended.[7] Advantages are attributed to adhesive luting agents with a higher filler content, especially in terms of the removal of excess.

■ Conclusions

To achieve optimum bonding strength and hence a tight marginal seal of a restoration, the reaction time, the form of application, and the state of the tooth surface (wet or dry) must be closely observed when using adhesive systems.

As well as correct application of the adhesive system, the type of preparation also has an influence on bonding strength. The bond strength is better on a finished tooth surface than on a surface that has been prepared with a large-grit diamond. Laser preparation of the tooth surface generally causes a decrease in bond strengths. Therefore, an additional finishing is recommended.[4]

Product development in adhesive systems and adhesive luting agents is advancing very rapidly. This makes it difficult to choose a material, given that the choice should be based on sound long-term clinical results. The fact that manufacturers do not have to provide long-term data to obtain a license for their products is an added problem. If material constituents are used that have already been clinically tried and tested, in the majority of cases clinical trials can even be omitted prior to market launch. In some cases this means that products already available on the dental market have to be recalled in the short term because they have not been clinically proven. The recommendation for dental practitioners is still to use adhesives and adhesive luting agents with successful long-term data until verified data are available proving that a newer, simplified system yields equivalent results.

References

1. Bindl A, Lüthy H, Mörmann WH. Strength and fracture pattern of monolithic CAD/CAM-generated posterior crowns. Dent Mater 2006;22:29–36.
2. Buonocore MG. A simple method of increasing the adhesion of acrylic filling materials to enamel surfaces. J Dent Res 1955;34:849–853.
3. Cantoro A, Goracci C, Papacchini F, Mazzitelli C, Fadda GM, Ferrari M. Effect of pre-cure temperature on the bonding potential of self-etch and self-adhesive resin cements. Dent Mater 2008;24:577–583.
4. Cardoso MV, Coutinho E, Ermis RB, Poitevin A, Van Landuyt K, De Munck J, Carvalho RC, Van Meerbeek B. Influence of dentin cavity surface finishing on micro-tensile bond strength of adhesives. Dent Mater 2008;24:492–501.
5. Frankenberger R, Lohbauer U, Schaible RB, Nikolaenko SA, Naumann M. Luting of ceramic inlays *in vitro*: Marginal quality of self-etch and etch-and-rinse adhesives versus self-etch cements. Dent Mater 2008;24:185–191.
6. Hanning M, Reinhardt KJ, Bott B. Self-etching primer vs phosphoric acid: an alternative concept for composite-to-enamel bonding. Oper Dent 1999;24:172–180.
7. Krämer N, Sindel J, Petschelt A. Einfluss des Füllkörpergehaltes von Hybridkompositen auf die Filmschichtstärke. Dtsch Zahnärztl Z 1996;51:166–168.
8. Meng X, Yoshida K, Atsuta M. Influence of ceramic thickness on mechanical properties and polymer structure of dual-cured resin luting agents. Dent Mater 2008;24:594–599.
9. Piwowarcyk A, Bender R, Otti P, Lauer HC. Long-term bond between dual-polymerizing cementing agents and human hard dental tissue. Dent Mater 2007;23:211–217.
10. Radovic I, Monticelli F, Goracci C, Vulicevic ZR, Ferrari M. Self-adhesive resin cements: a literature review. J Adhes Dent 2008;10:251–258.
11. Taschner M, Frankenberger R, Garcìa-Godoy F, Rosenbusch S, Petschelt A, Krämer N. IPS Empress inlays luted with a self-adhesive resin cement after 1 year. Am J Dent 2009;22:55–59.
12. Van Landuyt KL, Kanumilli P, De Munck J, Peumans M, Lambrechts P, Van Meerbeek B. Bond strength of a mild self-etch adhesive with and without prior acid-etching. J Dent 2006;34:77–85.
13. Van Meerbeek B, De Munck J, Yoshida Y, Inoue S, Vargas M, Vijay P, Van Landuyt K, Lambrechts P, Vanherle G. Buonocore memorial lecture. Adhesion to enamel and dentin: current status and future challenges. Oper Dent 2003;28:215–235.
14. Yoshiyama M, Matsuo T, Ebisu S, Pashley D. Regional bond strengths of self-etching/self-priming adhesive systems. J Dent 1998;26:606–616.

14 Direct restorative technology

Brigitte Zimmerli, Matthias Strub, and Simon Flury

■ Introduction

Placement of restorations made of composite resin materials is currently the standard technique for direct restorations. Restorations made of modern composite resin materials show similar survival rates to amalgam restorations.[17] It is advisable to place direct restorations because of the greater amount of tooth substance preserved and the lower cost to patients. However, composite resin materials are subject to polymerization shrinkage, which results in various clinical problems: enamel cracks, marginal leakage, marginal discoloration, secondary caries, fracture of thin restoration margins, and postoperative hypersensitivity. Material modifications and different application techniques are being used in an attempt to counteract polymerization shrinkage and to increase long-term survival of composite resin restorations.

■ Composite resin materials

Composite resin materials can be classified into groups based on the size of the filler particles, the matrix components, or the viscosity of the material. There is a trend towards the use of smaller filler particles in composites. The products on the market nowadays are almost exclusively nano-filled hybrid composites and nanocomposites. The classification based on viscosity uses three categories: "packable", "conventional", and "flowable"; but this provides only limited information about material properties. This is why more significance is now attached to the classification based on the matrix components (Table 14-1).

Table 14-1 Classification of resorative composite resin materials based on the matrix components

Matrix	Fillers	Chemical system	Group	Example
Conventional matrix	Glass, quartz, silicon dioxide	Methacrylates	Hybrid composites, nanocomposites	Tetric EvoCeram®, Filtek supreme XT®
Inorganic matrix	Glass, quartz, silicon dioxide	Inorganic poly-condensates	Ormocers	Admira®, Definite®
Acid-modified methacrylates	Fluorosilicate glass	Polar groups	Compomers	Dyract eXtra®
Ring-opening epoxides	Glass, quartz, silicon dioxide	Cationic polymerization	Siloranes	Filtek Silorane®

Composite resin

These materials are made up of a methacrylate matrix, inorganic fillers, and coupling agents. The matrix mainly comprises bis-GMA (bisphenol-A-glycidyl dimethacrylate) and shorter-chain monomers such as UDMA (urethane dimethacrylate), TEGDMA (triethylene glycol dimethacrylate), and TEGMA (triethylene glycol methacrylate). There has been ample discussion of the leaching of monomers out of the restorative materials, yet a few patients are sensitized to individual monomers. A high filler content is important in order to minimize polymerization shrinkage and guarantee material strength.[14] The admixture of very small filler particles like nanoparticles makes fine polishing easier.[19] Today, composite resins are used for all classes of restoration.

Compomers

This group of materials is composed of composite resin and glass ionomer cement technology. As well as the conventional monomers, the matrix also contains carbonic acids with polymerizable double bonds. The polymerization is mainly due to polymerization of the monomers; an acid-base reaction only takes place at the interfaces. Fluorosilicate glasses are added as fillers. Although fluoride release is modest,[12] it is sufficient to have an inhibiting effect on caries formation in the adjacent tooth, according to an *in vitro* study.[15] Compomers are particularly suitable for restorations in primary teeth. Compomers are contraindicated in the esthetic region because of the tendency to marginal discoloration. In addition, abrasion stability is low, which is why the material should not be used for extensive restorations.[10,25,26] Pretreatment of the tooth surface with an adhesive is necessary to maximize the bond strength of compomer materials.[8,20]

Ormocers

The term "ormocer" is an acronym for *or*ganically *mo*dified *cer*amic. Ormocers differ from composite resins as they contain an inorganic network as well as the organic components of the matrix. The inorganic component is bound to the organic monomers with silane molecules. This represents an attempt to counteract polymerization shrinkage.[27] Furthermore, the inorganic network is supposed to reduce the elutability (release into a solvent) of the monomers and hence reduce the cytotoxicity.[21] Ormocers can be used for all classes of restoration.

Siloranes

The matrix of this substance group contains ring-shaped monomers which reduce polymerization shrinkage by opening the ring structure during chain formation. Siloranes are highly hydrophobic, therefore it is necessary to use a specific adhesive system that allows bonding between the restoration and the dental surface. The stability of the material in a variety of media is very good because of the low water absorption.[11] Filtek Silorane® is currently the only product from this group that is available on the market. In view of the limited color palette available, application is restricted to the posterior teeth for the moment. Radiopacity is in the lower range but is expected to be improved further by the manufacturer.

Direct restorative technology

■ Clinical application

Creating an optimal operating field

Creating an absolutely dry operating field increases the quality of all adhesively luted dental restorations. Using a rubber dam is the most reliable way to achieve this. Rubber dam application also improves the view into the operating field and can optimize the longevity of the restoration in patients whose cooperation is limited (Fig 14-1). Not least, many patients who are sensitive to gag reflux find a rubber dam acceptable after a certain amount of persuasion. This is because they have less feeling of restriction, they do not have to swallow as much cooling water, and sensitive parts, such as the dorsal edge of the tongue, are not touched. Numerous shapes of rubber dam are today available which are ideally suited to different situations. As a supportive measure, the rubber dam can be affixed to the gingiva with Histoacryl® (Fig 14-2), or a "liquid rubber dam" made of polymerizable resins can be applied in addition to create a dry operating field (Opaldam®). For creation of a relative dry operating field or extensive anterior restorations, a cheek retractor (Optragate®) might also be useful (Fig 14-3).

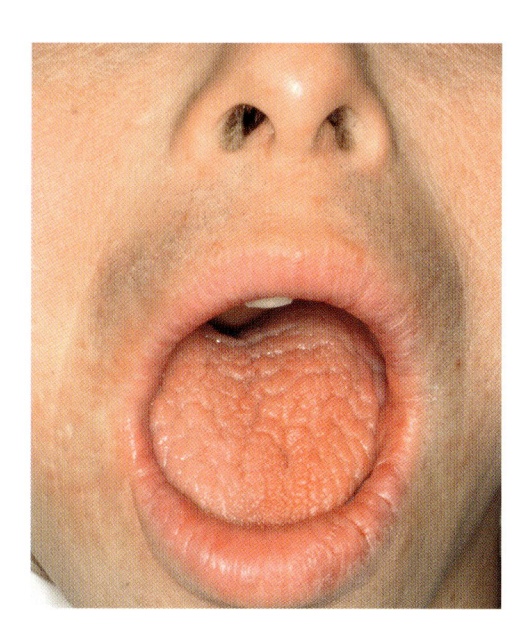

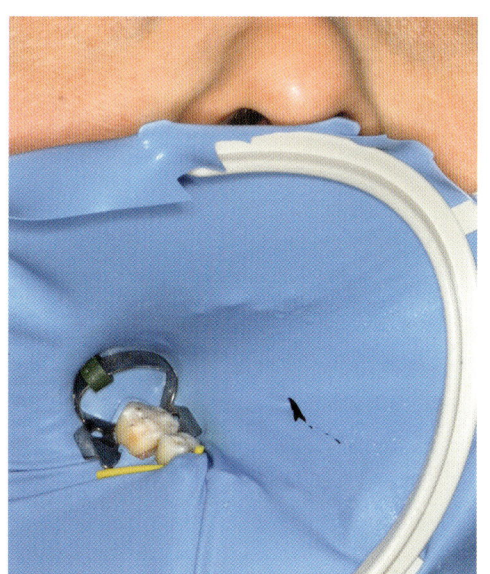

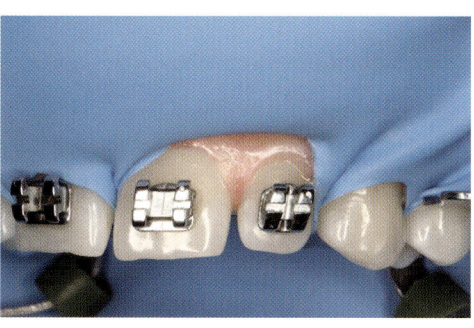

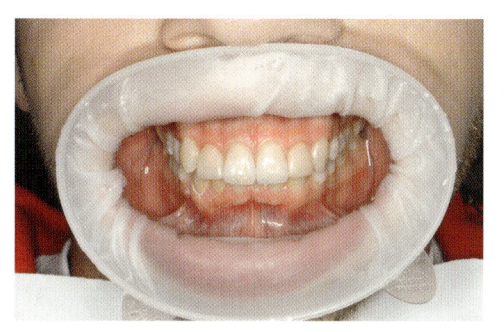

Fig 14-1 Top right and left: rubber dam application makes it possible to create a dry field in initially "impossible" cases. Even patients with a strong gag reflex perceive the application of a rubber dam as comfortable because neither water spray nor instruments will touch the oral mucosa.

Fig 14-2 Bottom left: creation of an absolutely dry field using a rubber dam during treatment to widen the left maxillary lateral incisor with composite resin. To guarantee an optimum view and exclude interference with the rubber dam during the tooth widening, the rubber dam was "attached" to the gingiva at the central and lateral incisors using Histoacryl.

Fig 14-3 Bottom right: in certain cases it can be advantageous to place the restoration with only a relatively dry field. In this example, both maxillary lateral incisors were enlarged with composite resin. Owing to the application of Optragate, cheek and lip parts do not have to be additionally retracted.

Rubber dam application allows controlled creation of a dry operating field. The overall view, protection of the patient (especially against aspiration of small parts and against disinfectant solutions during root canal treatment), and patient compliance can all be improved by the use of rubber dams.

Auxiliary instruments

Good matrix technique is crucial to the success of a restoration. In the posterior region, the use of preformed sectional matrices has become an established technique. Polymerization when using metal matrices is the same as that used for transparent matrices. Simple shaping of a sufficient contact point is possible with sectional matrix systems by the application of wedges and separating rings (Fig 14-4). In this connection it has been shown that using separating rings is more efficient than using wedges alone.[16] Transparent matrices are suitable for anterior restorations. For extensive restorations, these matrices can be individually molded using a temporary composite resin (Telio CS Inlay/Onlay); they also greatly facilitate the shaping of restorations (Fig 14-5).

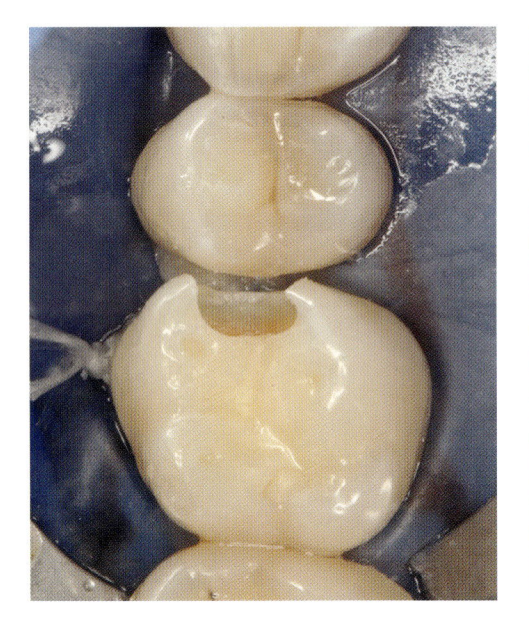

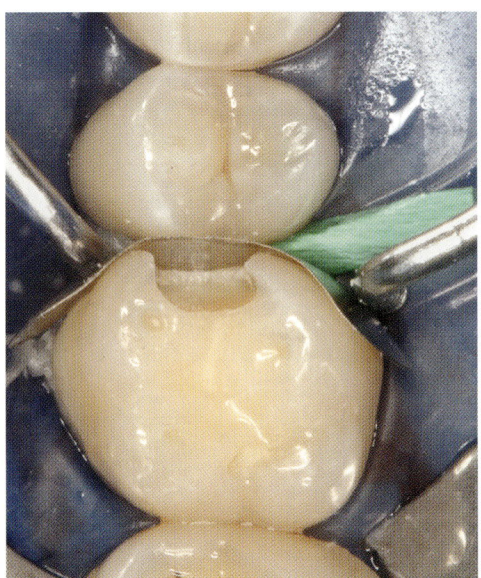

Fig 14-4 Top left: in the right maxillary first molar, a Class II cavity is prepared mesially.
Top right: a molded sectional matrix made of metal is used for matrix placement. After wedging with a wooden wedge, the separating ring is applied. As a result, the interdental space is widened and the matrix is perfectly fitted to the tooth.
Bottom: the view after placement of the restoration shows how perfectly the restoration can be shaped with the aid of this matrix technique.

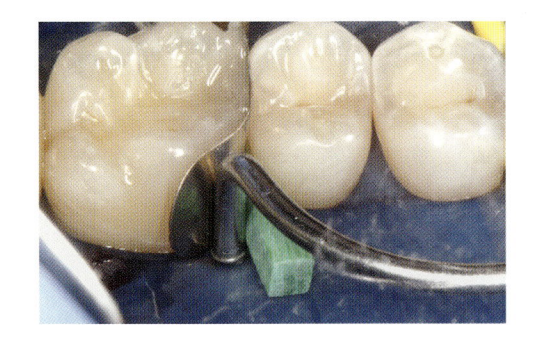

Direct restorative technology

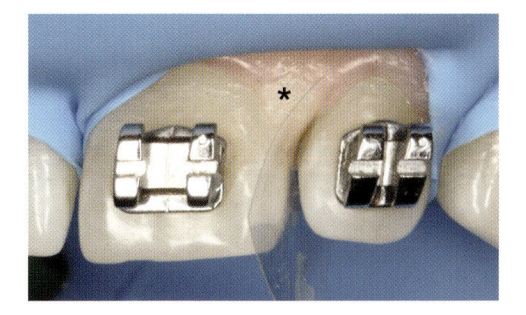

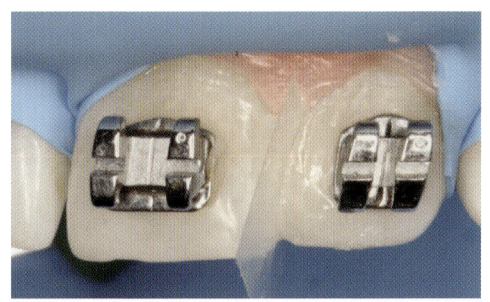

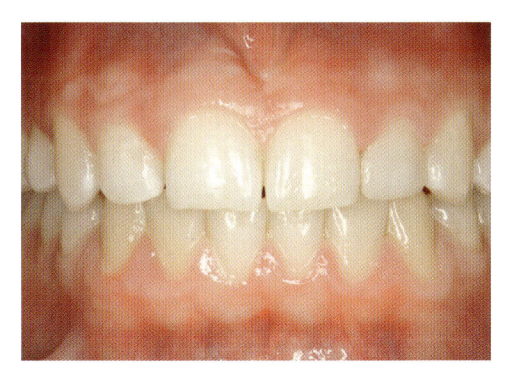

Fig 14-5 Top left: a transparent matrix is placed in the sulcus of the left maxillary lateral incisor, which is being widened. The temporary resin material (*) is adapted to the adjacent tooth so that the matrix is perfectly shaped. While the temporary resin material sets, the central and lateral incisors are separated slightly with a spatula.
Top right: thanks to the optimized matrix technique, widening of the lateral incisor is then relatively easy to perform.
Bottom: final documentation after completion of the orthodontic treatment. The restoration mesial to the right maxillary lateral incisor integrates well into the overall picture.

Sectional matrices and separating rings make it far easier to shape the contact point in interdental restorations in the posterior region. In the anterior region, the wedging and contouring of the resin matrix can be individualized with the aid of a temporary resin material.

Layering technique

The use of a layering technique improves the quality of a resin restoration because it allows polymerization shrinkage to be controlled more closely. The configuration of a cavity (C-factor) determines whether shrinkage stress will develop. The more a restoration surface is bound to the tooth or restoration margin, the more stress will develop.[7]

The horizontal layering technique can be used for small cavities (Fig 14-6 top left). This technique involves placing horizontal layers on top of each other and polymerizing them individually. The occlusal relief is contoured with the final layer. This technique is very simple, but it can complicate occlusal shaping.

By contrast, the occlusal anatomy can be contoured easily using the oblique layering technique. However, this can lead to problems in the homogeneous adaptation of the separate layers (Fig 14-6 top right). Where the individual layers converge at a relatively narrow angle, especially at the bottom of the cavity, there is a greater risk of heterogeneities (air enclosure).

The use of the centripetal layering technique is advisable (Fig 14-6 bottom). This technique involves converting the Class II cavity into a Class I cavity. It is important that the first layer touching the matrix is placed very thinly. In large cavities, two layers can be placed one after another so that the first layer extends from the buccal side along the matrix to the mid-

Fig 14-6 *Top left: schematic diagram of the horizontal layering technique. Buccal view. The increments are layered from an apical to a coronal direction.*
Top right: schematic diagram of the oblique layering technique. Approximal view. The first layer can be placed horizontally. The subsequent layers run obliquely from the cavity wall to the floor of the cavity.
Bottom: schematic diagram of the centripetal layering technique. Buccal view. The first layer is placed thinly along the matrix. The Class II cavity is thereby reshaped into a Class I cavity. The subsequent layers are added horizontally or obliquely.

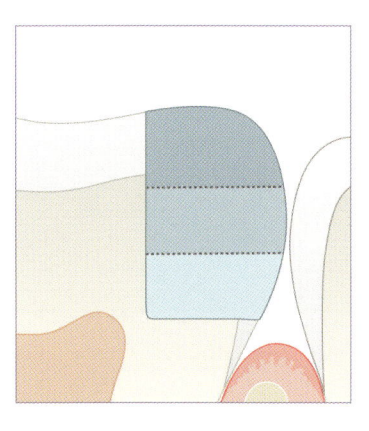

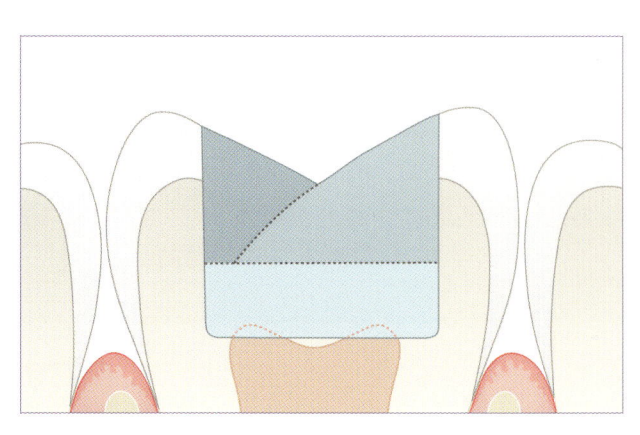

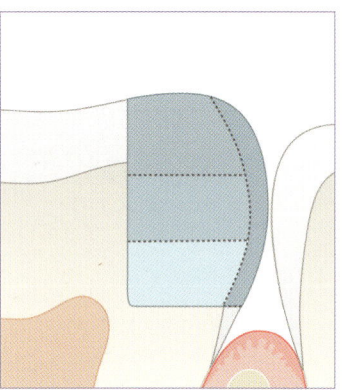

dle of the cavity and the second layer covers the remaining matrix wall from the middle to the oral limit of the cavity. Given efficient creation of a dry operating field and optimum oral hygiene by the patient, at this stage the matrix can be removed, giving a better overall view and simplifying the shaping of the restoration.

It is a matter of debate whether a flowable composite resin should be used for the first layer in order to ensure optimum coverage of the cavity and create a tight marginal seal. In addition, such a layer is thought to act as a stress breaker. If a filled adhesive system is used, application of a flowable composite resin is not necessary. When a flowable composite resin is used, it is essential to apply the layer very thinly. If the layer is too thick, it increases the probability of marginal leakage; this is because a low-filled flowable composite resin is subject to considerable polymerization shrinkage.

Where there are several adjacent restorations, any temptation to treat all cavities simultaneously with the adhesive system then restore them one after another should be resisted. However, it has been shown that bond strength may be decreased if light curing of an adhesive system containing HEMA is delayed.[24] Thus the teeth should ideally be coated with the adhesive system and restored individually.

Possible layering techniques

Horizontal layering: only for very small cavities or as the first layer in deep cavities
Oblique layering: simplifies contouring of the occlusal relief
Centripetal layering: ideal for Class II cavities

Light polymerization

Sufficient light polymerization is important in terms of material stability. Furthermore it reduces the elutability of monomers from the material.[4,23] As well as quartz tungsten halogen curing units, plasma and LED devices are also used for light curing. In practice it is important to check the light intensity of the devices regularly. As a rule, the various test devices available on the market do not display the actual value correctly, but by using the same measuring device over a period of time it will be possible to see if there is any decrease in output. It makes sense to use protection sleeves for the light guide, as it has been shown that when light curing devices are used in dental practices, light guides are frequently contaminated with adhesive or composite resin residues.[6] For composite polymerization, the curing light should reach a minimum intensity of 400 mW/cm^2. Curing luting agents for indirect restorations and posts, should be at least 800 mW/cm^2. Sufficient light curing is based on the correct interaction between curing device, type of light source, and restoration (Fig 14-7). In the case of LED devices, another decisive factor is that the spectrum of the light emission covers the absorption range of the initiator. Camphor quinone (absorption peak $\lambda = 468$ nm) is commonly used as a photoinitiator, and some composite resins, particularly those that are very light in color, may also contain Lucerin (absorption peak $\lambda = 380$ nm) or other initiators.

Polymerization strategy

- Polymerization device ↔ Light exposure
  - Output
  - Spectrum
  - Light guide
  - Time
  - Program
  - Distance from restoration
- Restoration
  - Layer thickness
  - Color
  - Photoinitiator

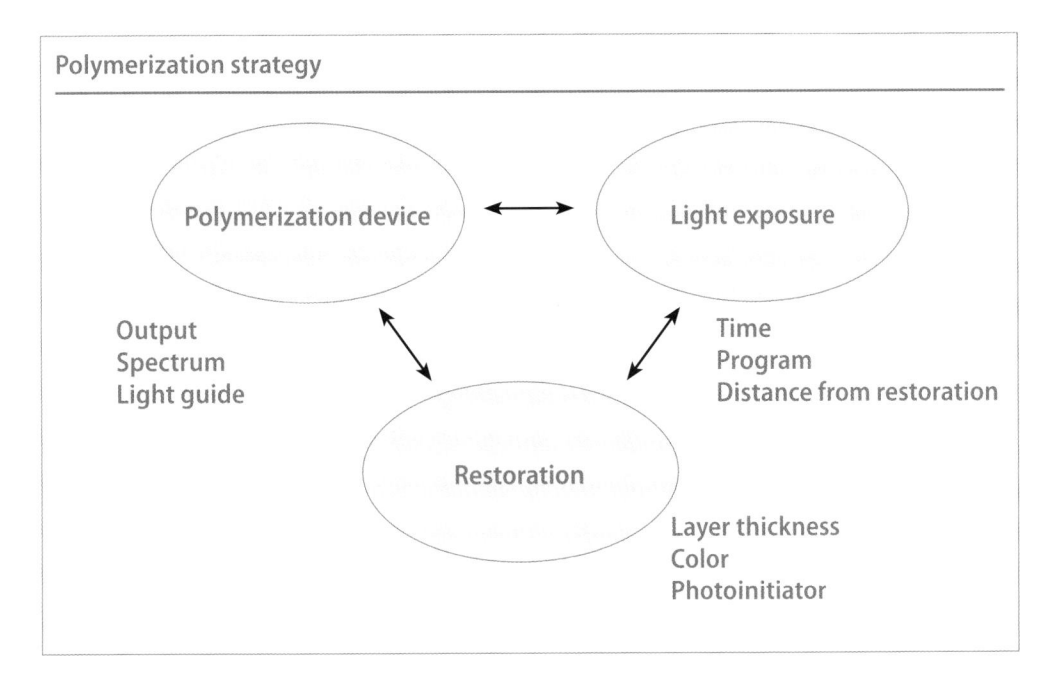

Fig 14-7 The polymerization strategy must be based on the three parameters of polymerization device, light exposure, and restoration.

Required light intensity

≥ 400 mW/cm²   for polymerization of direct composite resin materials
≥ 800 mW/cm²   for polymerization of adhesive luting agents for indirect restorations and post cementation

Positioning the light guide close to the restoration being cured is necessary to ensure the quality of the polymerization. The only way to check this rigorously is to use protective glasses or a protective shield that allow the user to look directly into the blue light. If there is no visual control, the light guide is usually not held close enough to the surface of the restoration and the restoration is not exposed to enough light. Insufficient polymerization of the restorative material will reduce the longevity of the restoration.

In practice it is important to check the consistency of the light intensity of the light curing unit. The light guide can be protected against contamination by using a protective sleeve.

Final finishing and polishing

Composite resin restorations must be finished and polished as well as possible. This is partly because plaque retention and accumulation, which can lead to gingivitis or secondary caries, can be prevented by correct polishing. However, insufficiently polished restorations can also cause discomfort to patients, and they become discolored more quickly, which results in esthetic losses.[3,5,13] The fact that composite resin is composed of ingredients of unequal hardness and size leads to problems in the surface polishing.[22] On the one hand, the organic matrix is less abrasion-resistant than the fillers and so can be selectively removed by polishers. On the other hand, filler particles can be dislodged from the matrix during polishing.

Polishing with discs coated with abrasive particles (usually aluminum oxide) produces very good results because the smooth, flat form of the discs polish the fillers and organic matrix evenly.[1,2,18] However, it is not usually possible to reach every part of a restoration using these discs. Occlusal reliefs can only be adequately polished using polishing points, cups, or brushes. These polishing instruments are mainly silicone or rubber polishers containing abrasive silicon carbide, aluminum oxide, or diamond particles. In the case of brushes, the bristles are coated with abrasive material.

Polishers are usually supplied by manufacturers as sets, the individual instruments differing in their hardness and grit size. Combination sets with different polishing pastes are also available on the market. The individual polishers in such multiple-step systems are coordinated with each other and matched to the composite resin types. Omitting intermediate steps in order to save time is not generally recommended. In particular, a fine-grit polisher or a brush might not be adequate to remove large areas of unevenness or grooves prior to the final polishing. The use of multiple-step polishing systems yields more reliable results than single-step polishing systems.

Other factors that play a role in the quality of finishing include the type of composite resin used and the handling of the instruments by the dental practitioner. Although the greatest polishing effect is achieved within the first 5 seconds, depending on the restorative material and polishing system, more than 1 minute of pure polishing time might be required to achieve an optimum surface.[9] The contact pressure also plays a role: polishing discs should only be used with a little pressure. They are used at rotary speeds of between 10,000 and 30,000 rpm and require no water cooling. A speed of 10,000 rpm is sufficient for brushes with polishing pastes, which are also used dry. Felt polishers, on the other hand, are first moistened in combination with pastes, and polishing instruments of the silicone or rubber type and polishing brushes are used with water cooling. For these, the recommended speed seldom exceeds 20,000 to 30,000 rpm, based on manufacturers' instructions. Working is again done with only light pressure. The excessive production of heat during polishing can damage composite resin surfaces, resulting in more fillers being leached out or organic matrix brushed out.

Amalgam restorations have, as a matter of course, to be repolished during recall appointments. Restorations made from composite resin materials similarly require regular aftercare in order to guarantee the longevity of the restoration.

Polishing of restorations
The use of polishing sets is recommended. The polishers should be applied only with slight pressure.

■ Summary

The use of composite resin materials for direct restorations is today regarded as standard. The material properties necessitate certain adjustments during the course of composite resin placement compared with an amalgam restoration. Sound knowledge of the different composite resin materials makes it easier to use them correctly as restorative materials.

All light-curing composite resin materials should be processed under dry conditions. To achieve this, it has proved beneficial to use a rubber dam because the cheek and tongue can be effectively retracted at the same time. It is not only the patient who tends to find treatment more stress-free with a rubber dam, but also the dental practitioner.

The use of sectional matrices and separating rings makes it far easier to shape sufficient approximal contact points.

The problems of polymerization shrinkage can be controlled by using an appropriate layering technique and correct light curing of the resin material. Regular testing of the curing light intensity will guarantee consistent quality of the restoration.

Yesterday retention – today adhesion?

The final finishing of a restoration is important to the long-term success of the restoration. During recall appointments, composite resin restorations should be repolished because thin-layer residues of adhesive materials often do not become visible until follow-up. If left in place, these residues can cause discoloration of the restoration margins.

The procedure for the fabrication of a composite resin restoration is illustrated step by step in Figs 14-8 to 14-31.

Case 1: Figs 14-8 to 14-16

Fig 14-8 Initial situation with caries mesial to the left maxillary first molar.

Fig 14-9 Preparation with rotary instruments, leaving the approximal enamel wall in place to minimize damage to the adjacent tooth.

Fig 14-10 Fully excavated cavity. The enamel margins are beveled in the approximal area. Preparation of the mesial enamel ridge is performed with preparation instruments which spare the adjacent tooth (oscillating files in the Prepcontrol head, front end cutting diamond preparation burs [tc-b]) (see Chapter 11).

Fig 14-11 Application of sectional matrix. The matrix is fixed in the interdental space with a wooden wedge. The separating ring is adapted for additional adaptation of the matrix and better separation.

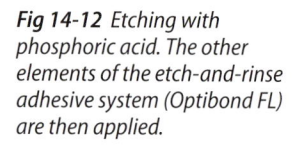

Fig 14-12 Etching with phosphoric acid. The other elements of the etch-and-rinse adhesive system (Optibond FL) are then applied.

Fig 14-13 The centripetal layering technique is employed. This involves placing the first layer along the matrix. This layer is kept very thin.

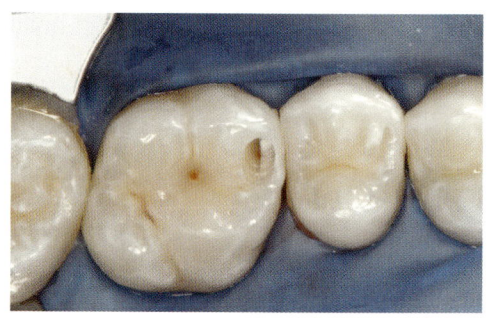

Fig 14-8

Fig 14-9

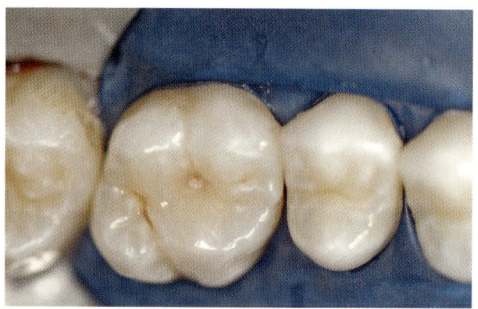

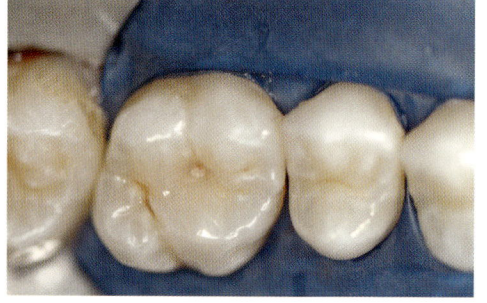

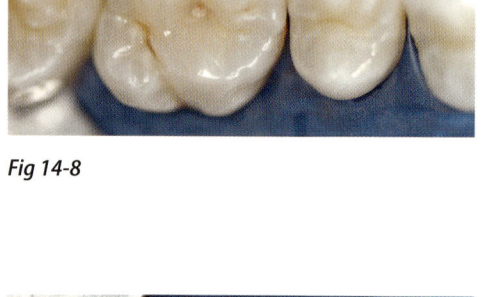

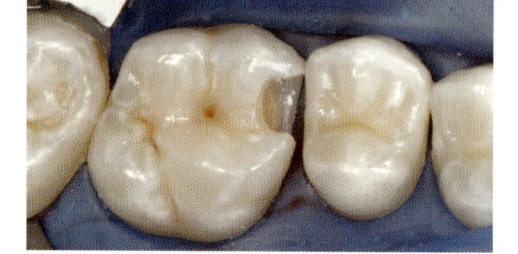

Fig 14-10

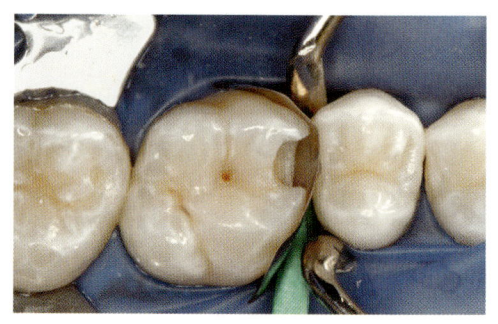

Fig 14-11

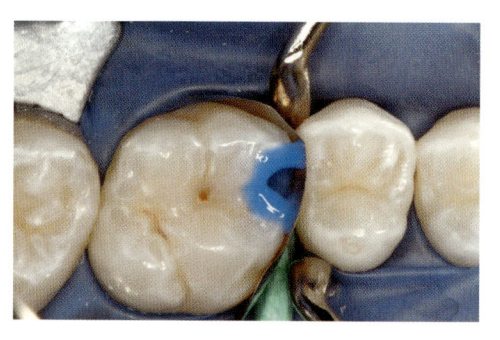

Fig 14-12

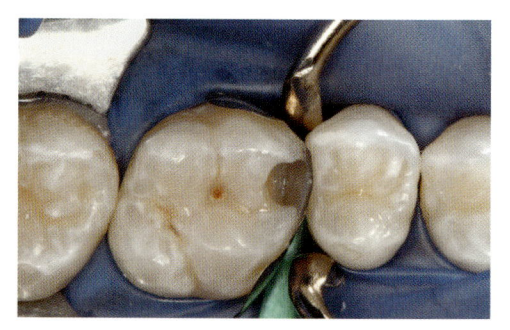

Fig 14-13

14
Direct restorative technology

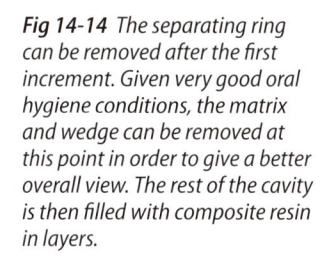

Fig 14-14 The separating ring can be removed after the first increment. Given very good oral hygiene conditions, the matrix and wedge can be removed at this point in order to give a better overall view. The rest of the cavity is then filled with composite resin in layers.

Fig 14-15 Thanks to good adaptation of the matrix and an appropriate layering technique, the material excess is kept within limits.

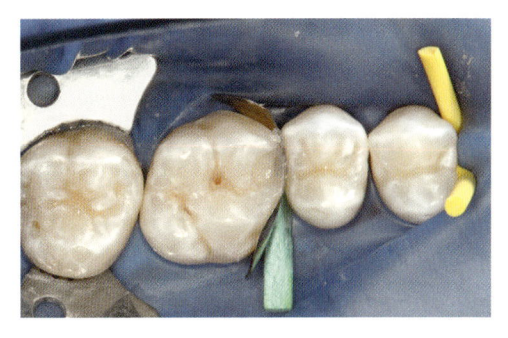

Fig 14-14

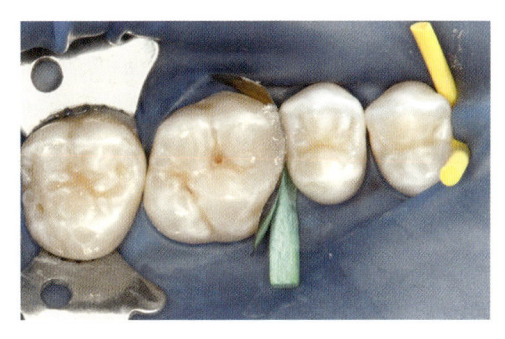

Fig 14-15

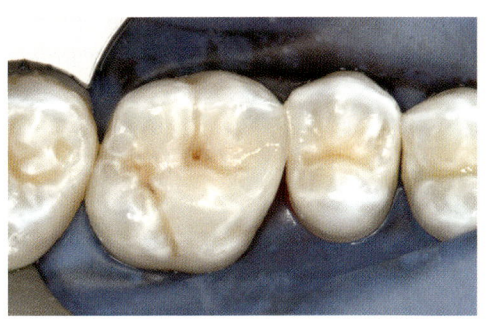

Fig 14-16 The fully finished restoration. The approximal contact is present and the approximal ridge is perfectly shaped.

Fig 14-16

Case 2: Figs 14-17 and 14-18

Fig 14-17 The left maxillary central incisor had undergone root canal restoration and was treated with a composite resin restoration in the incisal third. The patient was troubled by the esthetics.

Fig 14-18 After bleaching using the walking bleach technique, the composite resin restoration was renewed. The restoration integrates harmoniously into the overall picture, not least because of improved imitation of the surface texture.

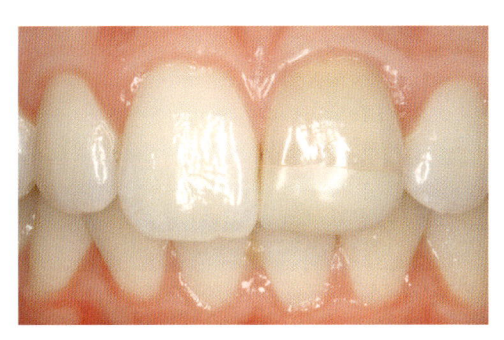

Fig 14-17

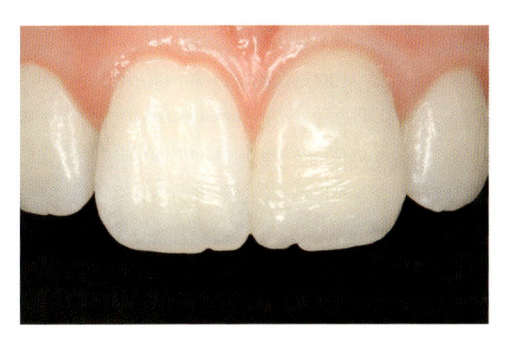

Fig 14-18

VI Yesterday retention – today adhesion?

Case 3: Figs 14-19 and 14-20

Fig 14-19 The color choice for the enamel material is made at the incisal margin of the cleaned tooth.

Fig 14-20 The color choice for the dentin material is made in the cervical region of the tooth.

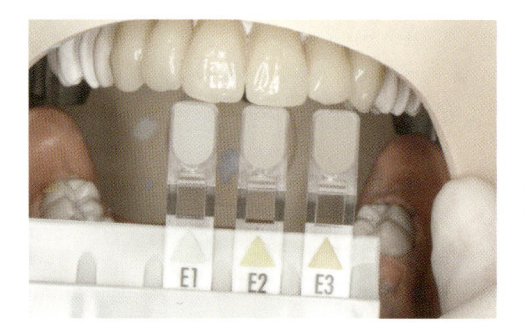

Fig 14-19

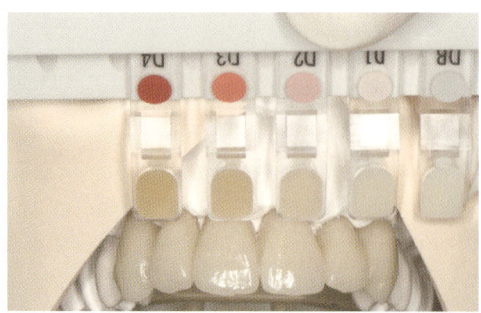

Fig 14-20

Case 4: Figs 14-21 to 14-29

Fig 14-21 For larger defects, it is worth preparing a silicone key over the waxup or mock-up. The key is cut to size using a scalpel or Japanese knife so that it accurately accommodates the incisal edge.

Fig 14-22 Silicone key trimmed to fit. The first premolars are enclosed, the incisal margin of the anterior teeth is cut to fit, and gingival supports of the key are removed. At the site of the defect, a little enamel material is then placed in the key as the first layer, adapted to the tooth, then allowed to set. This gives rise to a palatal enamel wall which facilitates further shaping of the anterior restoration.

Fig 14-23 The correct layer thickness is checked with a mirror. The different dentin shades are applied in an overlapping fashion from cervical (darker material) to coronal (lighter material). A thin layer of enamel is finally laid over the dentin material. The enamel layer is slightly thicker incisally and tapers off in a cervical direction.

Fig 14-24 Restoration margins and restoration surface are first smoothed with oscillating instruments.

Fig 14-25 Longitudinal grooves can simply be incorporated using a bevel-shaped file in a gentle wiping

Fig 14-26 The surface is further smoothed with silicone polishers.

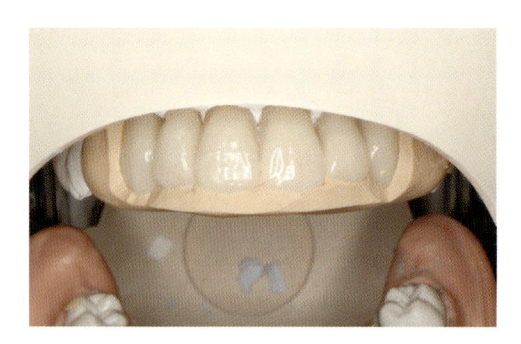

Fig 14-21

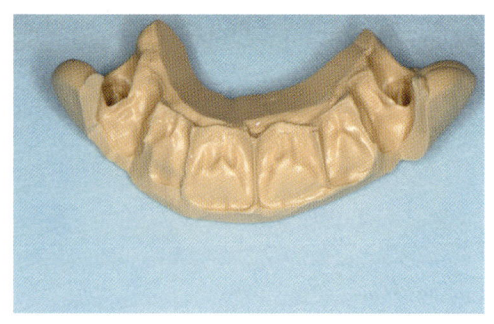

Fig 14-22

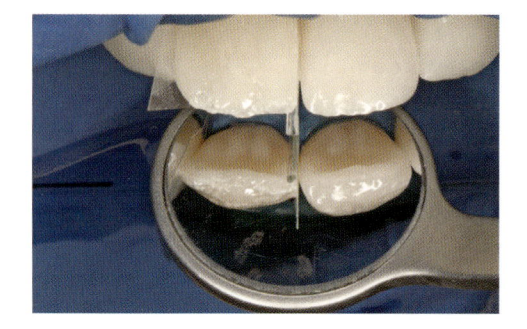

Fig 14-23

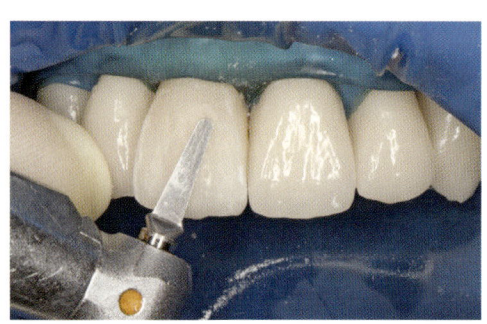

Fig 14-24

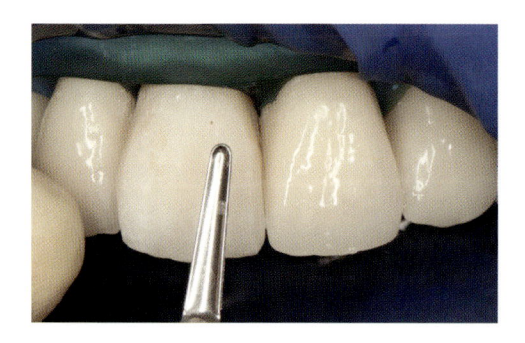

Fig 14-25

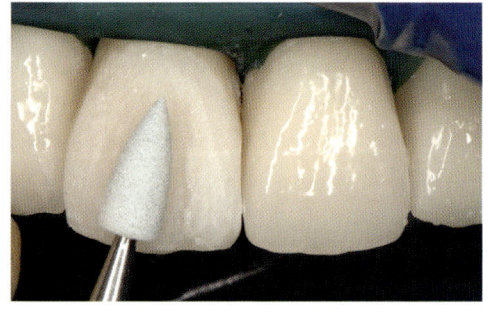

Fig 14-26

Direct restorative technology

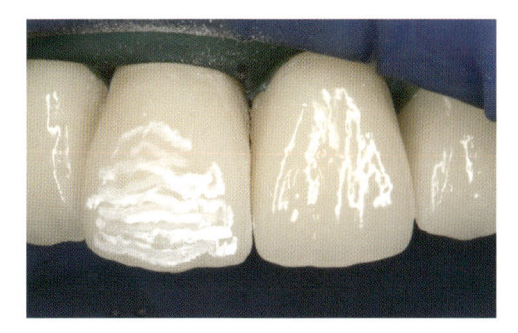

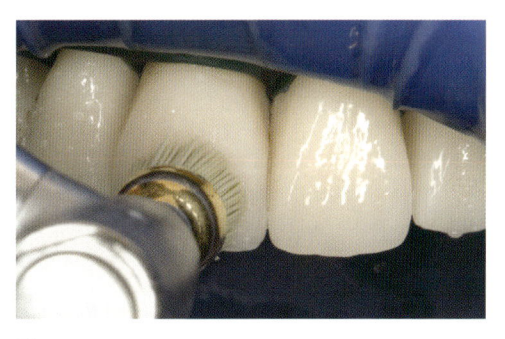

Fig 14-27

Fig 14-28

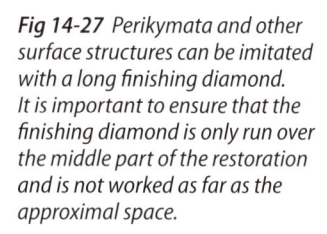

Fig 14-27 Perikymata and other surface structures can be imitated with a long finishing diamond. It is important to ensure that the finishing diamond is only run over the middle part of the restoration and is not worked as far as the approximal space.

Fig 14-28 After application of the finest silicone polisher, the restoration surface can be polished to a high-glaze finish with an Occlubrush or a combination of brush and polishing paste.

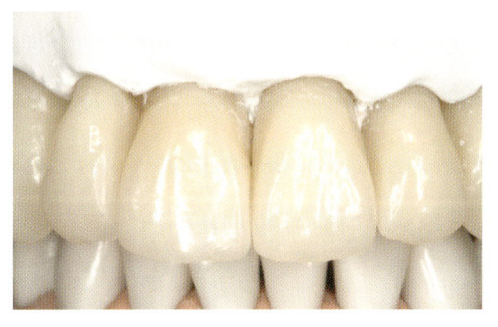

Fig 14-29

Fig 14-29 The imitation of surface characteristics means that light on the surface of the restoration is naturally refracted.

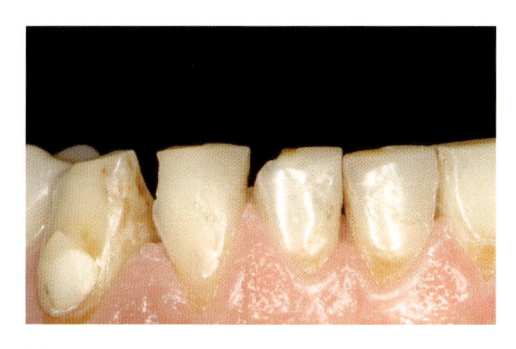

Fig 14-30

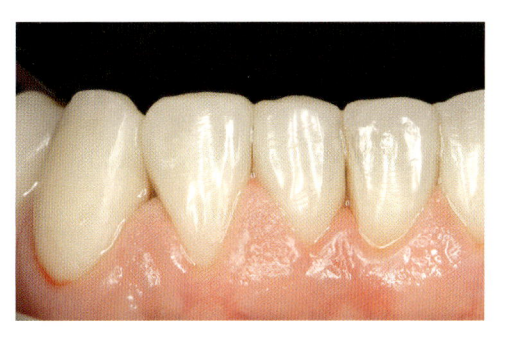

Fig 14-31

Case 5: Figs 14-30 and 14-31

Fig 14-30 Situation in a patient who had severe erosion resulting from reflux. The thickness of the enamel is markedly reduced; furthermore, restoration losses have occurred in the interdental spaces.

Fig 14-31 Direct composite resin veneers with build-up of incisal edge. The individual surface structures are noticeable and give the teeth a natural and youthful appearance.

■ References

1. Barbarosa SH, Zanata RL, Navarro MFDL, Nunes OB. Effect of different finishing and polishing techniques on the surface roughness of microfilled, hybrid and packable composite resins. Braz Dent J 2005;16:39–44.
2. Berastegui E, Canalda C, Brau, E Miquel C. Surface roughness of finished composite resins. J Prosthet Dent 1992;68:742–749.
3. Bollen CML, Lambrechts P, Quirynen M. Comparison of surface roughness of oral hard materials to the threshold surface roughness for bacterial plaque retention: A review of the literature. Dent Mater 1997;13:258–269.
4. Caughman WF, Caughman GB, Shiflett RA, Rueggeberg F, Schuster GS. Correlation of cytotoxicity, filler loading and curing time of dental composites. Biomaterials 1991;12:737–740.
5. Chan KC, Fuller JL, Hormati AA. The ability of foods to stain two composite resins. J Prosthet Dent 1980;43:542–545.

6. Ernst CP, Busemann T, Kern T, Willershausen B. Feldtest zur Lichtemissionsleistung von Polymerisationsgeräten in zahnärztlichen Praxen. DZZ 2006;9:466–471.

7. Feilzer AJ, De Gee Aj, Davidson CL. Setting stress in composite resin in relation to configuration of the restoration. J Dent Res 1987;66:1636–1639.

8. Folwaczny M, Loher C, Mehl A, Kunzelmann KH, Hickel R. Class V lesions restored with four different tooth-colored materials - 3-year results. Clin Oral Investig 2001;5: 31–39.

9. Heintze SD, Forjanic M, Rousson V. Surface roughness and gloss of dental materials as a function of force and polishing time *in vitro*. Dent Mater 2006;22:146–165.

10. Hse KM, Wei SH. Clinical evaluation of compomer in primary teeth: 1-year results. J Am Dent Assoc 1997;128:1088–1096.

11. Ilie N, Hickel R. Macro-, micro- and nano-mechanical investigations on silorane and methacrylate-based composites. Dent Mater 13 Epub ahead of print (2009).

12. Itota T, Carrick TE, Yoshiyama M, McCabe JF. Fluoride release and recharge in giomer, compomer and resin composite. Dent Mater 2004;20:789–795.

13. Jones CS, Billington RW, Pearson GJ. The *in vivo* perception of roughness of restorations. Br Dent J 2004;196: 42-45.

14. Kim KH, Ong JL, Okuno O. The effect of filler loading and morphology on the mechanical properties of contemporary composites. J Prosthet Dent 2002;87:642–649.

15. Lennon AM, Wiegand A, Buchalla W, Attin T. Approximal caries development in surfaces in contact with fluoride-releasing and non-fluoride-releasing restorative materials: an *in situ* study. Eur J Oral Sci 2007;115:497–501.

16. Loomans BAC, Opdam NJM, Roeters JJM, Bronkhorst EM, Burgersdijk RCW. Comparison of proximal contacts of class II resin composite restorations *in vitro*. Oper Dent 2006;31:680–685.

17. Manhardt J, Chen H, Hamm G, Hickel R. Buonocore Memorial Lecturer. Review of the clinical survival of direct indirect restorations in posterior teeth of the permanent dentition. Oper Dent 2004;29:481–508.

18. Marigo L, Rizzi M, La Torre G, Rumi G. 3-D surface profile analysis: different finishing methods for resin composites. Oper Dent 2001;26:562–568.

19. Mitra SB, Wu D, Holmes BN. An application of nanotechnology in advanced dental materials. J Am Dent Assoc 2003;134:1382–1390.

20. Moodley D, Grobler SR: Compomers: adhesion and setting reactions. SADJ 2003;58:24–28.

21. Polydorou O, König A, Hellwig E, Kümmerer K. Long-term release of monomers from modern dental-composite materials. Eur J Oral Sci 2009;117:68–75.

22. Pratten DH, Johnson GH. An evaluation of finishing instruments for an anterior and posterior composite. J Prosthet Dent 1988;60:154–158.

23. Sideriou ID, Achilias DS: Elution study of unreacted Bis-GMA, TEGDMA; UDMA, and Bis-EMA from light-cured dental resins and resin composites using HPLC. J Biomed Mater Res Part B: Appl Biomater 2005;74B:617–626.

24. Van Landuyt KL, Snauwaert J, De Munck J, Coutinho E, Yoshida Y, Suzuki K, Lambrechts P, Van Meerbeek B. Origin of interfacial droplets with one-step adhesives. J Dent Res 2007;86:739–744.

25. Wucher M, Grobler SR, Senekal PJ. A 3-year clinical evaluation of a copomer, a composite and a compomer/composite (sandwich) in class II restorations. Am J Dent 2002;15:274–278.

26. Yap AU, Chung SM, Chow WS, Tsai KT, Lim CT. Fracture resistance of compomer and composite restoratives. Oper Dent 2004;29:29–34.

27. Yap AU, Soh MS. Post-gel polymerization contraction of "low shrinkage" composite restoratives. Oper Dent 2004;29:182–187.

15 Restoration repairs

Brigitte Zimmerli and Matthias Strub

■ Introduction

Dental practitioners spend a large part of their working time replacing existing restorations.[19] The main problems leading to failure of a primary restoration are secondary caries and fractures.[5,6] Other reasons for failure include discoloration and debonding. Repaired restorations have been shown to be more susceptible to secondary caries than replaced restorations.[9] Replacement of a restoration will always enlarge the original cavity,[8] and there is a possibility of pulpal irritations triggered by the preparation trauma. The thinner the remaining dentin wall, the more pronounced the pulpal inflammation caused by bacteria and the deeper the penetration of free monomers into the pulpal tissue.[3] Thus the placement of repairs rather than a replacement increases the life-span of the tooth.[20] Repairs are usually easy to perform and are therefore ideal for patients who are more difficult to treat, such as the elderly[7] and children.[4]

■ Composite resin restoration repair

It is almost impossible for the dental practitioner to determine exactly what material was used for the original restoration if no note on the material appears in the patient's records.[21] However, it has been shown that the quality of the restoration does not depend on whether the same composite resin material or a different one is used for the repair.[11,18]

Looking at bond strengths, a repair achieves around 20% to 99% of the bond strength of a nonrepaired composite resin.[15,23–26] Use of etchants alone cannot increase the bond strength of repairs.[1,10,17,22] Mechanical pretreatment appears to play an important role in repairs,[1,2,24] but the bond strength will be insufficient after purely mechanical pretreatment of the surface.[16] Air-abrasive polishers, diamond finishers, or carborundum stones can be used for further surface treatment. The CoJet™ system, in particular, seems to yield good results.[22] In practice it is important to wait until the CoJet system has been applied before placing the acid etching process so that the etching pattern is preserved on the tooth surface.[12] Furthermore, a number of studies have reported an improvement in bond strength after application of a silane.[2,13,14] In the process, contamination of the tooth surface with silanes has no adverse effect on the adhesive bond.[12]

Composite resin repair
- Blasting with aluminum oxide or silicon oxide
- Tooth conditioning
- Silanization
- Applying the adhesive system

■ Ceramic restoration repairs

Ideally, when ceramic inlays are being repaired a small undercut is prepared. The application of hydrofluoric acid provides reliable conditioning of the material surface. However, the use of hydrofluoric acid in the mouth is controversial and should only be undertaken with adequate rubber dam application and sufficient safety precautions (protective glasses for the dental team and the patient). It is not necessary to use hydrofluoric acid if tribochemical pretreatment (CoJet) with silicon-coated aluminum oxide particles is carried out. These particles are placed onto the ceramic surface under pressure and fuse with it, resulting in a silicatized layer. If parts of the metal coping are exposed, these are pretreated with silanes and covered with opaquers. If composite resin alone is applied, it is not possible to prevent the metal coping from shining through in most cases and the subsequent restoration will have a grayish appearance. An attractive result can usually be achieved by this repair technique, at least in the acute situation (Figs 15-1 and 15-2). Unfortunately, there are currently no long-term data available on the success of ceramic repair restorations.

Ceramic repair
- Blasting with silicon oxide
- Tooth conditioning
- Silanization
- Applying the adhesive system

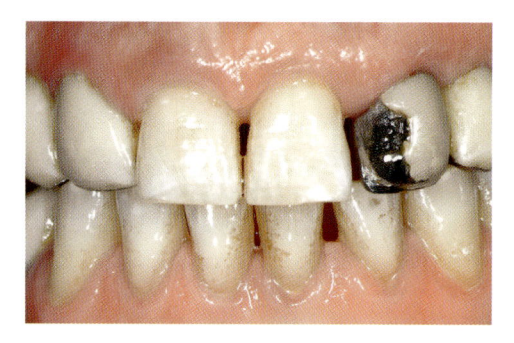

Fig 15-1 Ceramic fracture of a metal-ceramic restoration at the maxillary left lateral incisor. A new restoration cannot be placed at the present time.

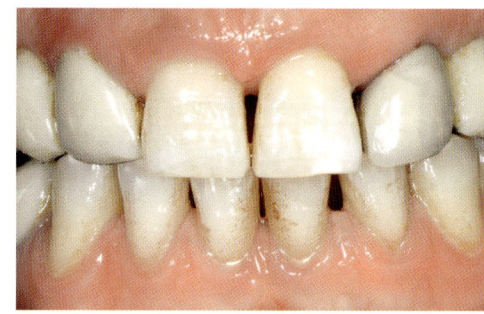

Fig 15-2 The restoration surface was conditioned using the methods described. The metal coping was covered with opaquer and composite resin was then applied.

■ Amalgam restoration repairs

Amalgam restorations can, of course, continue to be topped up or repaired with amalgam. Although corrosive processes may take place at the interface between two amalgam restorations, this technique is acceptable. The popularity of using composite resin materials for repair restorations has grown with the concept of the amalgam-free dental practice and is justifiable as an alternative therapeutic approach. Lack of adhesion to the amalgam can be compensated for by means of retentive preparation. In addition, the amalgam restoration can be blasted with aluminum oxide and pretreated with a silane. Adhesive techniques are employed on the tooth itself.

Amalgam repair
- Blasting with aluminum oxide
- Tooth conditioning
- Applying the adhesive system

■ Metal restoration repairs

If possible, an undercut is prepared in the precious metal restoration. The surface is then silicatized by being blasted with silicon oxide (CoJet) in order to facilitate an adhesive bond. After conditioning of the tooth surface, the silane is applied to the metallic surface. The adhesive system and the repair composite resin are then applied. If a metal coping has to be masked, an opaquer should be applied before the resin composite.

Metal repair
- Blasting with silicon oxide
- Tooth conditioning
- Silanization
- Applying the adhesive system

■ Summary

Repairs are regarded as a fully valid therapeutic approach in tooth preservation. Repair of the defective part of an extensive restoration can certainly yield better long-term results than complete replacement. Furthermore it has been shown that replacement is always associated with a much greater additional loss of dental hard tissue than repair. Repair of a restoration can enhance the comfort of treatment in patients whose cooperation is limited, such as the elderly or children. The end result of a repair can definitely be better than that of a replacement. It is important to ensure that there is a sufficient adhesive bond between tooth, old restorative material, and repair material. This demands correct conditioning of both the old restorative material and the tooth surface.

■ References

1. Bonstein T, Garlapo D, Donarummo J Jr, Bush PJ. Evaluation of varied repair protocols applied to aged composite resin. J Adhes Dent 2005;7:41–49.
2. Brosh T, Pilo R, Bichacho N, Blutstein R. Effect of combinations of surface treatments and bonding agents on the bond strength of repaired composites. J Prosthet Dent 1997;77:122–126.
3. Camps J, Déjou J, Rémusat M, About I. Factors influencing pulpal response to cavity restorations. Dent Mater 2000;16:432–440.
4. Croll TP. Repair of Class I resin-composite restoration. ASDC J Dent Child 1997;64:22–27.
5. Deligeorgi V, Wilson NH, Fouzas D, Kouklaki E, Burke FJ, Mjör IA. Reasons for placement and replacement of restorations in student clinics in Manchester and Athens. Eur J Dent Educ 2000;4: 153–159.
6. Deligeorgi V, Mjör IA, Wilson NH. An overview of reasons for the placement and replacement of restorations. Prim dent Care 2001;8:5–11.
7. Ettinger RL. Restoring the ageing dentition: repair or replacement? 1990;40:275–282.
8. Gordan VV, Mondragon E, Shen C. Replacement of resin-based composite: evaluation of cavity design, cavity depth, and shade matching. Quintessence Int 2002;33:273–278.
9. Gordan VV, Shen C, Riley J 3rd, Mjör IA. Two-year clinical evaluation of repair versus replacement of composite restorations. J Esthet Restor Dent 2006;18:144–153.
10. Gregory WA, Pounder B, Bakus E. Bond strengths of dissimilar repaired composite resins. J Prosthet Dent 1990;64:664–668.
11. Gregory WA, Berry S, Duke E, Dennison JB. Physical properties and repair bond strength of direct and indirect composite resins. J Prosthet Dent 1992;68:406–411.
12. Hannig C, Hahn P, Thiele PP, Attin T. Influence of different repair procedures on bond strength of adhesive filling materials to etched enamel in vitro. Oper Dent 2003;28:800–807.
13. Hannig C, Laubach S, Hahn P, Attin T. Shear bond strength of repaired adhesive filling materials using different repair procedures. J Adhes Dent 2006;8:35–40.
14. Hisamatsu N, Atsuta M, Matsumura H. Effect of silane primers and unfilled resin bonding agents on repair bond strength of a prosthodontic microfilled composite. J Oral Rehabil 2002;29:644–648.
15. Kallio TT, Lastumäki TM, Vallittu PK. Bonding of restorative and veneering composite resin to some polymeric composites. Dent Mater 2001;17:80–86.
16. Kamann WK, Gängler P. Filling repair and repair fillings. Schweiz Monatsschr Zahnmed 2000;110: 1054–1071.
17. Miranda FJ, Duncanson MG Jr, Dilts WE. Interfacial bonding strengths of paired composite systems. J Prosthet Dent. 1984 Jan;51(1):29-32.
18. Mitsaki-Matsou H, Karanika-Kouma A, Papadoyiannis Y, Theodoridou-Pahine S. An *in vitro* study of the tensile strength of composite resins repaired with the same or another composite resin. Quintessence Int 1991;22: 475–481.
19. Mjör IA. Placement and replacement of restorations. Oper Dent 1981;6:49–54.
20. Mjör IA. Repair versus replacement of failed restorations. Int Dent J 1993;43:466–472.
21. Pappacchini F, La De Castro F, Goracci C et al. An investigation of the contribution of silane to the composite repair strength over time using a double sided microtensile test. International Dentistry SA 2006;8:54–63.
22. Papacchini F, Dall'Oca S, Chieffi N et al. Composite-to-composite microtensile bond strength in the repair of a microfilled hybrid resin: effect of surface treatment and oxygen inhibition. J Adhes Dent 2007;9:25–31.

23. Shahdad SA, Kennedy JG. Bond strength of repaired anterior composite resins: an *in vitro* study. J Dent 1998 Nov;26(8):685–694.
24. Söderholm KJ, Roberts MJ. Variables influencing the repair strength of dental composites. Scand J Dent Res 1991;99:173–80.
25. Swift EJ Jr, LeValley BD, Boyer DB. Evaluation of new methods for composite repair. Dent Mater 1992;8:362–365.
26. Swift EJ Jr, Cloe BC, Boyer DB. Effect of a silane coupling agent on composite repair strengths. Am J Dent 1994;7:200–202.

16 Post systems

Brigitte Zimmerli and Matthias Strub

■ Introduction

Today we have moved away from the previous, mechanical approach of reinforcing a tooth by the post-and-core method towards a biomimetic approach. The inserted post should have properties as similar to natural teeth as possible. Furthermore, post anchorage is only used when it is necessary for retention of built-up restorations because post insertion always leads to weakening of the root. Quite a lot has also changed with regard to the materials used. While gold-cast cores were seen as the method of choice for a long time, metallic posts have now been replaced by nonmetallic materials. The reason for this lies in the growing use of all-ceramic restorations, which require a tooth-colored build-up because of their higher translucency. Furthermore, a post-and-core made of metal usually has to be anchored deep in the root canal, which increases the risk of perforation or root fractures. Another disadvantage of the post-and-core method is the stiffness of the material, which makes nonrepairable failures more likely. This is why zirconium but particularly fiber posts are now gaining in significance. However, zirconium has not become established as a standard material because of unfavorable material properties (high modulus of elasticity) and poor revisability. This review therefore focuses on the adhesive luting of fiber posts.

The adhesive cementation of posts poses special problems for dental practitioners:
- It is difficult to get a clear view into the canal.
- The canal walls are contaminated with root canal sealant and gutta-percha remnants.
- The histology of the root canal changes from the coronal to the apical: a relatively large number of tubules are encountered coronally, whereas atubular fibrodentin is increasingly found apically.
- It is difficult to monitor the application of adhesive and cement in the root canal.
- The root canal has an unfavorable configuration factor (c-factor): the luting cement shows hardly any free surface, which leads to high stress during the setting process.
- Light polymerization of the luting agent is made difficult. Fiber posts conduct light poorly in an apical direction.

Indications

The indications for post-and-core restorations are clearly reduced nowadays. Whenever possible, an attempt is made to restore the endodontically treated tooth using adhesive techniques without post retention.

The position of the tooth in the dental arch, the anatomy of the pulp cavity, the existing residual hard tissue, and, not least, the prosthetic restoration are important factors in the decision on whether or not a post has to be placed (Table 16-1). Despite adhesive luting of the fiber post in the root canal, the indications for post placement cannot be expanded: a circular ferrule in the dentin of around 2 mm must be guaranteed for the success of a post-and-core.[11,14] If this is not the case, crown lengthening, extrusion of the root, or tooth extraction must be planned.

Table 16-1 Relative indications for post placement

	Post "yes"	Post "no"
Position in dental arch	Anterior tooth, premolar	Molar
Forces acting	Horizontal	Vertical
Pulp cavity	Small, narrow	Large, wide
Dental hard tissue	Markedly minimized	> 2 existing tooth walls
Prosthetic restoration	Bridge abutment, denture retention	Single-tooth restoration

If the decision is made in favor of a post restoration, only a single post per tooth is now inserted into the anatomically most suitable root. It is not necessary for a post to be cemented in every root canal in a molar.

Nowadays posts are used very sparingly and only serve to anchor build-up restorations.

Post systems

Table 16-2 gives an overview of the advantages and risks of individual post systems. Gold-cast core restorations have today receded into the background, mainly because of esthetic demands and the desire for nonmetallic restorations. It should nevertheless be noted that gold-cast core build-ups show good long-term results. The desire for modern post materials led from the carbon post to the zirconium and then the fiber post. Carbon posts are no longer popular because of their dark color. Zirconium posts are in use, but they do have a number of significant drawbacks. First, the posts are very rigid, which increases the likelihood of root

Table 16-2 Comparison of different types of post

	Fiber post	Zirconium post	Metal post/gold core
Elasticity modulus	+ (similar to dentin)	– (stiff)	– (stiff)
Esthetics	+	+	–
Adhesion	+	–	–
Radiopacity	+/–	++	++
Temporary	Not necessary	Not necessary	Necessary
Revisability	+	–	+/–
Experience	+/–	+/–	+
Failures	Debonding, post fracture (correctable)	Post fracture, root fracture (not correctable)	Loss of retention (correctable), root fracture (not correctable)

+: good/favorable property; +/–: moderate/average property; –: poor/unfavorable property

and/or post fractures. Second, revision of the root canal filling is almost impossible. To do this, the zirconium post has to be completely drilled out of the root canal, which can additionally weaken the root or lead to perforation. Glass fiber posts are an interesting alternative, especially since the build-up restoration is placed immediately after cementation of the post and hence the risky phase of the temporary post (ie, leakage, root fracture) can be avoided.

The relevant working steps for adhesive post luting are outlined below. An overview of the individual working steps is given in Table 16-3.

> Fiber post systems are routinely utilized nowadays. Post placement and restoration build-up can therefore be completed in a single session without a temporary phase.

■ Root canal preparation

The root canal filling material is removed to the desired post length (Figs 16-1 and 16-2). It is important to make sure that there are no cement or gutta-percha residues left on the walls of the root canal. This is not easy to check and an operating microscope can prove valuable. Additional widening of the canal should be avoided so that the smallest possible post can be inserted. Furthermore, a sufficiently long apical seal must be retained. A minimum seal length of 4 mm is required, but it can certainly be left longer than that. The post length in the root canal should roughly correspond to the height of the planned build-up. In addition, it is important to ensure that part of the root segment bearing the fiber post is embedded in bone, which can sometimes be difficult in cases of advanced periodontal disease.

Table 16-3 Chronological sequence of working steps in fiber post placement

Working step	Content	Notes
1. Root canal filling	Sufficient root canal filling, tight temporary seal	Observe setting time of the sealant: wait until completely set before cementing the post. Fill root canal by vertical filling technique only as far as the intended post length.
2. Preparation of the root canal	Removal of sealant and gutta-percha to the desired post length	An operating microscope makes it easier to check the cleaning of the canal walls.
3. Root canal irrigation	Removal of the smear layer with EDTA irrigant	If irrigated with NaOCl, an ascorbin solution should be used as a follow-on irrigant. CHX (0.2 %) as the final irrigant has a positive effect on bond strength.
4. Post pretreatment	Silanization of the post surface	Silanization is a matter of controversy, but it certainly has no negative effect. Other methods may also be used for post pretreatment (eg, sandblasting).
5. Cementation	Placement of the luting agent immediately followed by post placement	Application of the adhesive system with microbrushes; remove excess with a paper point; luting agent should ideally be applied with a syringe directly into the canal.
6. Light curing	Polymerization of the luting agent	Choose a sufficiently long light exposure time; hold light guide as close as possible to the root canal entrance.
7. Building up restoration	Application of the build-up restoration material, grinding back of the build-up	The fiber post must be entirely covered with composite resin.

EDTA: ethylene diamine tetra-acetate, NaOCl: sodium hypochlorite, CHX: chlorhexidine

In anticipation for post placement, the root canal is prepared as little as possible. An apical seal of 4 mm or more must be left in place. The post length in the root canal should roughly correspond to the height of the build-up restoration.

The canal should be thoroughly cleaned prior to cementation. It is imperative to remove the smear layer. Sodium hypochlorite leaves behind an oxygen-saturated root canal surface, which can inhibit the polymerization of resin luting agents.[12] To cancel out this negative effect, the root canal can be cleaned with ascorbic acid or sodium ascorbate.[9] The use of chlorhexidine (0.2 %) also has a positive effect on the bond strength of adhesive luting agents.[3]

Post systems

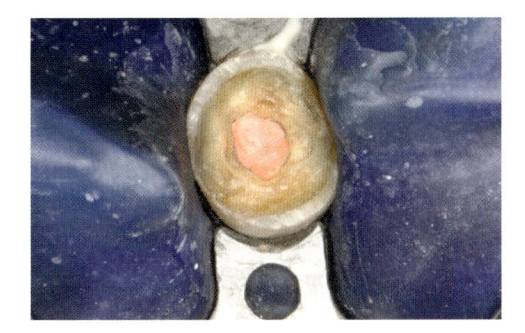

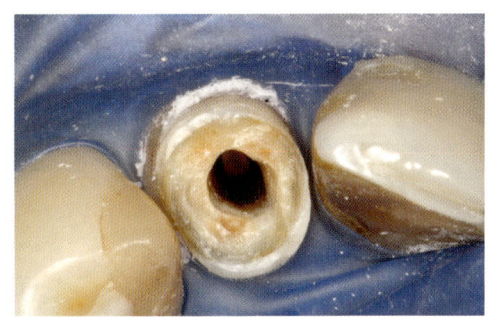

Fig 16-1 Maxillary right lateral incisor after completed root canal treatment.

Fig 16-2 The root canal filling is removed to the post insertion length. In the process, the root canal walls should be prepared as little as possible.

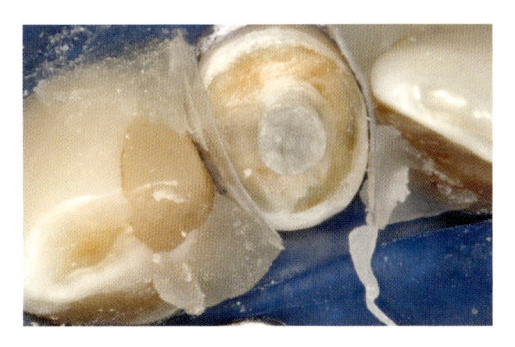

Fig 16-3 The shortened fiber post is cemented in the root canal. The transparent matrices were cemented with a temporary acrylic resin material (Telio CS®).

■ Post cementation

If an etch-and-rinse adhesive is used for cementation, it is essential to ensure that the reaction time of phosphoric acid in the root canal does not exceed 15 seconds.[7] The remaining adhesive components should be worked into the root canal surface using fine microbrushes. Ideally, a system for luting agent application that enables the dental practitioner to inject the cement directly into the canal through a thin cannula should be used. Luting agent application with a lentulo can result in air enclosures and inhomogenities (leakages) in the adhesive interface.[16]

Post pretreatment is a matter of intense debate: sandblasting, roughening with preparation tools, the application of silanes, or etching the outermost covering layer with hydrogen peroxide (24%) have all been considered. If silicatization with aluminum oxide (CoJet™) is undertaken, this pretreatment should be applied only briefly to avoid excessive weakening of the post's fiber matrix.[13] Silanization is usually found to improve bond strength.[1,8]

The results with regard to different luting agent systems are not clear-cut. The application of etch-and-rinse adhesive systems is difficult to control in the root canal. It is easier to handle self-etch systems, which is why they are used in most cases. The findings regarding self-adhesive cement systems have not yet been fully recorded. Until definite clinical results are available, these cement systems should not be used in the root canal. In every case, sufficient light curing of the luting agent is important because it markedly improves the conversion rate (polymerization degree) of the luting agent; the pure dark reaction of dual-cure luting agents is not adequate.[2] Shortening a post before cementation allows better access and a shorter distance between the light guide of the curing device and the luting agent (Fig 16-3).

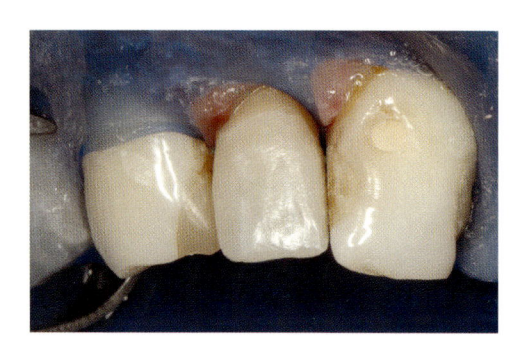

Fig 16-4 Finished composite resin build-up on the right lateral incisor. The restorations to adjacent teeth are then replaced for esthetic reasons.

If an etch-and-rinse adhesive is used, the phosphoric acid should not be applied for longer than 15 seconds. Self-etch adhesive systems are far simpler to apply in the root canal. The luting agent should be injected into the canal via a syringe.

■ Post-and-core restoration

A key aspect of a build-up restoration is that the post is entirely covered by composite resin (Fig 16-4). If this will not be the case, the post should be further shortened so that complete coverage becomes possible. Otherwise, the post can absorb moisture and direct this to the inside of the restoration, which can lead to disintegration of fiber and matrix and further lead to a debonding of the post.

The fiber post must always be fully covered by composite resin.

■ Conclusions

Nowadays, posts are only used for limited indications. In the molar region, post placement can usually be avoided for single tooth restorations due to the large area of the coronal pulpal cavity for adhesion. Molars that have been ground back as bridge abutments are exceptions. If a post is indicated, fiber posts and adhesive techniques are usually employed nowadays. The few long-term clinical data are certainly interesting.

The failure of a post-and-core is usually correctable in the case of fiber posts. The reported annual loss rates for fiber posts differ very widely, depending on the study: rates range from 0.3 % to 6.7 %.[5,6,10,15] When interpreting these values, however, it should be noted that 50 % of the losses are due to an endodontic failure. Quick and tight restoration of the endodontically treated tooth is important in preventing contamination of the freshly filled root canal. The root canal preparation and adhesive post luting should, of course, be performed with a rubber dam. Methods to help ensure a sufficient seal around the rubber dam in difficult situations are discussed in chapter 14.

In relation to post luting, some relatively new composite resin products are of interest: these can be used not only to cement the post in the canal, but also for the build-up restoration (eg, Multicore® Flow). The increased filler content of these systems, however, are controversially discussed.[4] There are still no clinical data on these new products and the literature needs to be monitored further before recommendations on these products can be made.

References

1. Aksornmuang J, Foxton RM, Nakajima M, Tagami J. Mictrotensile bond strength of a dual-cure resin core material to glass and quartz fibre posts. J Dent 2004;32:443–450.
2. Bitter K, Meyer-Lueckel H, Priehn K, Kanjuparambil JP, Neumann K, Kielbassa AM. Effects of luting agent and thermocycling on bond strengths to root canal dentin. Int Endod J 2006;39:809–818.
3. Erdemir A, Ari H, Gungunes H, Belli S. The effect of medications for root canal treatment on bonding to root canal dentin. J Endod 2004;30:113–116.
4. Ferrari M, Carvalho CA, Goracci C, Antoniolli F, Mazzoni A, Mazzoti G, Cadenaro M, Breschi L. Influence of luting material filler content on post cementation. J Dent Res 2009;88:951–956.
5. Ferrari M, Vichi A, Mannocci F, Mason PN. Retrospective study of the clinical performance of fibre posts. Am J Dent 2000;13:9B–13B.
6. Glazer B. Restoration of endodontically treated teeth with carbon fibre posts–a prospective study. J Can Dent Assoc 2000;66:614–618.
7. Hashimoto M, Ohno H, Endi K, Kaga M, Sano H, Oguchi H. The effect of hybrid layer thickness on bond strength: demineralized dentin zone of hybrid layer. Dent Mater 2000;16:406–411.
8. Magni E, Mazzitelli C, Papacchini F, Radovic I, Goracci C, Coniglio I, Ferrari M. Adhesion between fibre posts and resin luting agents: a microtensile bond strength test and SEM investigation following different treatments of the post surface. J Adhes Dent 2007;9:195–202.
9. Morris MD, Lee KW, Agee KA, Bouillaguet S, Pashley DH. Effects of sodium hypochlorite and RC-prep on bond strengths of resin cement to endodontic surfaces. J Endod 2001;27:753–757.
10. Naumann M, Blankenstein F, Kiessling S, Dietrich T. Risk factors for failure of glass fiber-reinforced composite post restorations: a prospective observational clinical study. Eur J Oral Sci 2005;113:519–524.
11. Pereira JR, De Ornelas F, Conti PC, do Valle AL. Effect of a crown ferrule on the fracture resistance of endodontically treated teeth restored with prefabricated posts. J Prosthet Dent 2006;95:50–54.
12. Rueggeberg FA, Margeson DH. The effect of oxygen inhibition on an unfilled/filled composite system. J Dent Res 1990;69:1652–1658.
13. Sahafi A, Peutzfeld A, Asmussen E, Gottfredsen K. Retention and failure morphology of prefabricated posts. Int J Prosthodont 2004;17:307–312.
14. Salameh Z, Sorrentino R, Papacchini F, Ounsi HF, Tashkandi E, Goracci C, Ferrari M. Fracture resistance and failure patterns of endodontically treated mandibular molars restored using resin composite with or without translucent glass fibre posts. J Endod 2006;32:752–755.
15. Signore A, Benedicenti S, Kaitas V, Barone M, Angiero F, Ravera G. Long-term survival of endodontically treated, maxillary anterior teeth restored with either tapered or parallel-sided glass-fiber posts and full-ceramic coverage. J Dent 2009;37:115–121.
16. Watzke R, Blunck U, Frankenberger R, Naumann M. Interface homogeneity of adhesively luted glass fiber posts. Dent Mater 2008;24:1512–1517.

17 The CEREC system

Domenico Di Rocco and Adrian Lussi

■ Introduction

Since CEREC technology was introduced in the early 1980s by Professor *W. Mörmann* and Dr *M. Brandestini* at Zurich University[11,12] the hardware and software have been continuously updated and refined. Today CEREC is regarded as a proven, comprehensive restorative system for the dental practice and laboratory. In everyday dental practice, all restorations can be designed and milled using CEREC, from simple inlays through to esthetically challenging anterior crowns.

Adhesively cemented inlays, onlays, and partial crowns offer a number of clinical advantages over metallic reconstructions: first, tooth substance can be preserved during preparation; second, the physical properties of CEREC ceramics are similar to those of enamel. Extensive studies of Vita Mark II ceramic in particular prove that its abrasion characteristics are similar to those of dental enamel.[6]

Correctly performed preparation, uniformly fine powdering, and a perfect optical image are decisive factors in achieving a durable and accurate CEREC restoration. Expertly carried out and placed CEREC reconstructions have an annual failure rate of less than 1%.[3,5,14,15] Thus the marginal gap, which is often unjustly criticized, does not play a significant role in adhesive cementation with composite resin. The longevity of a restoration can only be proved by means of clinical trials.

The same indications and contraindications apply to CEREC reconstructions as for indirectly fabricated ceramic reconstructions, which is why they are not listed here.

This chapter describes the preparation guidelines, an amalgam replacement with inlay and overlay, the rehabilitation of a root-treated tooth with an endo-crown, and a case of anterior rehabilitation with veneers.

Preparation guidelines for fabrication of a ceramic restoration

The preparation advice listed in Table 17-1 applies to all direct and indirect ceramic restorative methods – irrespective of the material chosen.

Table 17-1 Preparation guidelines for fabrication of a ceramic restoration

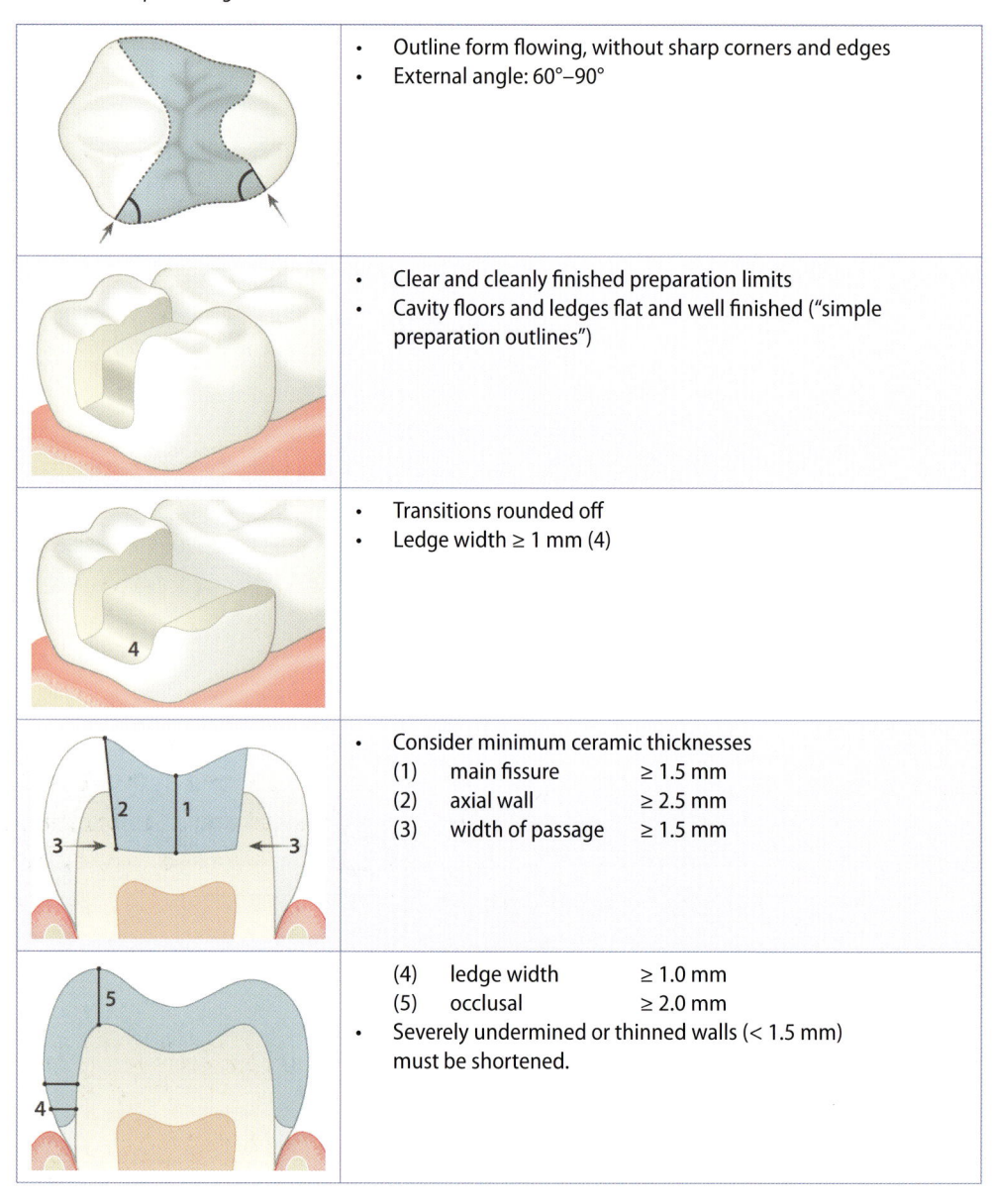

	• Outline form flowing, without sharp corners and edges • External angle: 60°–90°
	• Clear and cleanly finished preparation limits • Cavity floors and ledges flat and well finished ("simple preparation outlines")
	• Transitions rounded off • Ledge width ≥ 1 mm (4)

	• Consider minimum ceramic thicknesses
	  (1) main fissure ≥ 1.5 mm
	  (2) axial wall ≥ 2.5 mm
	  (3) width of passage ≥ 1.5 mm

	(4) ledge width ≥ 1.0 mm (5) occlusal ≥ 2.0 mm • Severely undermined or thinned walls (< 1.5 mm) must be shortened.

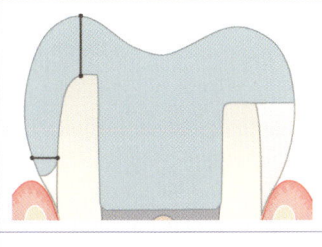	• Restore endodontically treated teeth in the molar region as an "endo-crown" or with conventional CEREC crown; in the premolar region: conventional restoration.
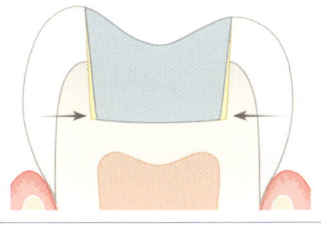	• Slight undercuts (up to max. 0.5 mm, →←) in the passage area are permitted. During insertion they are sealed with composite resin (yellow). • Larger undercuts must be blocked out (immediate dentin sealing, IDS), the cusps are shortened if there are very thin walls.
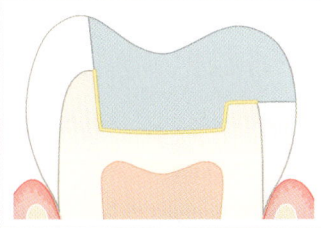	• After preparation the dentin surface must be treated using IDS (yellow line) and the enamel margins redefined. The IDS protects the pulp against bacteria, toxins, and other noxae → less postoperative pain.

■ Case studies

Case 1 – Amalgam replacement

This case study describes the treatment of a patient with CEREC inlays and overlays (Vita MK II).

History-taking and findings

A 55-year-old patient in good general health presented because he wanted to have his amalgam restorations in the fourth quadrant replaced by ceramic restorations (Fig 17-1). Furthermore, his right mandibular second premolar displayed typical clinical symptoms of cracked tooth syndrome. Extraoral as well as intraoral examination revealed no pathological findings. All the teeth were CO_2-positive and caries-free.

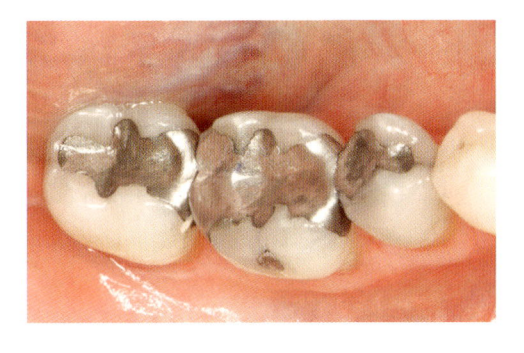

Fig 17-1 Pretreatment situation: the patient has requested amalgam replacement.

Treatment planning and procedure

After history-taking and discussion with the patient, the treatment was tackled with Vita MK II ceramic. Vita MK II is a pure feldspar ceramic with very enamel-like abrasion behavior[6] and a biaxial fracture strength of approximately 120 MPa.

In a single session the amalgam restorations were removed under rubber dam and the definitive preparations were fabricated (Fig 17-2). As the cusps of the second premolar showed marked infraction lines labially and lingually, a classic overlay preparation was selected for that tooth. The first and second molars were prepared for two- and three-layer inlays. After the preparations were completed, the dentin surfaces were sealed with an adhesive layer (dentin and enamel bonding). Owing to the oxygen inhibition layer, the adhesive was set with the aid of a transparent glycerol gel. The adhesive (Optibond Fl, Kerr) was placed and subsequently cleaned, using 25 μm aluminum oxide powder to abrade some substance.[7,8,16] After the optical impression and the CEREC-supported fabrication, the reconstructions were characterized and glazed at the patient's request (Fig 17-3).

Under rubber dam the IDS (immediate dentin sealing) was cleaned with 25 μm aluminum oxide powder; the dentin should not be exposed, if at all possible. The reconstructions were then adhesively placed according to the conventional cementation protocol. In this case, the reconstructions were cemented with Variolink II (Fig 17-4), then fully finished. The provision of the three reconstructions took just under 4 hours.

At the 2-year follow-up the reconstructions had margins that clinically could not be probed (Fig 17-5). The reconstruction on the second premolar was too light in color in comparison with the other inlays. However, the patient did not perceive this as a problem.

Fig 17-2 The finished preparations.

Fig 17-3 Individualized Vita MK II restorations.

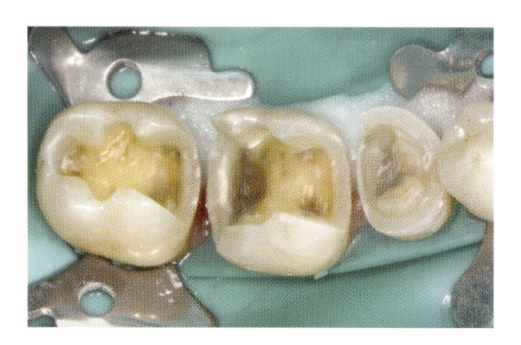

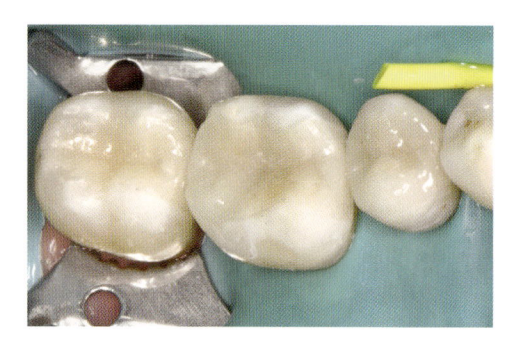

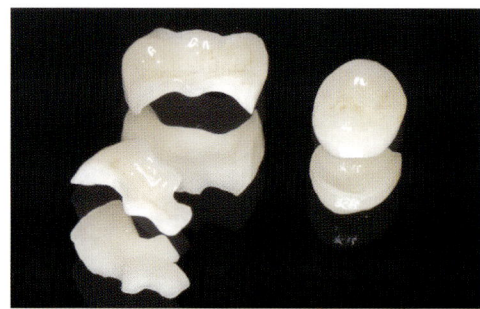

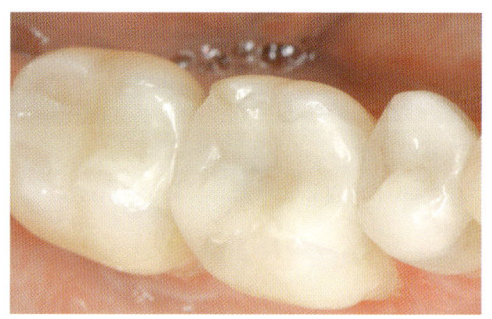

Fig 17-4 Inserted restorations.

Fig 17-5 Check-up after 2 years.

Case 2 – Endo-crown

The term "CEREC endo-crown" was coined by Dr. A. Bindl and Professor W. Mörmann.[1] CEREC endo-crown denotes the restoration of a devitalized tooth with an overlay or a crown, whereby the restoration usually has what is known as a canal inlay in the area of the pulp cavity (Fig 17-6).

In the case of devitalized molars and premolars, the cusps should be shortened and built up with the restoration in order to avoid subsequent cusp fracture.[4]

While the classic and the reduced crown preparation in the molar and premolar region are associated with similarly good results, the reconstruction of devitalized premolars with a classic endo-crown (epi-gingival crown stump with canal inlay) leads to far more failures than in the molar region.[2] Premolars should therefore be treated with an endo-overlay or, where residual dental tissue is reduced, by means of a classic post-and-core using a CEREC crown (Fig 17-7).

History-taking and findings

A 28-year-old patient in good general health without any specific medical risks presented with a request to have a fractured left mandibular first molar built up. The clinical findings showed a profound carious lesion in the distal area. The CO_2-negative first molar was root-treated in a student operation and provisionally restored (Fig 17-8).

Treatment planning and procedure

In consultation with the patient, restoration of the tooth with an IPS e.max CAD endo-crown was planned for stability reasons. IPS e.max CAD is a lithium disilicate ceramic which has a markedly increased biaxial fracture strength of 350 to 360 MPa relative to the "conventional" CEREC ceramics, such as Vita MK II or IPS Empress CAD. However, processing is done on the lithium metasilicate precursor, the so-called blue block. This ceramic precursor has a lower biaxial fracture strength, approximately 130 MPa, hence the reconstruction can be fitted *in situ* and adjusted before fabrication.

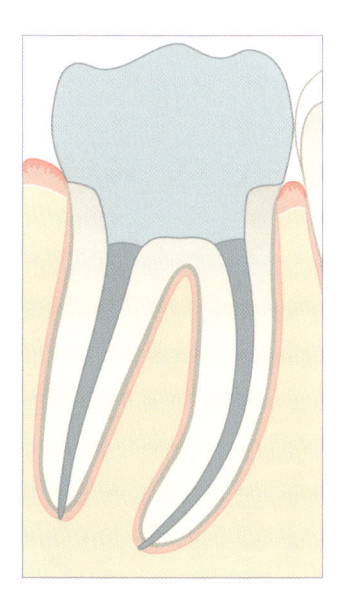

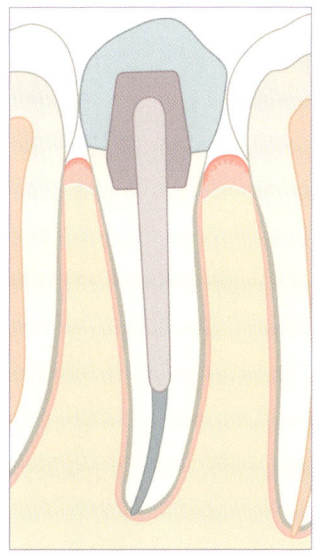

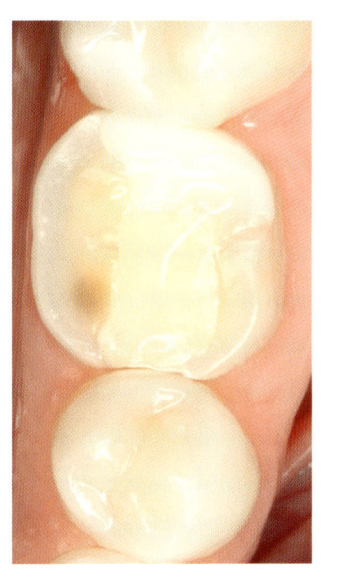

Fig 17-6 CEREC endo-crown with canal inlay.

Fig 17-7 Conventional post-and-core with glass fiber post and composite resin.

Fig 17-8 Pretreatment situation: status after root filling and provisional restoration.

Before preparation, all the temporary materials were first removed. The cusps were then shortened and the transitions were rounded off and finished (see Table 17-1). In the area of the previous crown cavity, peg-shaped widening of the preparation was performed for the so-called canal inlay (Fig 17-9). The purpose of this step is to enlarge the adhesive surface and increase the mechanical retention of the reconstruction (Fig 17-6). If the canal inlay is very deep, the pulp cavity should be blocked out with composite resin beforehand so that a maximum depth of 3 mm is not exceeded and complete polymerization of the light-cured luting composite resin is guaranteed. Alternatively, dual-cure composite resins may be used. An IDS was then applied to the dentin surface. Adhesive residues on the enamel were removed, a centric bite registration carried out, and optical images of the bite record and the preparation were made. The shape of the reconstruction was calculated using the CEREC tooth database. The proposed restoration could then be individually adapted with the aid of the tools in the Design window.

The lithium metasilicate reconstruction (which took about 25 minutes' milling time) was tried in and the occlusion was checked and adjusted. The reconstruction was then pre-polished using suitable rubber polishers and fixed onto the object holder with a special putty firing paste. The endo-crown was individualized using the system's stains (IPS e.max CAD Crystall Stains and Shades) and it was covered with a thin layer of glaze (IPS e.max CAD Crystall Glaze). The glaze can be applied in spray form or prior to staining in paste form. Finally, the lithium metasilicate crown was annealed under vacuum and a specific two-stage firing at 850 °C (known as *Oswald* maturation). The finished crown was tried in and checked before cementation.

Lithium disilicate reconstructions can be inserted using adhesive, self-adhesive, or conventional methods, but adhesive fixation is preferable in every case. Cementation with a

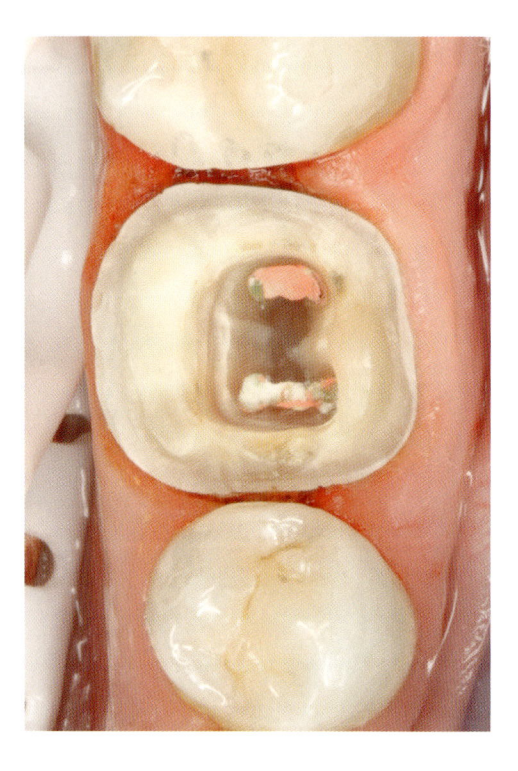

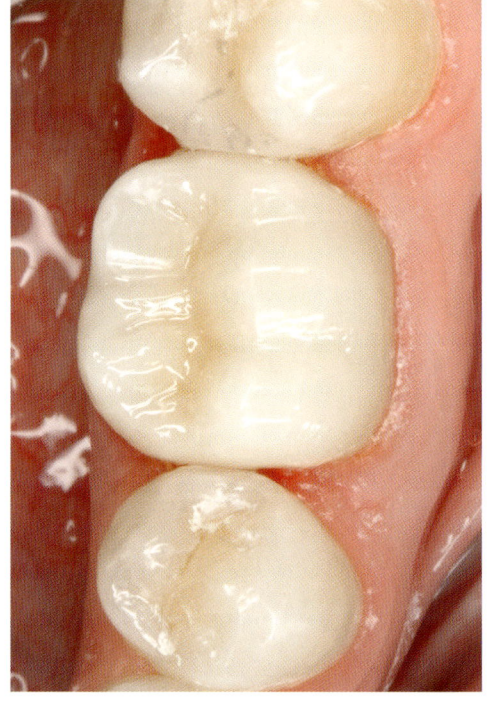

Fig 17-9 Finished preparation with canal inlay.

Fig 17-10 Final image of the individualized and glazed IPS e.max CAD-LT endo-crown.

dual-cure composite resin is recommended for endo-crowns because of the increased ceramic dimensions. In this case study, the endo-crown was adhesively luted with a dual-cure composite resin cement (Fig 17-10). To do this, the ceramic was first etched with hydrofluoric acid for 20 seconds, thoroughly rinsed, then coated with a silane. After cleaning with aluminum oxide powder, the residual tooth substance was pretreated with phosphoric acid and an appropriate bonding agent. After removal of the composite resin residues, the occlusion is checked once again and adjusted, if necessary.

Case 3 – Anterior rehabilitation with veneers

Esthetic rehabilitation in the anterior region using full-ceramic reconstructions continues to place extremely high demands on dentists and dental technicians and is associated with high costs for the patient. The CEREC system offers an affordable and relatively straightforward means of fabricating esthetic reconstructions for the anterior region. For any major change in the area of the anterior teeth, it is advisable to arrange for a waxup incorporating the planned tooth positioning and tooth form (Fig 17-11). The waxup is then used to produce a mock-up *in situ*, which helps the dental practitioner and patient to assess the planned tooth position and tooth form.

History-taking and findings

A 46-year-old patient in good general health presented with a request to have the position of her maxillary anterior teeth corrected. She was disturbed by the slightly retroclined central incisors and wanted correction of the slight overlapping of these teeth (Fig 17-13). She rejected orthodontic treatment for reasons of time and because she was afraid that a speech defect that had been corrected during a lengthy course of treatment might return. As a basis for the treatment planning, study casts and a diagnostic waxup were fabricated (Figs 17-11 and 17-12).

Treatment planning and procedure

After the pretreatment phase with waxup and mock-up had been completed and after the patient had given her consent, the central incisors were subjected to minimally invasive preparation because of their retroclined position (Fig 17-14). No dentin sealing (IDS) was required because there had never been any exposure of the dentin.

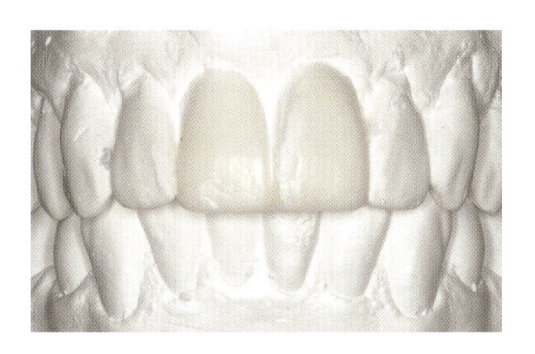

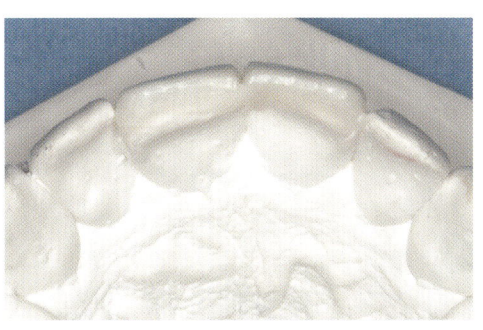

Fig 17-11 Waxup to assess the planned tooth position and tooth form.

Fig 17-12 Positional correction in the waxup of the retroclined maxillary central incisors.

Fig 17-13 Pretreatment situation: observe the overlapping of the central incisors.

Fig 17-14 Minimally invasive preparation of the central incisors.

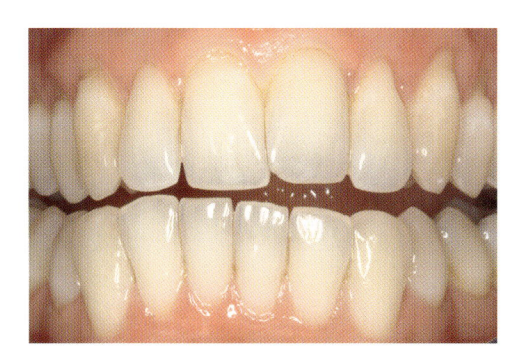

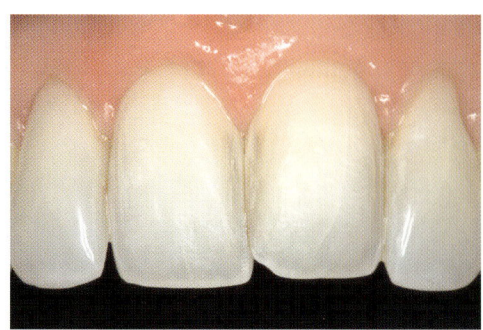

The design mode chosen for the veneers was the correlation method. The waxup was first scanned in, then an optical record of the preparation was taken. (An existing, correctly shaped reconstruction that needs to be replaced can also be used as the correlate.) After entry of the preparation limit and correction of the equator or the copying line, the system calculated a proposed reconstruction. Where necessary, this was altered and adjusted using the Design tools. The veneers were then milled from IPS Empress CAD multi-A2 blocks, fitted in the mouth, and annealed in the ceramic furnace with the glaze spray from the system (IPS Empress Universal Glaze Spray).

After the glaze firing, the reconstructions were tried in and, with the patient's consent, were prepared for seating. The ceramic was etched with 5% hydrofluoric acid and cleaned in an ultrasonic bath. After complete drying of the ceramic surface, a silane was applied (Ivoclar Vivadent Monobond S). At the same time, the teeth were dried under rubber dam and cleaned with 25 μm aluminum oxide powder. A purely light-cured composite resin (eg, Variolink Veneer) lends itself to cementation of a translucent leucite-reinforced glass ceramic reconstruction. After the veneers had been positioned on the prepared teeth, the composite resin residues were removed using foam pellets and Superfloss. The composite resin in the area of the reconstruction borders was briefly illuminated, then covered with a transparent glycerol gel and completely light cured both labially and palatally.

Finally, the composite resin residues still remaining were carefully removed by pressure-free scraping with a scalpel or a narrow, straight Proxoshape file. The palatal contacts were checked and, where necessary, corrected. The use of scalers or curettes to remove composite resin residues is not recommended because of the increased risk of chipping the ceramic.

At the first check-up (Figs 17-15 and 17-16), which took place shortly after insertion and was mainly for the purpose of removing any subgingival composite resin residues,[9,10] the patient stated that her wishes had been satisfied in every respect.

This case study shows that the CEREC system can be used successfully in the anterior region under practice conditions.

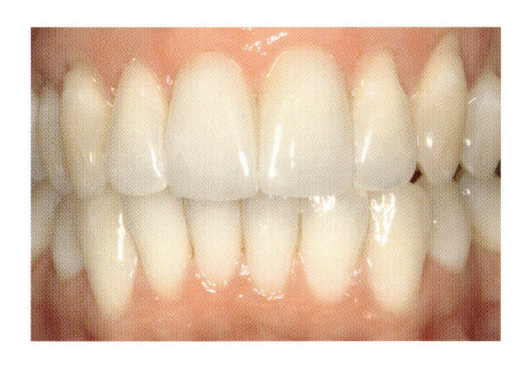

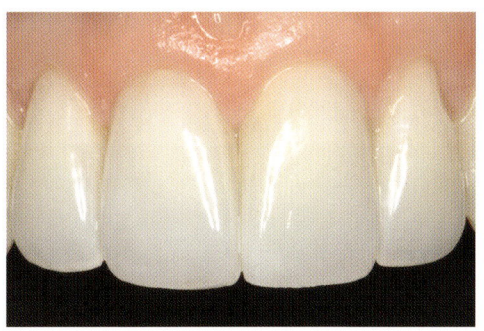

Fig 17-15 Check-up a few days after insertion of the restoration.

Fig 17-16 Close-up of the reconstructed teeth.

Cases 1 to 3 – Aftercare

In all three case studies the patient's wishes were successfully fulfilled with metal-free reconstructions. The reconstruction margins were assessed at the check-ups and reworking was found not to be necessary in any of the three cases. The gingiva also showed no signs of inflammation in any of the cases. The patients were entered into 6-month recall regimes.

■ Discussion and final evaluation

CEREC reconstructions in the posterior region are widely described in the scientific literature and can be regarded as high-quality, durable restorations.[3,13–15,17] The case studies presented here show that, with the CEREC system, esthetically demanding and high-quality full-ceramic restorations can be fabricated and inserted easily and efficiently in everyday practice.

The ceramic materials currently available make it possible to do esthetically sound and lasting restorative work on vital and devitalized posterior as well as anterior teeth using the CEREC system.

Depending on ceramic dimensions, purely light-curing or dual-cure composite resins are recommended for luting CEREC reconstructions. One exception is the IPS e.max CAD ceramic because of its material strength. As well as adhesive luting, which is preferable in every case, fixation with a self-adhesive composite resin or even with a conventional cement may also be considered for IPS e.max CAD reconstructions.

Careful rechecking of the reconstruction margin during aftercare and the inclusion of patients in a regular recall system are always advisable.

References

1. Bindl A, Mörmann WH. Clinical evaluation of adhesively placed Cerec endo-crowns after 2 years – preliminary results. J Adhes Dent 1999;1:255–265.
2. Bindl A, Richter B, Mörmann WH. Survival of ceramic computer-aided design/manufacturing crowns bonded to preparations with reduced macroretention geometry. Int J Prosthodont 2005;18:219–224.
3. Fasbinder DJ. Clinical performance of chairside CAD/CAM restorations. J Am Dent Assoc 2006;137:22S–31S.
4. Hannig C, Westphal C, Becker K, Attin T. Fracture resistance of endodontically treated maxillary premolars restored with CAD/CAM ceramic inlays. J Prosthet Dent 2005;94:342–349.
5. Hass M, Arnetzl G et al. CEREC vs. Laboratory inlays; CAD/CAM in aesthetic dentistry. Quintessence, Berlin 1996:299–312.
6. Krejci I. Wear of CEREC and other restorative materials; Quintessence Publishing Co. Chicago 1991:245–251.
7. Magne P. Immediate dentin sealing: a fundamental procedure for indirect bonded restorations. J Esthet Restor Dent. 2005;17:144–155.
8. Magne P, Kim TH, Cascione D, Donovan TE. Immediate dentin sealing improves bond strength of indirect restorations. J Prosthet Dent 2005;94:511–519.
9. Mansour YF, Pintado MR, Mitchell CA. Optimizing resin cement removal around esthetic crown margins. Acta Odontol Scand 2006;64:231–236.
10. Mitchell CA, Pintado MR, Geary L, Douglas WH. Retention of adhesive cement on the tooth surface after crown cementation. J Prosthet Dent 1999;81:668–677.
11. Mörmann WH, Brandestini M, Ferru A, Lutz F, Krejci I. Marginale Adaptation von adhäsiven Porzellaninlays *in vitro*. Schweiz Mschr Zahnmed 1985;95:1118–1129.
12. Mörmann WH, Brandestini M, Lutz F, Barbakow F. Chairside computer-aided direct ceramic inlays. Quintessence Int 1989;20:329–339.
13. Otto T, Schneider D. Long-term clinical results of chairside Cerec CAD/CAM inlays and onlays: a case series. Int J Prosthodont 2008;21:53–59.
14. Reiss B. Long-term clinical performance of CEREC restorations and the variables affecting treatment success. Compend Contin Educ Dent 2001;22:14–18.
15. Reiss B. Clinical results of Cerec inlays in a dental practice over a period of 18 years. Int J Comput Dent 2006;9:11–22.
16. Stavridakis MM, Krejci I, Magne P. Immediate dentin sealing of onlay preparations: thickness of pre-cured Dentin Bonding Agent and effect of surface cleaning. Oper Dent 2005;30:747–757.
17. Zimmer S, Göhlich O, Rüttermann S, Lang H, Raab WH, Barthel CR. Long-term survival of Cerec restorations: a 10-year study. Oper Dent 2008;33:484–487.

Bleaching

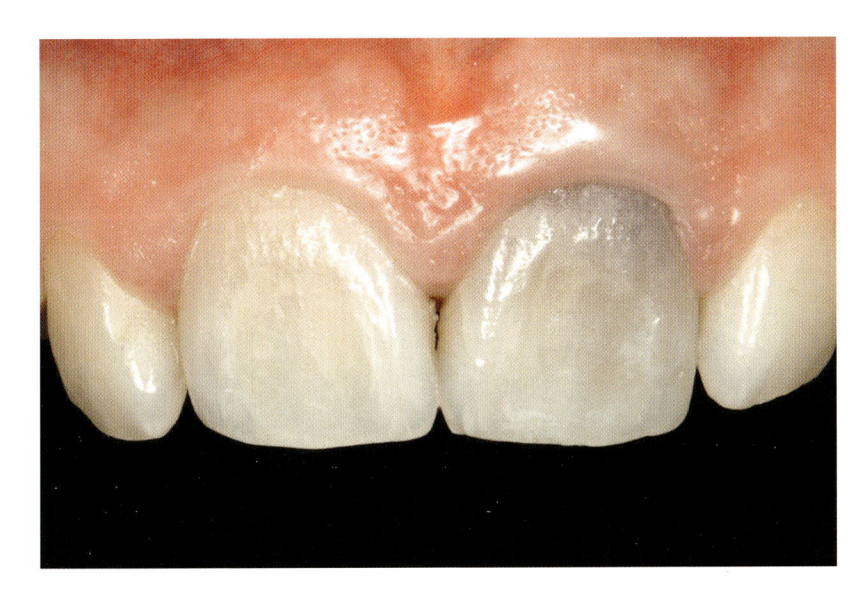

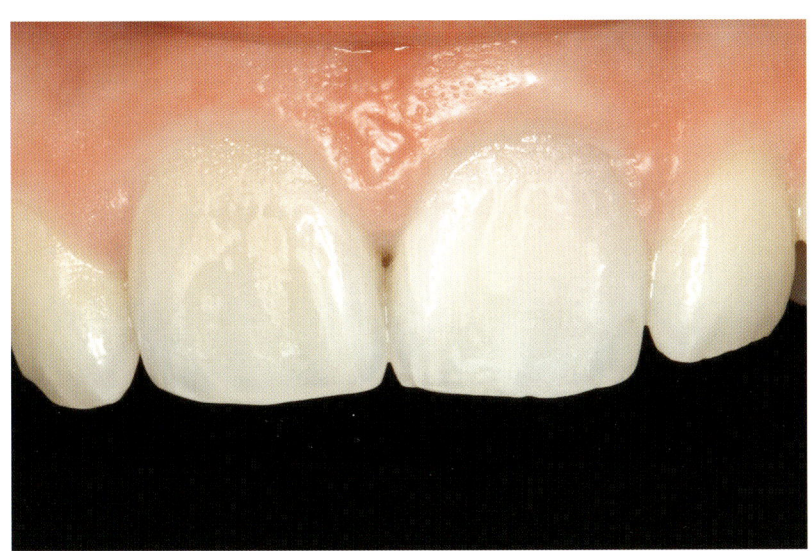

VII

18 Bleaching

Brigitte Zimmerli and Anne Grüninger

■ Introduction

White teeth stand for youth, health, and success. In fact, the natural perception of tooth color is increasingly being distorted by advertising and magazines (Fig 18-1). The use of cosmetic corrections is now becoming less and less restrained. This became apparent recently from a survey in Switzerland where one in three women said they were thinking of having some form of cosmetic surgery. The teeth were rated as the most important part of the body (91%) for esthetics (source: independent advice centre for plastic surgery, Acredis, 2008).

This trend means that the demand for (snow-)white teeth is relatively high. In a representative survey in the UK, 3,215 people were questioned about the color of their teeth: 50% of the people surveyed claimed to have a normal tooth color; 6% found their teeth distinctly too dark; the remainder stated that they had slight to moderate tooth discoloration. In this study, people's perception of the color of their own teeth was strongly associated with gender, age, income, and history of smoking.[1]

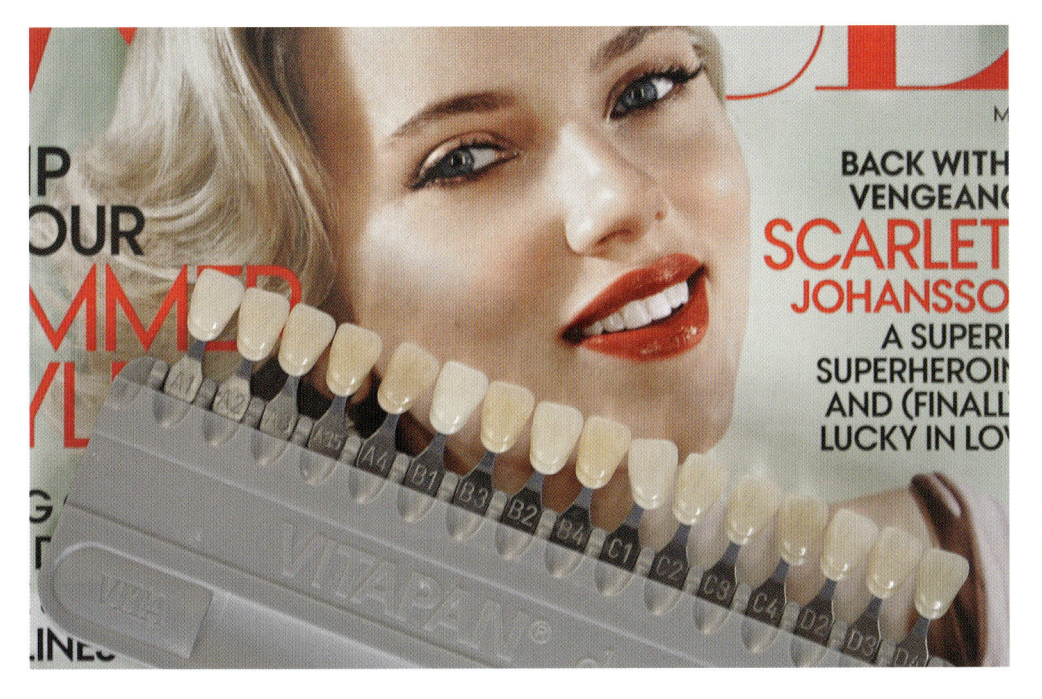

Fig 18-1 The teeth of the cover girl are much whiter than the normal tooth colors on the VITA color scale. The common use of editing covers of magazines can change patients' perceptions regarding "normal" tooth color.

■ Etiology of discolored teeth

Discoloration arises as a result of the formation and deposition of chemically stable chromogenic products. The color pigments are made up of long-chain carbon molecules. Discolorations can arise extrinsically or intrinsically (Table 18-1).

As in the past, discolorations caused by metallic ions (silver posts, amalgam restorations) still cannot be reliably bleached using the techniques currently available.[18] Tetracycline stains (Fig 18-2) have also long been regarded as nonbleachable. However, 6 months' bleaching treatment with a splint has produced some good results.[16]

Table 18-1 Reasons for tooth discoloration (from Plotino et al[18])

Extrinsic factors	Intrinsic factors (systemic)	Intrinsic factors (local)
• Food and beverages (wine, coffee, tea, carrots, oranges) • Tobacco • Mouthwashes • Plaque	• Medicines (tetracycline) • Metabolism (fluorosis) • Genetics (hyperbilirubinaemia, amelogenesis and dentinogenesis imperfecta)	• Pulp necrosis • Intrapulpal bleeding • Remaining pulp tissue after root canal treatment • Restorative material • Root resorption • Age

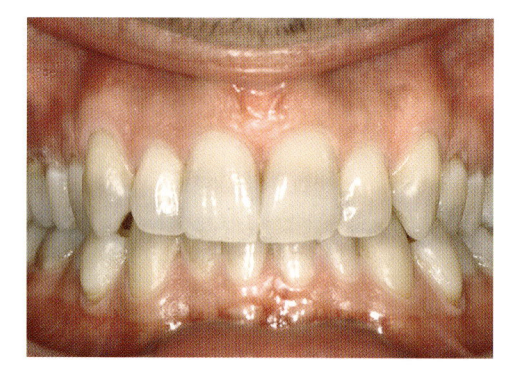

Fig 18-2 Generalized tetracycline stains. These stains can be lightened by long-term bleaching splint therapy.

■ Mechanism of bleaching

During bleaching, the color pigments deposited in the tooth are oxidized. In the process, they are split into smaller, lighter molecules. During the course of bleaching, the long-chain carbon molecules are converted into carbon and water and given off, together with the oxygen that is released from the peroxide of the bleaching agent.

In Europe, bleaching agents containing a maximum of 6% hydrogen peroxide or an equivalent quantity of other oxygen-releasing agents can be purchased directly by patients. Products with a higher percentage are licensed solely for professional use.

Hydrogen peroxide (H_2O_2), sodium perborate in the form of mono-, tri- ($NaBO_2 \cdot H_2O_2 \cdot 3H_2O$), or tetrahydrate as well as carbamide peroxide ($CH_4N_2O \cdot H_2O_2$) are used as bleaching agents. All bleaching agents release oxygen radicals, which initiate the bleaching reaction. In dentistry, a variety of methods are used for the application of bleaching agents. The most popular methods are described below.

The effects of bleaching agents on tooth structure and restorative materials is a matter of intense debate.[2] Some *in vitro* studies reveal measurable changes, eg, a decrease in the microhardness of the dental enamel.[4] In a review article, however, it was stated that bleaching agents do not promote the development of erosion or carious lesions nor do they increase abrasion.[13]

■ Bleaching procedure

Before any bleaching therapy is started, the following treatment steps should be carried out:
- Tooth cleaning and a general dental check-up (including tooth vitality test).
- Dental photographs with shade guide.
- Information to patient: costs, risks, expectations about the results of bleaching.

When bleaching has been carried out, the final result should also be photographed for inclusion in the patient's records.

■ Home bleaching

In the case of home bleaching, the bleaching agent is applied to the row of teeth in a specially prepared thermoformed splint (Fig 18-3) or a prefabricated tray (Fig 18-4). Ideally, the bleeching agent is applied for 1 to 2 hours. However, if the product is worn overnight, the bleaching outcome is not enhanced and there is a possibility that the bleaching agent might be swallowed.

Various studies regarding local and systemic toxicity have classified dental bleaching agents as relatively safe therapeutic products.[19] The teeth might be slightly oversensitive during the therapy. This hypersensitivity subsides again after cessation of the bleeching therapy.

Whether the bleaching splint is prepared with a final groove, with special reservoirs, or is in direct contact with the tooth does not appear to be important with regards to the outcome of the treatment.[12,15] The application of a 15% carbamide peroxide gel during the course of a home bleaching treatment for 2 weeks produced a better immediate result than 10% carbamide peroxide gel. However, at the six-week follow-up, the difference in concentration no longer had a significant effect on the bleaching outcome.[14]

VII Bleaching

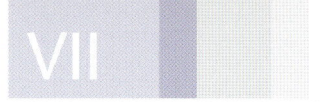

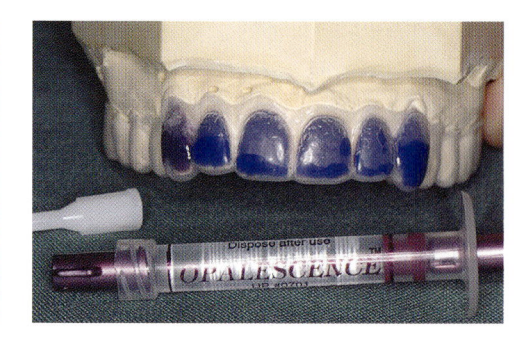

Fig 18-3 Top left: young patient with generalized "yellowish" teeth.

Top right: thermoformed splint with reservoirs for the maxillary incisors to be bleached, labial view.

Bottom left: the excess bleaching agent is removed with a cotton bud. Opalescence® 10 % is used as the bleaching agent.

Bottom right: after 2 weeks' home bleaching, there has been pronounced lightening of the maxillary anterior teeth compared with the mandibular anteriors.

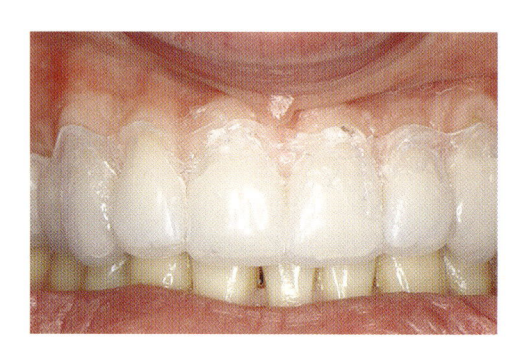

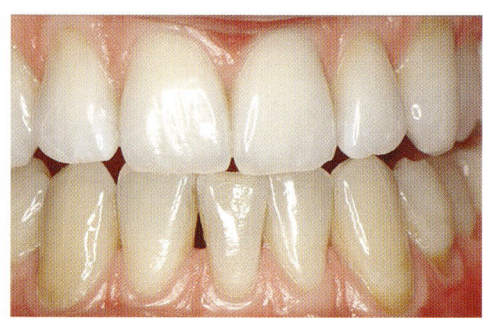

Fig 18-4 Top left: an individually prepared thermoformed splint can be dispensed with by using prefabricated trays (Très White Supreme, Ultradent).

Top right: the prefabricated splints comprise a green plastic tray and a transparent film onto which the viscous bleaching gel is applied.

Bottom left: the splints are placed on the teeth by the patient. After pressing well in place, the green tray is removed.

Bottom right: a strip containing bleaching agent remains adhered to the teeth. The film only lies imprecisely on the teeth and can slip. Furthermore, the cervical area of the teeth is only incompletely wetted by the bleaching agent. Wearing comfort is limited. However, the bleaching effect is entirely satisfactory.

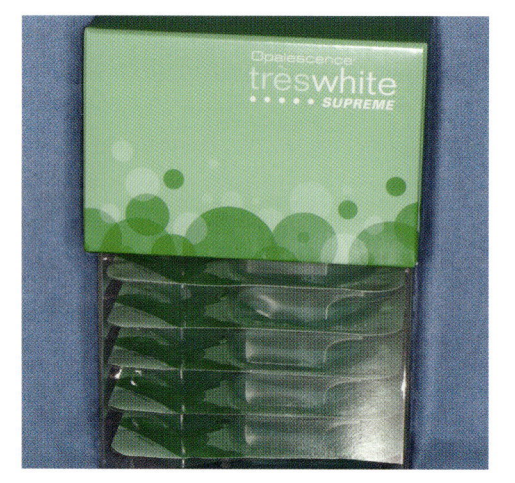

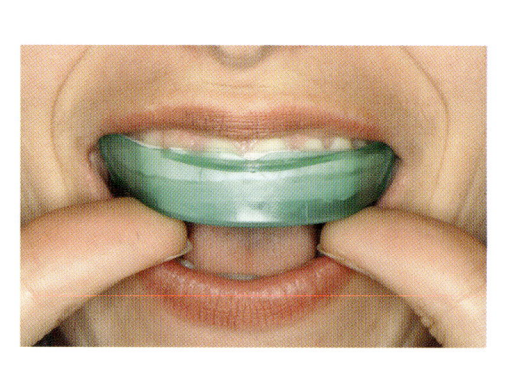

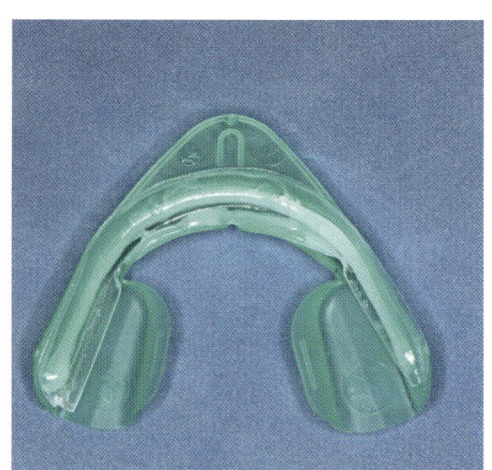

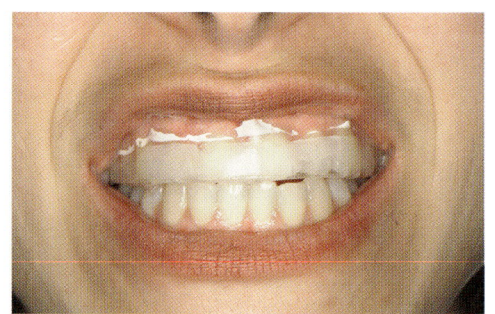

Home bleaching

The bleaching agent is applied at home in a tray or a splint. An exposure time of 1 to 2 hours a day is sufficient.

Patient information for home bleaching

- The bleaching result is not predictable.
- Hypersensitivity of teeth is common during bleaching.
- Store the bleaching agent in the refrigerator, out of the reach of children.
- Store the splint in a dry place, clean it with neutral liquid soap, do not boil.
- Pour just a little bleaching agent into the splint (maximum 1/4 height of the splint).
- Wear time: 1 to 2 hours a day.
- Do not consume any strongly colored foods immediately after bleaching.
- Existing restorations might appear dark after bleaching and might have to be renewed.

■ Walking bleach technique

The walking bleach technique is the most popular method for lightening endodontically treated teeth (Fig 18-5). It has been used in dentistry for 50 years. Before beginning the treatment, existing root canal fillings and all restorations present in the teeth should be tight and adequate. The root canal filling is removed to about 2 mm subgingivally in order to prevent any persistence of cervical discoloration. The root canal filling material is sealed with a cavity base (eg, resin-modified glass ionomer cement). The bleaching agent (sodium perborate mixed with water or proprietary bleaching agent) is then placed in the pulp cavity and the coronal area of the tooth (Fig 18-6). Prior etching of the pulp cavity or heating of the bleaching agent is contraindicated. The access is tightly closed with a provisional restoration. Ideally, the provisional is sealed with an adhesive, provided that a composite resin is not chosen as the temporary material. After 3 to 5 days, the bleaching result is re-evaluated and the bleaching agent is reapplied if necessary. Two to four applications are often required to lighten a severely discolored tooth (Fig 18-7). Unfortunately, the relapse rate for bleaching of nonvital teeth is relatively high:[6–8,11] after 5 years 25% of bleached teeth had again become darkened, and after 8 years the relapse rate was around 49%. Nevertheless, this method is a tooth substance-sparing therapy because bleaching often makes over-crowning unnecessary.

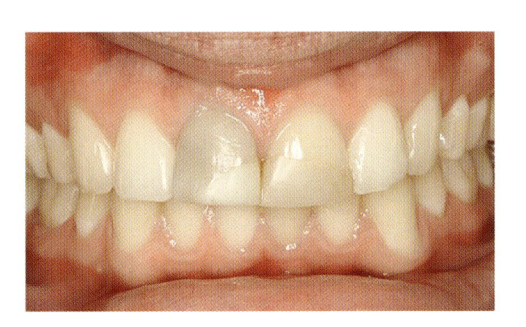

Fig 18-5 Status following anterior dental trauma. The maxillary central incisors are devitalized; the right central incisor has a gray discoloration and the left central incisor is slightly yellowish. Before restoration with veneers, both teeth are to be bleached.

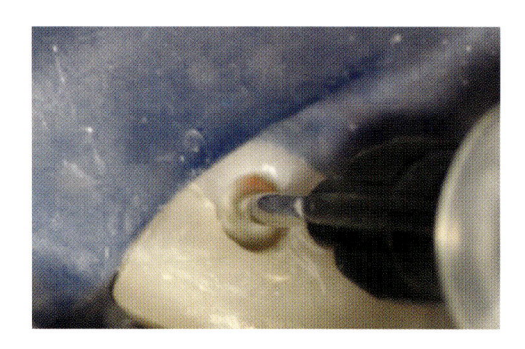

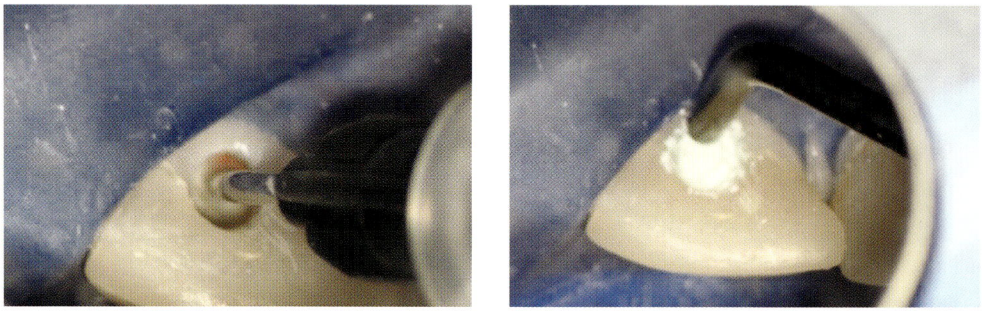

VII Bleaching

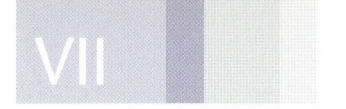

Fig 18-6 Left: application of the bleaching agent after prior sealing of the root canal filling with Vitrebond™.

Right: covering the bleaching agent with a layer of temporary restorative material.

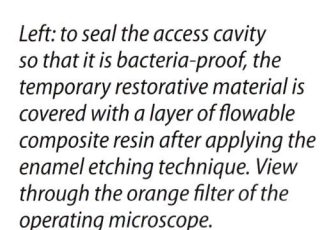

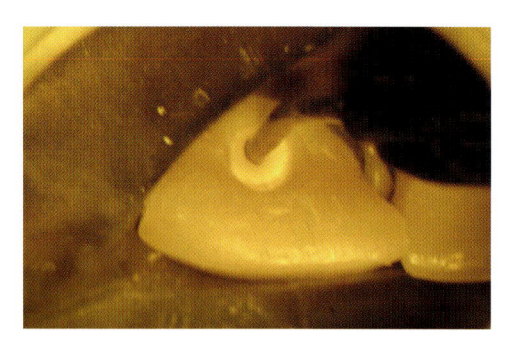

Left: to seal the access cavity so that it is bacteria-proof, the temporary restorative material is covered with a layer of flowable composite resin after applying the enamel etching technique. View through the orange filter of the operating microscope.

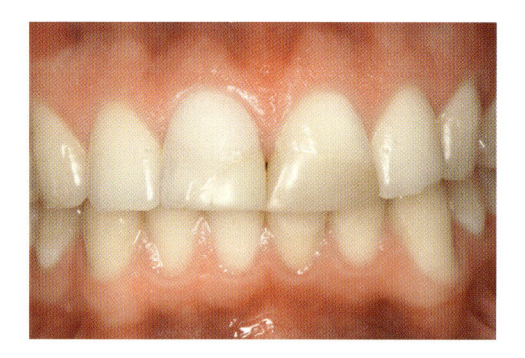

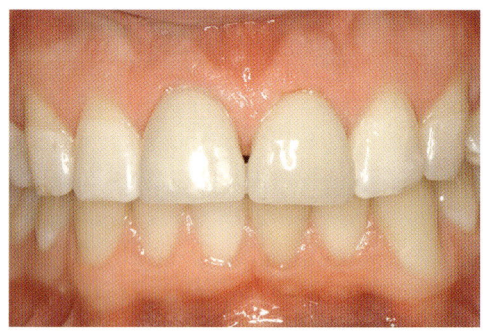

Fig 18-7 Left: status after the bleaching agent has been changed three times.

Right: status immediately after adhesive luting of the veneers onto the central incisors.

This risk of root resorption as a result of tooth bleaching is a constant topic of discussion. It should be noted that the resorption rates after walking bleach are correlated with high concentrations of bleaching agent (≥ 30 % hydrogen peroxide) and heat application.[7,10] Furthermore, nearly all the affected teeth had previously suffered a trauma.[10]

Walking bleach technique
The bleaching agent is placed in the pulp cavity and the coronal area of an endodontically treated tooth. The access is then temporarily sealed.

Patient information for walking bleach technique
- The bleaching result is not predictable.
- Re-darkening of the teeth is common.
- Teeth are susceptible to fractures during bleaching.
- Explanation of risk regarding cervical resorption.

In-office bleaching

In the case of in-office bleaching, the gingiva is tightly covered (rubber dam) after tooth cleaning. A highly concentrated bleaching gel (eg, Opalescence Boost 38%) is then applied to the teeth being treated (Fig 18-8 left). Depending on the product, application of heat or light is recommended. However, it has been shown that these supportive methods have no significant effect on the bleaching outcome. If necessary, the application of bleaching gel is repeated a second time.

This technique has limited indications. When bleaching several teeth, home bleaching has a better prognosis. This is because with in-office bleaching the greatest bleaching effect occurs as the teeth dry out; as a result, patients are often not satisfied with the outcome immediately after an in-office bleaching session and so the treatment has to be repeated two or three times.[5] The technique is best suited for bleaching single teeth. However, whether home bleaching or the walking bleach technique might produce better results still has to be determined.

Tight isolation of the gingiva poses another problem. Despite good rubber dam technique and the use of additional liquid isolating media, the bleaching agent can occasionally come into contact with the gingival tissue, causing a white gingival margin. While this will disappear within a short time, it does detract from the short-term result (Fig 18-8 right).

In-office bleaching
The highly concentrated bleaching agent is applied to the tooth in the dental surgery. The indications are limited.

Patient information for in-office bleaching
- The bleaching success is not detectable until the day after the bleaching has been carried out (drying out of the teeth).
- Despite isolating the teeth, areas of gingiva are often bleached at the same time.
- Hypersensitivity is common after bleaching, but reversible.

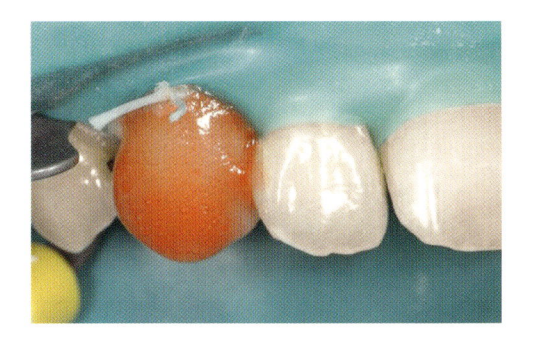

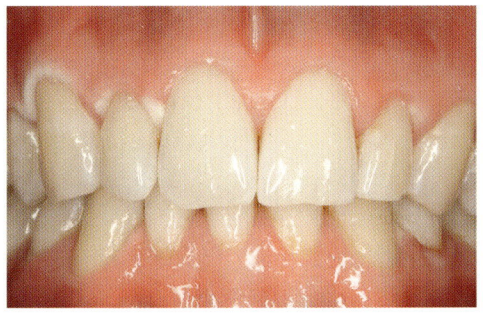

Fig 18-8 *Left: after isolation with rubber dam and ligature, the right maxillary canine is coated with Opalescence Ultra during in-office bleaching.*

Right: after removal of the rubber dam, a white gingival margin is visible. This is due to insufficient sealing during the bleaching procedure.

Over-the-counter products

Products for the application of bleaching agents are freely available on the market. Impregnated strips and solutions (paint-on products), which are applied directly to the tooth surface, are familiar products. Certain toothpastes are also recommended for lightening tooth color. A distinction needs to be drawn between products whose bleaching effect is achieved by a high abrasiveness factor of the paste (smokers' or anti-tartar toothpastes; eg, Rembrandt® Intense Stain™, Settima) and those that contain an increased concentration of bleaching agent (whitening toothpastes; eg, Swiss Dent, Pearl Drops®). The products may contain a maximum of 6% hydrogen peroxide. The effectiveness of over-the-counter products is not bad.[9] As the active ingredient is able to work over a prolonged period, these products are occasionally superior to in-office bleaching.[17] Hypersensitivity is less common because of the low hydrogen peroxide concentration. However, more severe gingival irritation has been reported with strips than with splint application.[3]

> **Over-the-counter products**
> These bleaching agents contain a maximum of 6% hydrogen peroxide. They are freely available to consumers.

Household products

Tips on lightening teeth using "household products" are exchanged in a variety of internet forums. The use of baking powder is a favorite. Tooth-lightening effects are also ascribed to lemon juice, salt, and tea tree oil. To some extent, patients should be advised against the use of these substances because they can have erosive effects if used regularly.

Conclusions

According to current knowledge, home bleaching should be preferred over other techniques as a method of lightening vital teeth. Vital bleaching by the home bleaching method can usually lighten by two shade levels without any problems (Fig 18-9). The walking bleach technique should be preferred for nonvital teeth. Stained teeth can often be lightened back to their original shade by walking bleaching (Fig 18-10). The other bleaching techniques can prove advantageous in specific cases.

The bleaching materials now available can be classified as relatively safe. Furthermore, swallowing of bleaching agent can be prevented by not wearing the bleaching splint overnight. In any event, good photographic documentation is necessary for all bleaching therapies in order to record the short-term and long-term success of the treatment. This is because patients often cannot remember the pretreatment situation due to the slow and continuous lightening process and might be dissatisfied with the result achieved.

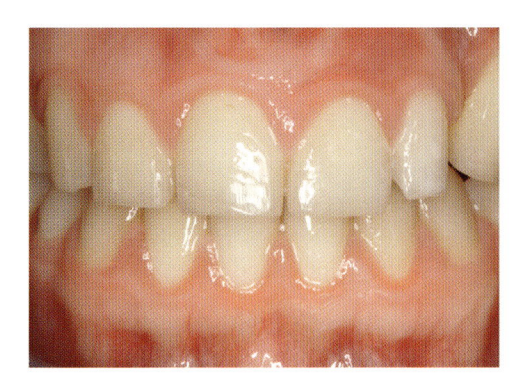

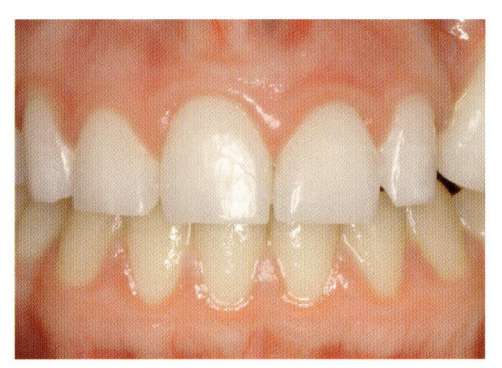

Fig 18-9 Left: this 18-year-old patient was referred by the orthodontist for space closure between the left maxillary lateral incisor and canine. In the planning discussion, the patient expressed a wish for "whiter teeth".

Right: after 2 weeks' home bleaching using an individual splint in the maxilla: the bleaching result is very satisfactory. Comparison with the mandibular teeth reveals the difference from the initial shade.

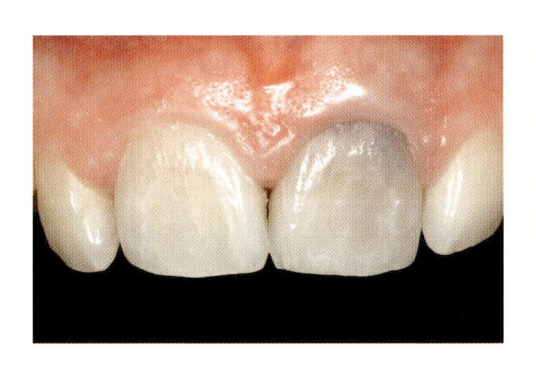

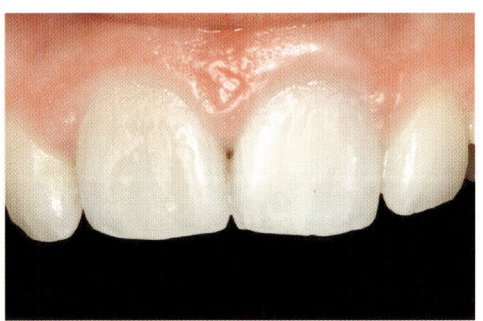

Fig 18-10 Left: a 24-year-old patient, who had suffered anterior dental trauma and root canal treatment to the right maxillary central incisor 5 years earlier. The patient was unhappy with the "gray tooth".

Right: after two applications of bleaching agent into the access cavity, the tooth is slightly lighter than the adjacent teeth.

References

1. Alkhatib MN, Holt R, Bedi R. Prevalence of self-assessed tooth discolouration in the United Kingdom. J Dent 2004;32:561–566.
2. Attin T, Hannig C, Wiegand A, Attin R. Effect of bleaching on restorative materials and restorations – a systematic review. Dent Mater 2004;20:852–861.
3. Auschill TM, Hellwig E, Schmidale S, Sculean A, Arweiler NB. Efficacy, side-effects and patients' acceptance of different bleaching techniques (OTC, in-office, at-home). Oper Dent 2005;30:156–163.
4. Chen HP, Chang CH, Liu JK, Chuang SF, Yang JY. Effect of fluoride containing bleaching agents on enamel surface properties. J Dent 2008;36:718–725.
5. De Silva Gottardi M, Brackett G, Haywood VB. Number of in-office light activated bleaching treatments needed to achieve patient satisfaction. Quintessence Int 2006;37:115–120.
6. Friedman S, Rotstein I, Libfeld H, Stabholz A, Heling I: Incidence of external root resorption and esthetic results in 58 bleached pulpless teeth. Endod Dent Traumatol 1988;4:23–26.
7. Friedman S. Internal bleaching: long-term outcomes and complications. J Am Dent Assoc 1997;128:26S–30S.
8. Glockner K, Hulla H, Eberleseder K, Städtler P: Five year follow-up of internal bleaching. Braz Dent J 1999;10:105–110.
9. Hasson H, Ismail AI, Neiva G. Home-based chemically-induced whitening of teeth in adults. Cochrane Database Sys Rev 2006;18:CD006202.
10. Heitersay GS, Dahlstrom SW, Marin PD. Incidence of invasive cervical resorption in bleached root-filled teeth. Aust Dent J 1994;39:82–87.
11. Holmstrup G, Palm AM, Lambjerg-Hansen H: Bleaching of discoloured root-filled teeth. Endod Dent Traumatol 1988;4:197–201.
12. Javaheri DS, Janis JN. The efficacy of reservoirs in bleaching trays. Oper Dent 2000;25:149–151.
13. Joiner A. Review of the effects of peroxide on enamel and dentin properties. J Dent 2007;35:889–896.

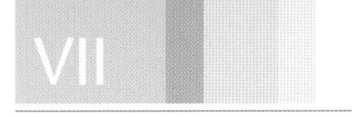

14. Matis BA, Mousa HN, Cochran MA, Eckert GJ. Clinical evaluation of bleaching agents of different concentrations. Quintessence Int 2000;31:303–310.

15. Matis BA, Hamdan YS, Cochran MA, Eckert GJ. Clinical evaluation of a bleaching agent used with and without reservoirs. Oper Dent 2002;27:5–11.

16. Matis BA, Wang Y, Eckert GJ, Cochran MA, Jiang T. Extended bleaching of tetracycline-stained teeth: a 5-year study. Oper Dent 2006;31:643–651.

17. Matis BA, Cochran MA, Eckert G. Review of the effectiveness of various tooth whitening systems. Oper Dent 2009;34:230–235.

18. Plotino G, Buono G, Grande NM, Pameier CH, Somma F. Nonvital tooth bleaching: a review of the literature and clinical procedures. J Endod 2008;34:394–407.

19. Schmalz G, Arenholt-Bindslev D. Bleichmittel in Biokompatibilität zahnärztlicher Werkstoffe. Urban & Fischer Verlag, München 2005; 277–280.

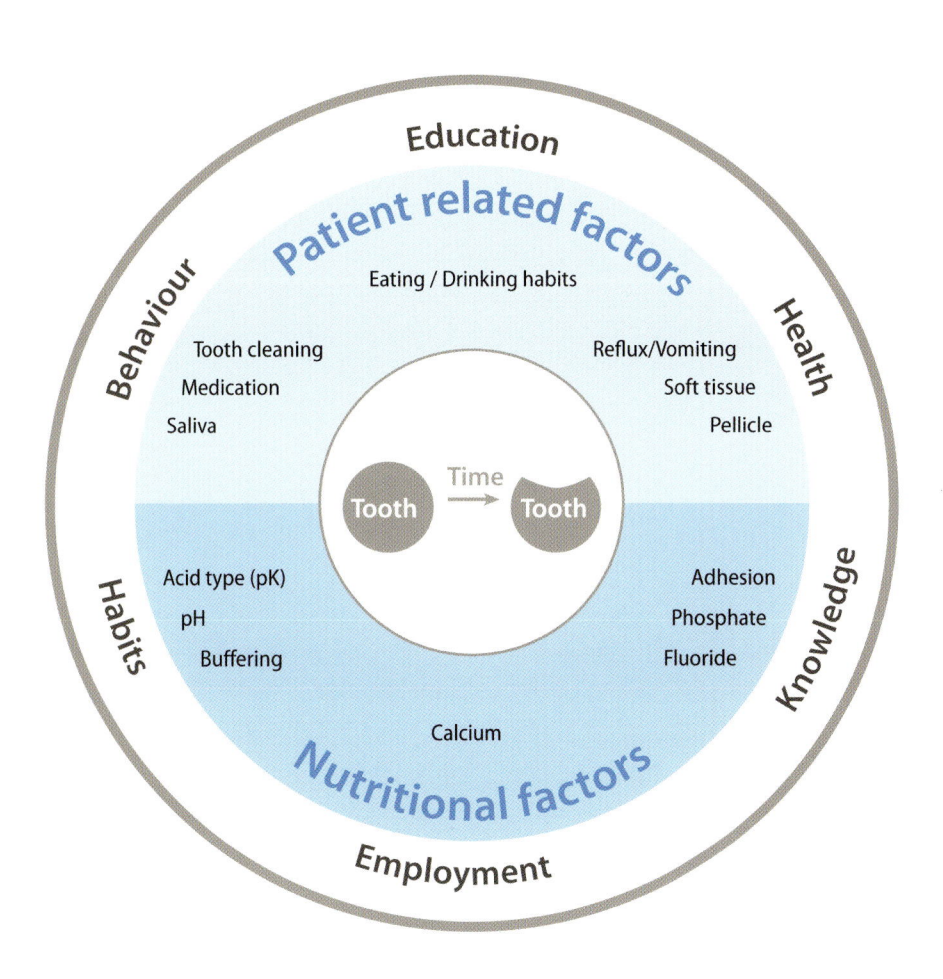

Dental erosion

VIII

Patient related factors
- Education
- Behaviour
- Health
- Eating / Drinking habits
- Tooth cleaning
- Medication
- Saliva
- Reflux/Vomiting
- Soft tissue
- Pellicle

Tooth → Tooth (Time)

Nutritional factors
- Habits
- Knowledge
- Employment
- Acid type (pK)
- pH
- Buffering
- Adhesion
- Phosphate
- Fluoride
- Calcium

19 Dental erosion

Adrian Lussi and Thomas Jaeggi

■ Introduction

There has been an increase in dental erosion in recent decades. This chapter looks at the clinical features of dental erosion, factors that protect against or promote its pathogenesis, and preventive measures.

It is important to distinguish whether a lesion primarily involves an erosive or an abrasive process, although these processes are often overlapped. History-taking, examination, and correct diagnosis are essential requirements for appropriate prevention. Analysis of a patient's dietary history calls for precise knowledge of the erosive potential of different drinks and foods as well as the symptoms associated with gastroesophageal reflux or anorexia/bulimia.

Other investigations, such as measurement of the flow rate, pH, and buffer capacity of the saliva, are valuable for identifying a patient's risk of erosion and making suitable prophylactic recommendations.

The treatment for erosion is not explored in detail here. A thorough account can be found in the book *Dental Erosion* by A. Lussi and T. Jaeggi (Quintessenz, 2011).

■ Diagnosis

Dental erosion is difficult to diagnose, especially in the early stages. This is because the enamel surface alters uniformly at the start. It is not until an advanced phase that pits are formed and/or dentin exposure occurs, at which point the lesions become clinically easily visible. Patients do not notice the lesions themselves until their teeth become "yellower" and "shorter" because of the thinner enamel layer or they suffer from hypersensitivity. This is exactly why it is important for clinicians to focus their diagnostic attention more keenly so that erosive lesions can be detected as early as possible and suitable preventive measures can be taken.

Characteristics of dental erosion
- Silky, glossy to matt surface
- Intact enamel ridge at the gingival margin
- Restorations are higher than the adjacent tooth substance
- Altered morphology of the teeth

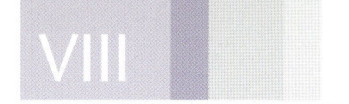

Depending on the localization of the erosive lesions, conclusions may be drawn about their cause(s). If acid damage mainly appears on the palatal surfaces of the maxillary anterior teeth and/or occlusal surfaces, exposure is probably caused by endogenous acids, eg, due to vomiting. Asymmetric occlusal erosion may be evidence of gastroesophageal reflux during the night. As patients often prefer to sleep on one particular side, any gastric acid collects on that side and the erosive defects are more pronounced there.

In terms of differential diagnosis, erosion must be distinguished from other defects of dental hard tissues. Different dental defects can appear simultaneously in the same dentition. Hence carious lesions might well exist alongside erosion. From a pathophysiological point of view, however, it is not possible for the defects to develop at the same time on the same tooth surfaces. While caries is formed by organized plaque, erosion arises due to direct exposure to acids. Other defects of the hard dental tissue, such as attrition and abrasion, also have to be distinguished from erosion. Such mechanically caused defects usually have sharply defined borders and arise because of the physiological and/or pathological impact of forces acting on the tooth surfaces (Fig 19-1). The clinical picture frequently shows some overlapping of erosion, abrasion, and attrition. This is understandable because loss of dental tissue happens more quickly when dental surfaces have already been damaged by erosion and are hence softened.[7,16,3] Figures 19-2 to 19-4 show erosion on the different tooth surfaces.

Fig 19-1 Diagram showing defects of dental hard tissue: caries (left), wedge-shaped defect (center), and dental erosion (right).

Fig 19-2 Early-stage labial erosion: surface defects are visible.

Fig 19-3 Early-stage occlusal erosion: pitting on the cusps with early dentin exposure, less than 50 % of the tooth surface is affected.

Fig 19-4 Advanced oral erosion with intact marginal enamel ridge. The dentin is extensively exposed.

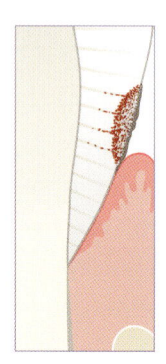

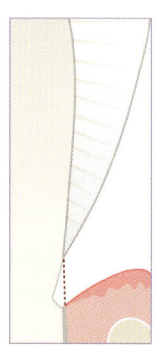

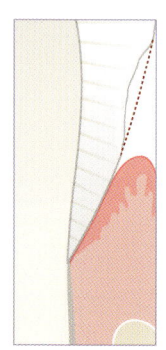

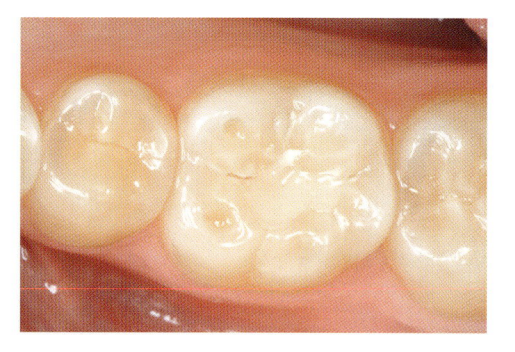

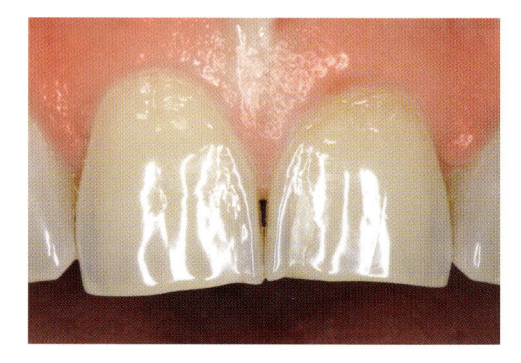

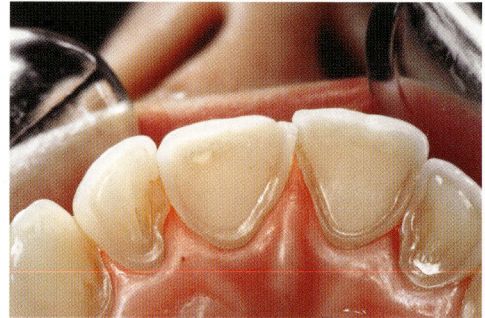

Basic Erosive Wear Examination (BEWE)

As soon as erosion is clinically detected or there are signs of an increased risk of erosion, a precise evaluation of a patient's risk should be carried out. The brief **B**asic **E**rosive **W**ear **E**xamination (BEWE) presented by Bartlett, Ganß, and Lussi[5] is well suited to quantifying erosion (Tables 19-1 and 19-2).

BEWE makes it possible to assess the acid damage to a dentition in a minimal amount of time. It is easy to learn and helps the examiner plan the ongoing management of the patient (Table 19-3). All the teeth (except the third molars) are examined for acid damage to labial, buccal, occlusal, and oral surfaces.

Table 19-1 BEWE: grading erosive wear

Grade[a]	Clinical appearance
0	No erosive tooth wear
1	Initial loss of surface texture
2[a]	Distinct defect, hard tissue loss < 50% of the surface area
3[a]	Hard tissue loss > 50% of the surface area

[a] Dentin is often involved in grades 2 and 3.

Table 19-2 BEWE assessment: in each sextant the highest grade value is marked and these are added to give a total score

Highest grade 1st sextant (17–14)	Highest grade 2nd sextant (13–23)	Highest grade 3rd sextant (24–27)	
Highest grade 6th sextant (44–47)	Highest grade 5th sextant (33–43)	Highest grade 4th sextant (37–34)	Total score

Table 19-3 Risk levels as a guide to clinical management

Risk level	Cumulative score of all sextants	Management
None	≤ 2	• Routine maintenance and observation • Repeat at 3-year intervals
Low	3–8	• Oral hygiene, dietary assessment, and advice • Routine maintenance and observation • Is reflux involved? Take photographs • Repeat every year
Moderate	9–13	• As above • Identify the main etiological factor(s) for tissue loss and develop strategies to eliminate respective impacts • Fluoridation measures or other strategies to increase the resistance of tooth surfaces • Minimally invasive restorations; monitoring of erosive wear with study casts, photographs, or silicone impressions • Repeat at 6- to 12-month intervals
High	≥ 14	• As above • Particularly for severe progression, consider special care, which may involve restorations/reconstructions • Repeat at 6- to 12-month intervals

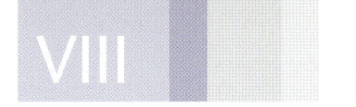

The recommendations on patient management are not strict guidelines because the opinions of experts differ widely in this area, and social aspects play an additional role.

The BEWE takes account of total loss of substance from the tooth surface. Although dentin is often exposed in severity levels 2 and 3, the assessment of "dentin exposure" that is commonly found in other indices is not included in the BEWE. This is because this assessment is difficult to do, and also because dentin involvement does not correlate with the severity of a defect in all cases due to the enamel layer not being a uniform thickness all over. In the cervical area or in the area of depressions, the dentin is exposed far more quickly. Omitting this assessment removes a source of error in the evaluation and makes it easier to compare the data of different investigators. Furthermore, in this way the index can be recorded from the actual patient as well as from casts or photographs.

The frequency with which the BEWE is repeated depends on the severity of the erosive lesions and on individual risk factors. For patients with major intrinsic and/or extrinsic acid exposure, it should be repeated every 6 months. An interval of 12 months or longer is adequate in the other cases.

■ Prevalence and incidence

The incidence and severity of dental erosion seems to have increased in recent years. However, it is very difficult to compare the various epidemiological studies with each other because often different assessment methods were used and the groups of patients studied are not consistent. Incidence studies are rare.[8,10,12,22,25] It is noticeable that the prevalence of dental erosion is frequently higher in younger populations than in study groups with a higher average age. Progression of the lesions must be anticipated with the advancing age of these still young patients. This in turn means that an increase in dental erosion in population groups of all ages must be assumed in future. Accordingly, early preventive measures need to be taken in order to prevent the onset and progression of dental erosion, if possible, or at least to slow down its progression. Table 19-4 gives an overview of the prevalence of dental erosion.

Table 19-4 Prevalence of erosion by age

Age group (years)	Prevalence (%)
2–5	6–50
5–9	14 (permanent dentition)
9–17	11–100
18–88	4–82

Localization in the dentition

Occlusal erosion is found frequently on the molars of both jaws, with the 6-year molars of the mandible being the most severely affected. Labial and buccal erosion mainly occurs in the canine-premolar region of the maxilla and mandible, followed by the maxillary anterior teeth and the molar surfaces in both jaws. Oral erosion, which is less common, very frequently affects the tooth surfaces of the maxillary incisors and canines.[11,17,21,22] The teeth most affected by erosion, classified by tooth surface, are summarized in Table 19-5, and the distribution of erosion on different tooth surfaces is shown in Figures 19-5 to 19-7.

Table 19-5 Teeth most affected by erosion, by tooth surface

Tooth surfaces	Teeth
Labial/buccal	Canines / premolars UJ/LJ
Occlusal	Molars LJ
Oral	Incisors UJ

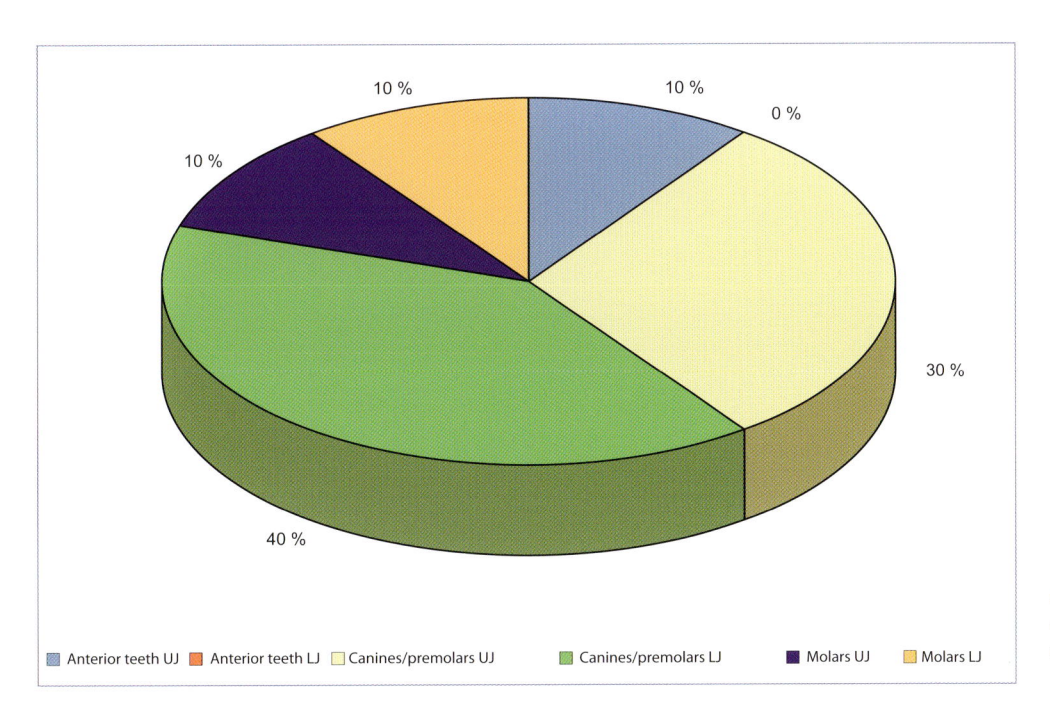

Fig 19-5 Distribution of labial and buccal erosion (in percentage) in patients aged between 18 and 63 years.[11,17,21,22]

VIII

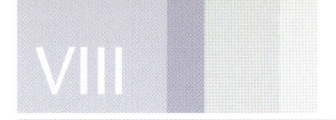

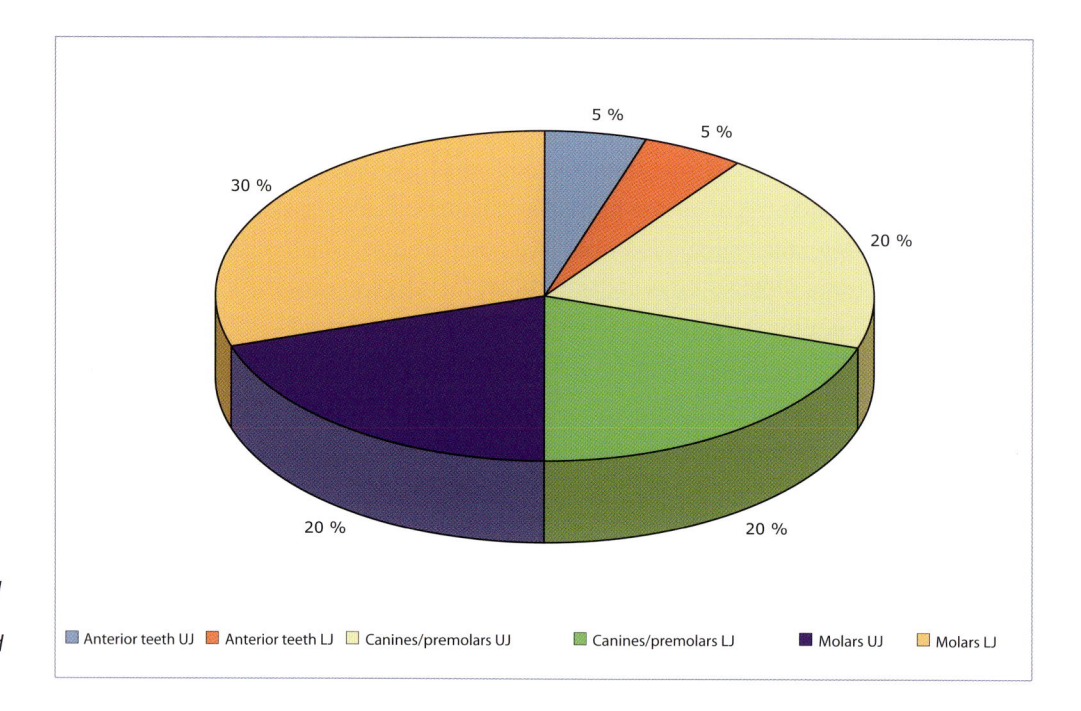

Dental erosion

Fig 19-6 Distribution of occlusal erosion (in percentage) in patients aged between 18 and 63 years.[11,17,21,22]

■ Anterior teeth UJ ■ Anterior teeth LJ ■ Canines/premolars UJ ■ Canines/premolars LJ ■ Molars UJ ■ Molars LJ

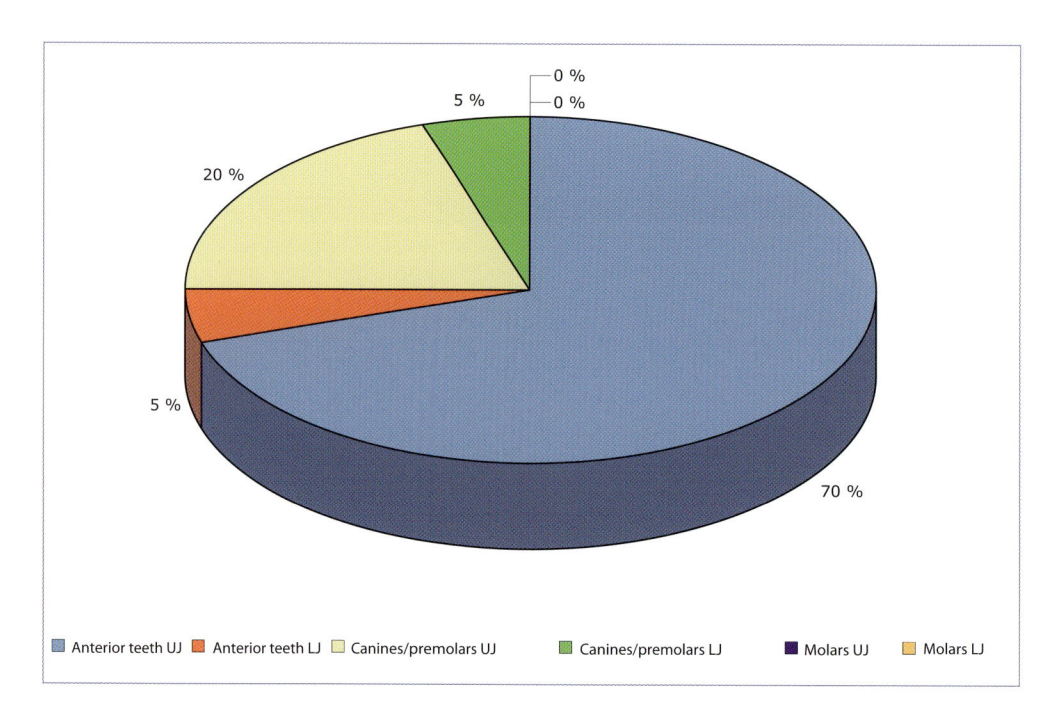

Fig 19-7 Distribution of oral erosion (in percentage) in patients aged between 18 and 63 years.[11,17,21,22]

■ Anterior teeth UJ ■ Anterior teeth LJ ■ Canines/premolars UJ ■ Canines/premolars LJ ■ Molars UJ ■ Molars LJ

Clinical case studies of the progression of erosion

Two clinical cases observed over a number of years are presented below. In all cases an attempt should be made to remove the cause of the acid damage after it has been diagnosed. The consumption of acidic food and drinks should be reduced, where necessary, and any endogenous causes that might exist treated by medication. Both the patients had a normal salivary flow rate, so no measures had to be taken with regard to this aspect. Regular applications of fluoride were recommended in order to build up a protective precipitate on the tooth surfaces.

Case 1: Male patient, comparison of the clinical situation at ages 21 and 23 years

Cause: Moderate gastroesophageal reflux; no excessive consumption of acidic food and drinks; salivary flow rates normal

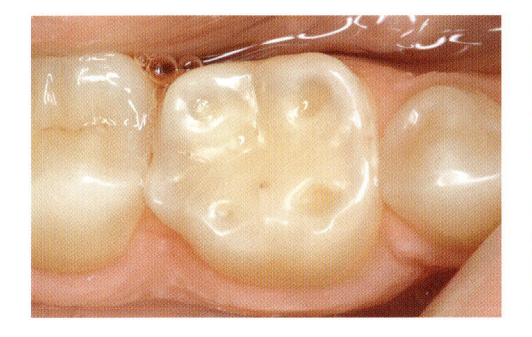

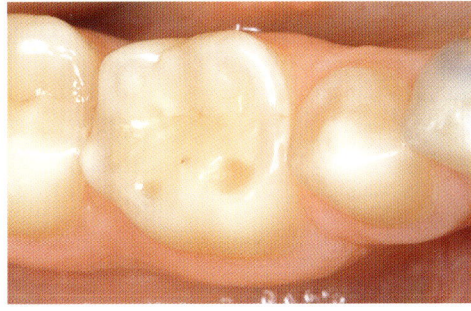

Fig 19-8 *Left: 21 years; right: 23 years.*

Case 2: Male patient, comparison of the clinical situation at ages 13½ and 18 years

Cause: Gastroesophageal reflux during the night, which was treated by medication; no excessive consumption of acidic foods and drinks; salivary flow rates normal

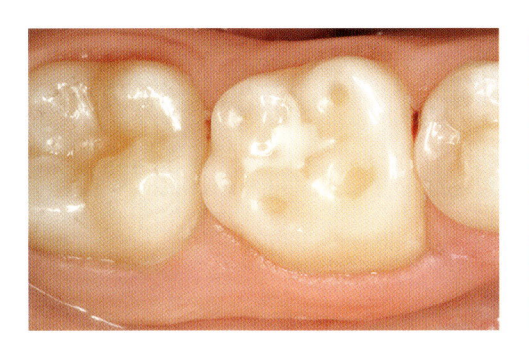

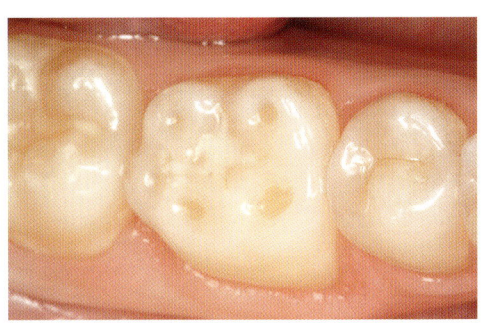

Fig 19-9 *Left: 13½ years; right: 18 years.*

Dental erosion

■ Etiology of erosion

Dental erosion, like caries, has a multifactorial etiology. Protective and promoting factors should be looked for. Figure 19-10 gives an overview of the patient-related and nutritional factors. The erosion process is modified by other general factors, which are shown in the outer circle.

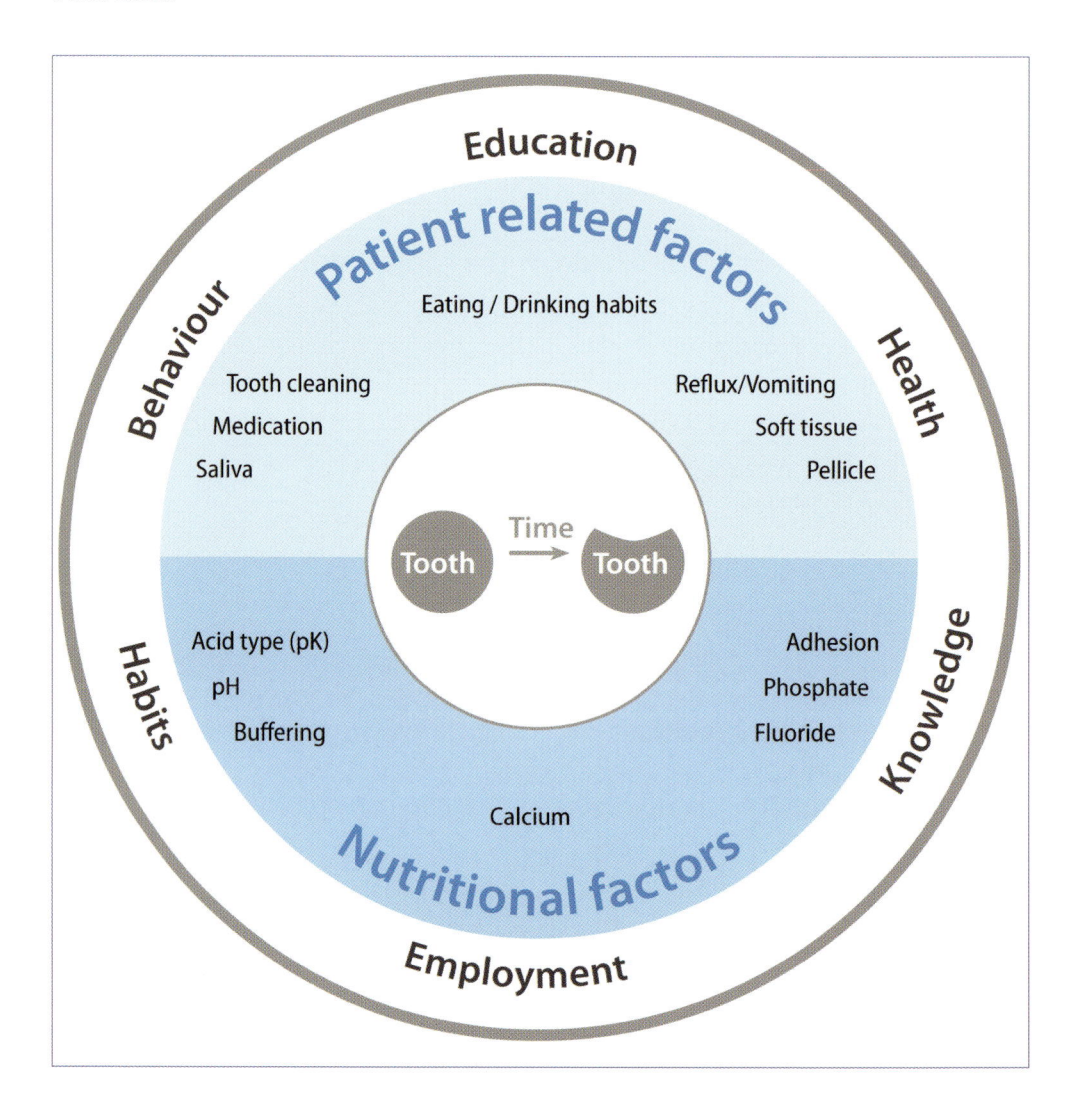

Fig 19-10 The various factors in the pathogenesis of dental erosion.

■ Patient-related factors

Eating and drinking habits
The way in which erosive foods or drinks are consumed (sipped, sucked in, with/without a straw) determines the duration and localization of the acid attack and hence the appearance of the erosion.[9,18,24] The frequency and duration of acid attacks are crucially important to the destruction of hard dental tissue and hence to the preventive measures that are taken. Teeth being in contact with acids during the night can also lead to erosion because of the reduced

production of saliva while asleep. For instance, the consumption of acid-containing sweet drinks, which many infants drink from their bottles during the night, will result not only in the formation of caries but also in massive erosive destruction of dental tissue.

Gastroesophageal reflux

When extrinsic causes have been excluded, mostly intrinsic factors, such as frequent vomiting or gastroesophageal reflux, are suspected as the cause of dental erosion.

Gastroesophageal reflux is one of the most common gastroenterology diagnoses, with a similar prevalence in children and adults. Roughly 7% to 10% of the population suffer from troublesome heartburn, acid reflux, or regurgitation on a daily basis. Even children at 12 months of age have reflux, with 8% affected.[26]

> Gastroesophageal reflux has a prevalence of around 10% in children and adults and often leads to erosive tooth damage.

Not every pathologically increased reflux will trigger symptoms. Over 50% of patients with gastroesophageal reflux do display erosive mucosal damage to the esophagus (reflux esophagitis), but 40% of these patients with reflux esophagitis report no clear reflux symptoms.[6,32,33] This shows that tissue damage in the upper gastrointestinal tract caused by reflux without typical symptoms is common. Characteristic reflux symptoms are listed in Tables 19-6 and 19-7.

Table 19-6 Possible symptoms of gastroesophageal reflux

Dental erosions
Acid, regurgitation
Heartburn
Epigastric pains, especially after certain foods and beverages (wine, citrus juices, vinegar, fatty foods, tomatoes, peppermint)
Acidic or bitter taste after waking up
Pain on swallowing (odynophagia) or uncomfortable sensations behind the breastbone (dysphagia)
Nausea
Vomiting
Cough
Chronic respiratory symptoms (asthma, dyspnea)

Table 19-7 Symptoms in patients with frequent vomiting in bulimia/anorexia

Dental erosions
Enlargement of the parotid gland
Redness in palate and pharynx
Formation of cracks in the lips (rhagades)
Skin and nail changes to the index and middle finger
Injuries/teeth marks on the back of the hands (signs of forced vomiting)

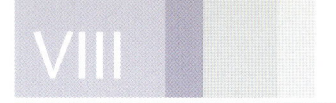

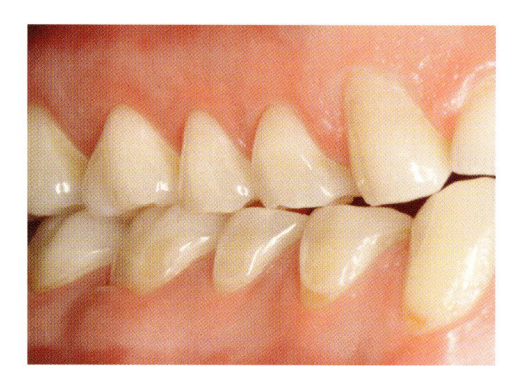

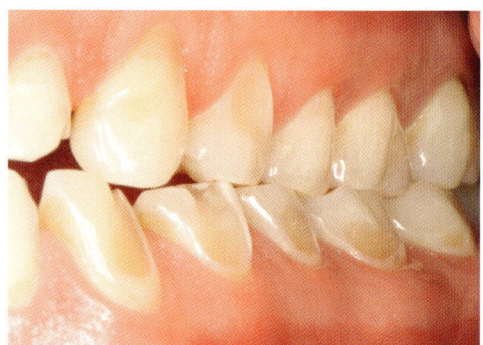

Fig 19-11 One-sided (left-right) distribution of erosion in a case of reflux, caused by sleeping on one side.

Gastroesophageal reflux with regurgitation during sleep can cause serious erosive lesions, which are often distributed on one side because of sleeping habits (Fig 19-11).

Asymmetrically distributed erosion points towards reflux.

Vomiting (bulimia, anorexia)

Other patient-related risk factors are anorexia nervosa, bulimia nervosa, and mixed forms with frequent vomiting. The prevalence of bulimia nervosa among 18 to 35-year-old women in the western industrialized countries is between 0.5% and 5% depending on the study – with an upward trend. Most patients suffering from anorexia nervosa are aged between 12 and 20 years. The prevalence of anorexia nervosa is 2% in this age group. Diagnosing is often straightforward in severely underweight anorexia patients. However, bulimia patients retain their normal weight in most cases, so that often several years may elapse before their condition is detected. Chronic vomiting usually leads to erosion in the area of the occlusal and oral tooth surfaces of the maxillary teeth, especially the incisors.[14,19,30]

Common symptoms in bulimia patients are oral and occlusal erosion affecting the maxillary teeth, enlargement of the parotid gland of metabolic origin, which can be painful, and sometimes enlargement of the submandibular salivary glands, xerostomia, erythema in the area of the pharyngeal and palatal mucosa, as well as painful redness and swelling of the lips, with scaling and the formation of rhagades.[1] The onset of these symptoms and a relevant medical and dietary history should cause dental practitioners to suspect a bulimic disease (Table 19-7). A dentist is often the first medical professional to recognize a case of bulimia. Clinical experience shows that bulimia is not always associated with erosion. This situation is closely linked to the hypersalivation that occurs before vomiting and is controlled by the "vomiting center" in the brain.[20]

Saliva, pellicle

The protective actions of saliva in response to acid attack include: acid dilution, acid neutralization, reduction of the dissolution of enamel by calcium and phosphate ions, remineralization, and pellicle formation. A pellicle is a diffusion barrier to acids and therefore offers some protection against erosion. Normal salivary flow rates are ≥ 0.25 ml/min (nonstimulated) or ≥ 1 ml/min (stimulated).

Tooth cleaning

Softened hard dental tissue is susceptible to processes of abrasion or attrition, which may cause overlapping of erosion, abrasion, and attrition. Markedly less enamel is abraded during teeth cleaning when there is no softening of the hard dental tissue than in people with pre-existing erosive damage.

■ Nutritional factors

pH, calcium, phosphate

Acidic soft drinks and fruit juices make up a steadily increasing proportion of total drinks consumption in Europe, and account for over 50% of nonalcoholic drinks consumed. The erosive nature of a drink or food is not only determined by the frequency of consumption and its pH, but also by its buffer capacity and chelating properties, and by other factors, such as calcium or phosphate content. The calcium and phosphate content of a drink or food has a decisive influence on how erosive it is. Immersion of enamel samples in a calcium-enriched, commercially available orange juice did not cause softening of the enamel surface. This orange juice (pH 4) can be recommended as a "functional food" for patients at risk of erosion. By contrast, orange juice without added calcium led to a decrease in enamel hardness. Yoghurt is another example of a food that does not normally cause erosion despite a low pH (approximately pH 4).

Isotonic sports drinks are often acidic and undersaturated in relation to enamel and dentin. It is not uncommon for them to cause erosion in sportspeople. Nonerosive sports drinks with added calcium are now available. Several studies have shown that the erosive potential of sports drinks can be reduced by the addition of calcium or casein phosphopeptide-stabilized amorphous calcium phosphate (CPP-ACP) (see chapter 6).[15,28,34] The safety of unflavored mineral water with regard to erosion has repeatedly been demonstrated.

Occupation and leisure activities

Regular contact with organic or inorganic acids at work can promote the onset and progression of erosion. The largest groups at risk of developing erosion in the workplace are workers in the chemicals and wine industries.

Sporting activities can lead to erosion as a result of erosive sports drinks or gastroesophageal reflux caused by strenuous training. However, it should be noted that in most cases other factors have to exist for erosion to develop.

Risk assessment

As soon as erosion is clinically detected or signs of an increased risk of erosion are present, a detailed discussion with the patient must take place. Simple questioning is usually not enough because patients are often unaware of their acid input. Therefore it is important to get patients to keep a detailed record of their diet for a few days (including a weekend). Key points in the risk assessment are given in Table 19-8.

Table 19-8 Factors to evaluate during risk assessment of erosion

Case history (medical, dental, dietary, behavioral)
Ask for a record of dietary intake for at least 4 days, including a weekend
Ask for risk factors not mentioned by the patient
Assess intake of citrus fruit, other fruit, berries, fruit juices, sports drinks, sugared drinks, tea infusions, alcohol, alcopops, pickled vegetables, raw vegetables, salad dressing, etc
Stomach problems: vomiting, sour taste, retrosternal presssure, signs of anorexia
Drugs: tranquilizers, vitamins, antihistamines, effervescent tablets
Dental hygiene: hardness of toothbrush, brushing habits (how? when? how often? how long?), abrasivity of dentifrice
Radiation therapy in the head area, salivary gland disease
Evaluation of non-carious tooth defects
Erosion index (BEWE), abrasions, attritions
Photographs, models (in order to determine progression)
Saliva analysis
Salivary flow rates, buffer capacity

Prevention of erosion

Based on the risk assessment, concrete advice on prevention can finally be given.

The aims of dietary education of patients is to reduce their acid intake and to alter any harmful habits. This is achieved on the one hand by decreasing the consumption of acid-containing food and drinks, and on the other hand by speeding up the consumption of erosive foods (to reduce the length of time they are in the mouth). Drinking in small sips and sucking the drink through the teeth are habits that promote erosion. Cheese can be recommended at the end of a meal because the high calcium and phosphate content as well as the proteins contained in some cheeses have a protective and/or remineralizing effect. Chilled acidic drinks are less erosive than nonchilled drinks.[4] Drinks and foods sweetened with xylitol seem to block the release of calcium from dental enamel and hence afford a certain protection against erosion.[2]

In reflux patients, investigation of the exact cause followed by treatment (medication/surgical) is paramount. Proton pump inhibitors are currently the best form of treatment for preventing reflux with the therapeutic aim of raising the pH above 4 for as long as possible.

In addition to the above measures already, it makes sense to instruct patients with active erosive lesions about proper oral hygiene. Erosion patients should be urged not to clean their teeth after acid exposure but beforehand. The waiting time of ½ to 1 hour before cleaning often quoted is not enough because the saliva needs significantly longer to repair softened hard dental tissue so that it can withstand tooth cleaning.

Furthermore, it should not be forgotten that caries is still the main problem in the population. In many countries, cleaning the teeth immediately after eating is correctly recommended for caries prevention. Instructing patients to wait for ½ to 1 hour is risky in health policy terms because it is likely that the teeth will not be cleaned at all. It is important that a healthcare professional gives the best possible preventive advice for the individual and checks periodically whether the advice is being followed. This is the only way to ensure that the appropriate preventive steps are being taken and continued.

In any event, a slightly abrasive dentifrice, a soft toothbrush, and a gentle brushing technique should be used. We recommend that patients with erosion rinse their mouths, eg, after vomiting, with a (stannous) fluoride rinse or with water. Various studies have shown increased effectiveness of highly concentrated fluoride if they were applied before, rather than after, the acid intake.[23,25] Through precipitation of a calcium fluoride-like mineral, a protective layer is formed. In conditions of decreased pH, this protective layer is decomposed before the underlying enamel is affected. To date, the question of the amount of time required for this calcium fluoride precipitate to be formed *in vivo* on tooth surfaces has not been resolved. However, it has been shown that *(1)* the calcium fluoride-like material is formed very quickly and *(2)* that slightly acidic pH stimulates precipitation.[27] It should be mentioned that products for dental hygiene that are slightly acidic but contain fluoride show no erosive potential.

Recent studies showed that TiF_4 and stannous-containing substances also exert a protective effect.[13] While TiF_4 discolors the teeth unpleasantly, this is less the case with Sn compounds. Stannous fluoride compounds form precipitates that are able to withstand acid attack and consequently, it protects teeth from erosion and/or its progression.[31]

The use of fluoride or stannous-containing fluoride rinse prior to acid attack is not always practical because very few people would be willing or able to apply fluoride deliberately before vomiting. On the other hand, it is simple to protect against erosion caused by nocturnal eructation by appropriate evening prophylaxis with fluoride. In addition, it should be noted that wearing a splint at night is contraindicated for reflux patients because, owing to the capillary forces between the teeth and the splint, which does not fit tightly everywhere, gastric acid can get under the splint. The time that acid is in contact with the teeth is thereby increased.

Xerostomia or hyposalivation can be induced by radiotherapy in the head and neck area and also by various drugs. If the latter is the case, it is advisable to consult the attending physician and arrange for a switch to a drug that does not have an adverse effect on saliva production.

Increasing the salivary flow rate by chewing gum protects the teeth[29] and reduces the postprandial reflux. Tooth-protecting chewing gums are the first choice for those with reduced salivary flow. Table 19-9 gives an overview of possible preventive measures when the risk of erosion is elevated.

Table 19-9 Proposed preventive measures

Controlling acid consumption
Reduce consumption of acidic foods, if possible, and restrict to few (main) meals as far as possible
Reducing acid exposure
Avoid drinking in sips, consume drinks quickly, do not suck them through the teeth. Cold drinks are less erosive!
End meals with cheese, use (sports) drinks/foods enriched with calcium
After vomiting, rinse with water or (stannous) fluoride mouthwash
Teeth-protecting chewing gums to stimulate the salivary flow rate
Controlling oral hygiene
Soft toothbrushes
Weakly abrasive dentifrice
Fluoride dentifrice
Gentle brushing technique
Regular application of (tin-containing) fluoride solution and/or more highly concentrated fluoride gels
For endogenous acid exposure
Initiation of causal therapy
Suspected reflux: refer to gastroenterologist
Anorexia/bulimia patients: arrange psychological or psychiatric consultation
Simple measures
Avoid reflux-promoting foods, eg, wine, citrus products, vinegary sauces, highly fatty foods, tomatoes, peppermint, coffee, black tea, chocolate
Small meals in the day and no large meal before going to bed
Tooth-friendly chewing gums after eating to reduce postprandial reflux
Medicinal measures
Acid blockers: proton pump inhibitors such as esomeprazole (Nexium®) 20 mg
Surgical measures
For severe reflux, surgical therapy (laparoscopic fundoplication) may be performed

References

1. Abrams RA, Ruff JC. Oral signs and symptoms in the diagnosis of bulimia. J Am Dent Assoc 1986;113:761–764.
2. Amaechi BT, Higham SM, Edgar WM. The influence of xylitol and fluoride on dental erosion *in vitro*. Arch Oral 1998;43:157–161.
3. Attin T, Buchalla W, Gollner M, Hellwig E. Use of variable remineralization periods to improve the abrasion resistance of previously eroded enamel. Caries Res 2000;34:48–52.
4. Barbour ME, Finke M, Parker DM, Hughes JA, Allen GC, Addy M. The relationship between enamel softening and erosion caused by soft drinks at a range of temperatures. J Dent 2006;34:207-213.
5. Bartlett D, Ganß C, Lussi A. Basic Erosive Wear Examination (BEWE): a new scoring system for scientific and clinical needs. Clin Oral Investig 2008;12:S65–68.
6. Buttar NS, Falk GW. Pathogenesis of gastroesophageal reflux and Barrett esophagus. Mayo Clin Proc 2001;76:226–234.
7. Davis WB, Winter PJ. The effect of abrasion on enamel and dentine and exposure to dietary acid. Br Dent J 1980;148:253–256.
8. Dugmore CR, Rock WP. The progression of tooth erosion in a cohort of adolescents of mixed ethnicity. Int J Paediatr Dent 2003;13:295–303.
9. Edwards M, Ashwood RA, Littlewood SJ, Brocklebank LM, Fung DE. A videofluoroscopic comparison of straw and cup drinking: the potential influence on dental erosion. Br Dent J 1998;185:244–249.
10. El Aidi H, Bronkhorst EM, Truin GJ. A longitudinal study of tooth erosion in adolescents. J Dent Res 2008;87:731–735
11. Ganß C, Schlechtriemen M, Klimek J. Dental erosions in subjects living on a raw food diet. Caries Res 1999;33:74–80.
12. Ganß C, Klimek J, Giese K. Dental erosion in children and adolescents – a cross-sectional and longitudinal investigation using study models. Community Dent Oral Epidemiol 2001;29:264–271.
13. Ganß C, Schlueter N, Hardt M, Schattenberg P, Klimek J. Effect of fluoride compounds on enamel erosion *in vitro*: a comparison of amine, sodium and stannous fluoride. Caries Res 2008;42:2–7.
14. Hellström I. Oral complications in anorexia nervosa. Scand J Dent Res 1977;8:71–86.
15. Hooper SM, West NX, Sharif N, Smith S, North M, De'Ath J, Parker DM, Roedig-Penman A, Addy M. A comparison of enamel erosion by a new sports drink compared to two proprietary products: a controlled, crossover study *in situ*. J Dent 2004;32:541–545.
16. Jaeggi T, Lussi A. Toothbrush abrasion of erosively altered enamel after intraoral exposure to saliva: an *in situ* study. Caries Res 1999;33:455–461.
17. Jaeggi T, Schaffner M, Bürgin W, Lussi A. Erosionen und keilförmige Defekte bei Rekruten der Schweizer Armee. Schweiz Monatsschr Zahnmed 1999;109:1171–1182.
18. Johansson AK, Lingström P, Imfeld T, Birkhed D. Influence of drinking method on tooth-surface pH in relation to dental erosion. Eur J Oral Sci 2004;112:484–489.
19. Jones RR, Cleaton-Jones P. Depth and areas of dental erosions and dental caries in bulimic women. J Dent Res 1989;68:1275–1278.
20. Lee M, Feldman M. Nausea and vomiting. In: Feldman M, Scharschmidt B, Sleisenger M, eds, Sleisenger and Fordstran's Gastrointestinal and Liver Disease: Pathophysiology, Diagnosis, Management 1998; 6th ed.: 117–127, Saunders Philadelphia.
21. Lussi A, Schaffner M, Hotz P, Suter P. Dental erosion in a population of Swiss adults. Community Dent Oral Epidemiol 1991;19:286–290.
22. Lussi A, Schaffner M. Progression of and risk factors for dental erosion and wedge-shaped defects over a 6-year period. Caries Res 2000;34:182–187.
23. Lussi A, Megert B, Eggenberger D, Jaeggi T. Impact of different toothpaste on the prevention of erosion. Caries Res 2008;42: 62–67.
24. Millward A, Shaw L, Harrington E, Smith AJ. Continuous monitoring of salivary flow rate and pH at the surface of the dentition following consumption of acidic beverages. Caries Res 1997;31:44–49.
25. Nunn JH, Rugg-Gunn A, Gordon PH, Stephenson G. A longitudinal study of dental erosion in adolescent girls. Caries Res 2001;35:296 (ORCA Abstract 97).

26. Osatakul S, Sriplung H, Puetpaiboon A, Junjana CO, Chamnongpakdi S. Prevalence and natural course of gastro-oesophageal reflux symptoms: a 1-year cohort study in Thai infants. J Pediatr Gastroenterol Nutr 2002;34:63–67.
27. Petzold M. The influence of different fluoride compounds and treatment conditions on dental enamel: a descriptive in vitro study of the CaF_2 precipitation and microstructure. Caries Res 2001;35:45–51.
28. Ramalingam L, Messer LB, Reynolds EC. Adding casein phosphopeptide-amorphous calcium phosphate to sports drinks to eliminate in vitro erosion. Pediatr Dent 2005;27:61–67.
29. Rios D, Honorio HM, Magalhaes AC, Delbem ACB, Machado MAAM, Silva SMB, Buzalaf MAR. Effect of salivary stimulation on erosion of human and bovine enamel subjected or not to subsequent abrasion: an *in situ/ex vivo* study. Caries Res 2006;40:218–223.
30. Robb N, Smith BGN, Geidrys-Leeper E. The distribution of erosion in the dentitons of patients with eating disorders. Br Dent J 1995;178:171–175.
31. Schlueter N, Duran A, Klimek J, Ganß C. Investigation of the effect of various fluoride compounds and preparations thereof on erosive tissue loss in enamel *in vitro*. Caries Res 2009;43:10–16.
32. Szarka LA, De Vault KR, Murray JA. Diagnosing gastroesophageal reflux disease. Mayo Clin Proc 2001; 76:97–101.
33. Vandenplas Y. Oesophageal pH monitoring for gastro-oesophageal reflux in infants and children. John Wiley & Sons, Chichester 1992.
34. Venables MC, Shaw L, Jeukendrup AE, Roedig-Penman A, Finke M, Newcombe RG, Parry J, Smith AJ. Erosive effect of a new sports drink on dental enamel during exercise. Med Sci Sports Exerc 2005;37:39–44.
35. Wiegand A, Egert S, Attin T. Toothbrushing before or after an acidic challenge to minimize tooth wear? An *in situ/ex vivo* study. Am J Dent 2008;21:13–16.

Endodontology

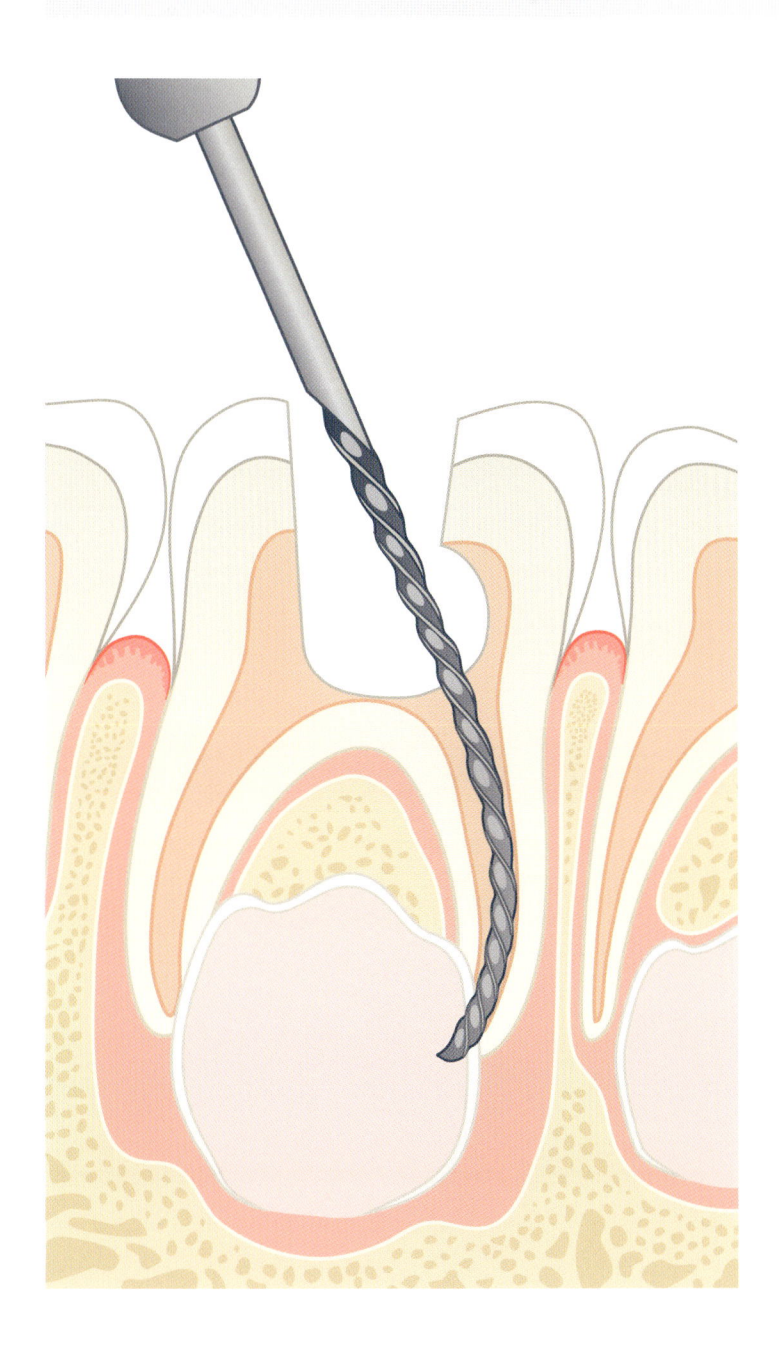

IX

20 Root canal preparation

Beat Suter

■ Risk analysis

Before any root canal treatment is undertaken, a risk analysis should be carried out. The purpose of this analysis is to inform the dental practitioner as well as the patient about the problems that might arise and the time and cost of the root canal treatment. The risk analysis can be used as a basis, if necessary, for the decision on whether the root treatment should be performed by a general dental practitioner (simple case), by an experienced clinician (moderately serious case), or by a specialist (because of considerable difficulties).

Where the limitations are drawn in this respect should be decided individually by each practitioner, based on a realistic self-assessment. Individuals' assessments can vary widely, depending on level of training, equipment, and personal preferences. For legal and ethical reasons, however, this assessment must not influence the indication for root canal treatment itself but only the decision about who will carry out the treatment and under what circumstances.

The risk analysis may serve as a foundation in a legal sense. In particular, any necessary added expense may be justified to the patient on the basis of the risk analysis.

Table 20-1 presents a checklist for the risk analysis. It is a broad simplification of a template produced by the Canadian Academy of Endodontics, which can be viewed online.[2]

Assessment of the anatomical variations to be encountered or knowledge about their frequency might also influence the risk evaluation and warn against unexpected difficulties.

Factors for assessment of risk and complications

Medical history
- Multiple medication
- Uncontrolled diabetes
- Possible consultation with the doctor

Endodontology

Local anesthesia
- History of anesthesia problems
- Acute pulpitis ("hot tooth")

Personal factors
- Limited capacity of mouth opening (where the incisal edge distance is less than approx 25 mm, root treatment is no longer possible)
- Retching (radiographs, rubber dam, etc)

Pulp cavity
- Calcifications, accessory root canals or additional roots make root canal treatment more difficult.

Canal anatomy
- The greater the canal curvature, the more difficult it is to treat.
- Mesial canals of lower molars are especially difficult because of multiple curvatures and merging of the root canals.
- Very short (< 13 mm) and very long canals (> 24 mm) pose greater problems.
- Teeth with C-shaped canals are very difficult to treat.
- Teeth with open apices require long-term treatment (apexification) or treatment with MTA (mineral trioxide aggregate).

Malpositioned teeth
- Rotated or tipped teeth can pose access problems, in some cases a straight line access can be difficult to achieve.
- Examples: buccally tipped maxillary second molars or malpositioned teeth under crowns and bridges.

Restorability
- The distance between the marginal edge of the reconstruction and the alveolar bone margin should be at least 2 to 3 mm.

Existing reconstructions
- Root canal treatments can be performed through existing reconstructions.
- It is important to bear in mind that the tooth underneath might be rotated or tipped.
- The reconstruction must be removed in case of secondary caries or loss of retention.

Retreatments, perforations, fractured instruments
- Retreatments are always risky or high-risk treatments.
- The treatment of perforations and the removal of fractured instruments are very difficult.

Other complications
- Trauma cases should generally be assigned to a higher risk level.
- Subgingival or subcrestal fractures can be difficult or impossible to treat.
- The same applies to internal resorptions which have penetrated through to the periodontium and to all external resorptions.
- Nonpenetrated internal resorptions are less difficult to treat.
- Treatment of a dens invaginatus or a double tooth formation is extremely difficult.
- Teeth with a reduced periodontal prognosis must be thoroughly evaluated. The outcome can be improved by cooperation between dental practitioners working on endodontic and periodontal aspects.

Table 20-1 Risk analysis in endodontology (based on: Canadian Academy of Endodontics, Standards of Practice, pp 4–52)

Risk factor	Points	Yes	Risk factor	Points	Yes
Significant medical problems	1		Pulp stones, markedly reduced pulp chamber	1	
Very severe systemic illness	3		Canal hardly visible clinically and radiologically	3	
Poor compliance, retching, limited mouth opening	1		Canal completely invisible clinically and radiographically	5	
Mouth opening < 25 mm, supine position impossible, uncertain diagnosis	3		Slight internal or apical resorption	1	
1st or 2nd molar or tipped/rotated tooth	1		Internal resorption with perforation, external marginal resorption	5	
3rd molar or severely tipped/rotated tooth	3		All other resorptions or perforations	3	
Rubber dam application difficult	1		Simple retreatment of a paste filling without canal transportation	1	
Rubber dam application only possible after time-consuming pretreatment	3		Fractured instrument, firmly cemented post/screw/gold core	5	
Molar with 3 canals, curved or difficult to access canals	1		All other retreatments	3	
4th canal, premolar with 3 canals, upper anterior tooth or premolar with 2 or more canals, type IV canal, C- or S-shaped canal, extremely short or extremely long canal	3		Trauma case (if not absolutely simple)	5	
Fusion of a tooth, dens invaginatus	5		Total risk points		

Root treatment with average risk (class 1):   < 2   points

Root treatment with high risk (class 2):   2–4   points

Root treatment with very high risk (class 3):   > 4   points

RESULT: Total: _____   Class: _____

Anatomy of root canals

To ensure that endodontic treatment is routinely successful in as many cases as possible, it is important for the practitioner to have comprehensive knowledge of all the anatomical variations. Anyone who has studied the anatomy of root canals in detail will be confronted with far fewer unpleasant surprises in everyday practice. For instance, the frequency of occurrence of three root canals for the maxillary first premolars is 5 %. This means that one in 20 maxillary first premolars will have three root canals; ie, it is not uncommon to come across this situation in practice. Dental practitioners should therefore have a clear three-dimensional idea of the anatomy of such a tooth, making it far easier for them to shape a correct access cavity and to locate all three canal orifices. If they do not, they will find it difficult to locate the canal orifices because they will not know where exactly to look.

Basically the anatomy of the endodontium reflects that of the periodontium to a certain extent. Improved knowledge of root canal anatomy is therefore also advantageous for periodontal therapy.

Table 20-2 gives an overview of the different types of root canals and the frequency of their occurrence, arranged by type of tooth. Figures 20-1 to 20-3 show selected clinical examples relevant to root canal anatomy.

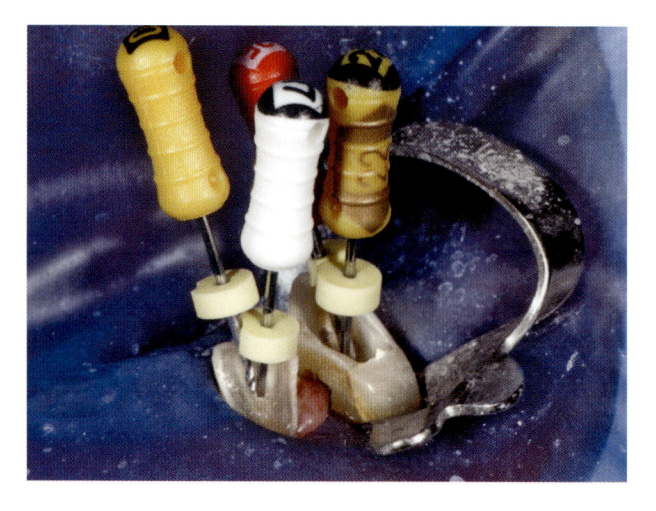

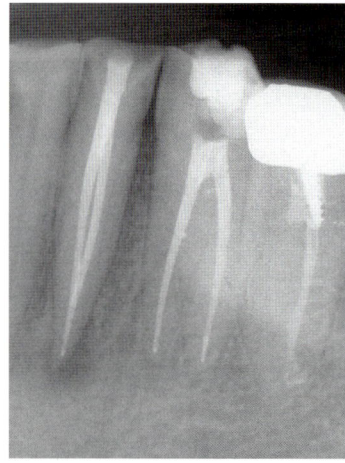

Fig 20-1 Left mandibular lateral incisor and canine each have two root canals (lateral incisor: canal type II; canine: two separate roots). The first premolar presumably has two root canals as well (type II or III).

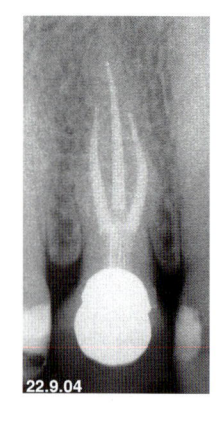

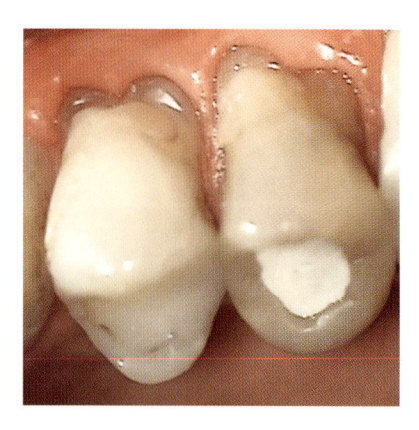

Fig 20-2 Left: right maxillary first premolar with three roots (each type I). Right: the buccal gingival contour on the left maxillary premolars indicates a situation with three roots (first premolar) or three root canals (second premolar).

20 Root canal preparation

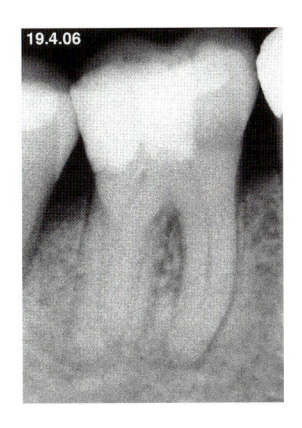

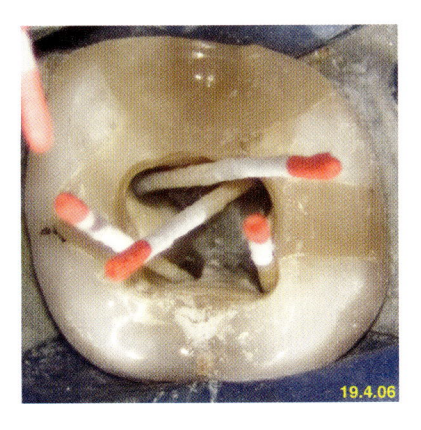

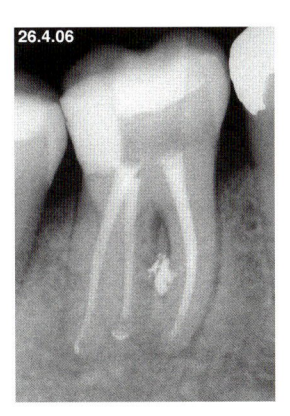

Fig 20-3 Initial radiograph (left), clinical situation (center), and final radiograph (right): right mandibular first molar with radix entomolaris. Note the widely divergent canals of the two distal roots.

Table 20-2 Anatomy of root canals (based on Peters[4–7])

Tooth/Root	Type I	Type II	Type III	Type IV	Type V	1√	2√	3√
UJ incisors	100%							
UJ canines	100%							
LJ incisors	75%	23%	2%					
LJ canines	75%	18%					7%	
UJ 1st premolar	8%	18%	69%		5%	40%	56%	4%
UJ 2nd premolar	48%	27%	24%		1%			
LJ 1st premolar	70%	4%		25%	1%			
LJ 2nd premolar	97%	rare		3%	rare			
UJ 1st molar, mb√	<40%	20–35%	10–40%					
UJ 2nd molar, mb√	57%	43%						
UJ 3rd molar	variable							
LJ 1st molar, m√	13%	30%	57%		isolated			
LJ 2nd molar, m√	58%	21%	21%					
LJ 3rd molar, m√	65%	18%	16%					
LJ 1st molar, d√	73%	13%	14%					
LJ 2nd molar, d√	94%	2%	4%					
LJ 3rd molar, d√	92%	4%	4%					
Isolated C-shaped LJ 2nd molar								

mb√ = mesiobuccal root; m√ = mesial root; d√ = distal root

Modern principles of root canal preparation

This section presents in sequential order the individual steps and considerations that are necessary for successful endodontic treatment. The description is based on many years of clinical experience in practice as well as on the evidence from scientific studies.

Precise knowledge of the principles outlined and their application facilitates the practitioners' daily work with root canals and significantly improves the results. In a manner of speaking, they are the recipe for success for root canal treatment.

Inlay-shaped access cavity

It is important to open the tooth wide occlusally (even if it is the dentist's own elegant work!). The preparation tends to be inlay-shaped (Fig 20-4). This involves sparing the dentin at the height of the canal orifice (ie, roughly at the height of the cementoenamel junction) and avoiding potential weakening of the crown margin. For this reason, round burs should be used exclusively for caries excavation; and otherwise they should only be considered for removing overhangs arising because of pulp horns. The outline of the access cavity should coincide with the canal anatomy, with each corner giving access to one canal. Crown and bridge preparing diamonds, Diamendo and ultrasonic abrasive instruments (Start-X® or KaVo SonicFlex Endo®) (Fig 20-5) are suitable instruments for preparing the access cavity.

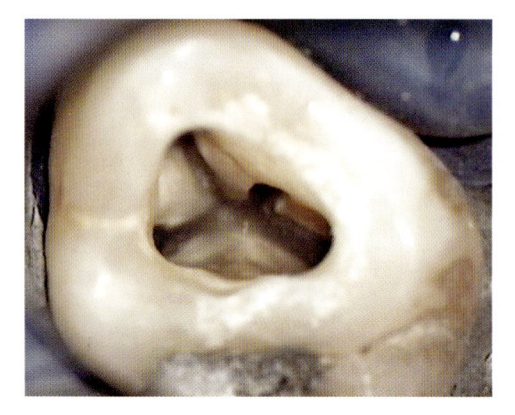

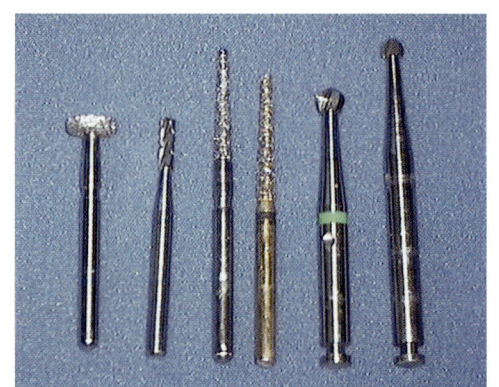

Fig 20-4 An endodontic access cavity should tend towards an inlay shape, with the canal orifices in the corners of the cavity.

Fig 20-5 Rotating instruments for the preparation of the endodontic access cavity.

Straight line access

With Start-X®, KaVo SonicFlex Endo®, or Gates Glidden burs (in descending order!), or Shaper X®, GT Accessory File®, Orifice Shaper®, *Hedström* files, or similar instruments, the canal orifice is straightened; ie, it is transported away from the furcation and towards the periphery (Fig 20-6). As a result, the initial canal curvature is eliminated and the root canal instrument can subsequently slide straight into the root canal (Fig 20-7). A lot of double curvatures can be eliminated from the outset using this method. Access to the canal is simplified and the risk of fracture of instruments is reduced.

Root canal preparation

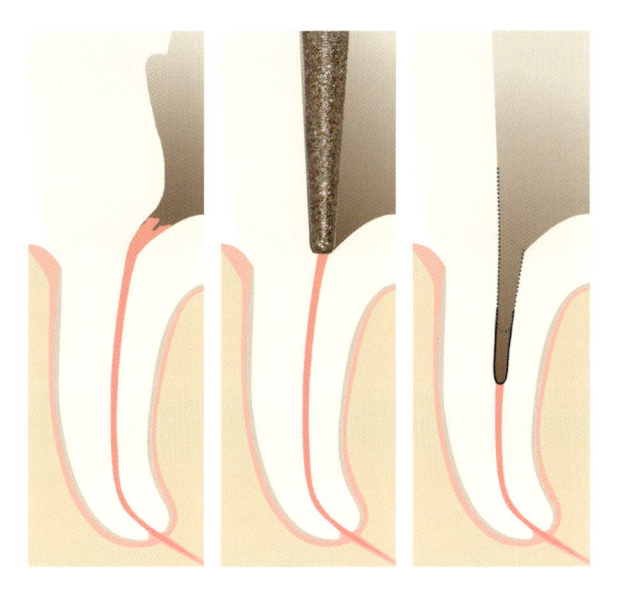

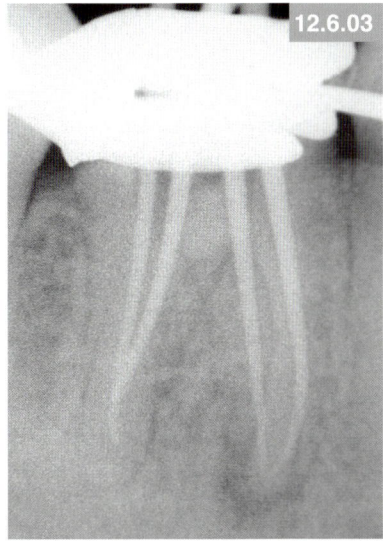

Fig 20-6 Schematic diagram of preparation of straight line access.

Fig 20-7 Right mandibular first molar, radiograph prior to root filling.

As a result of correct shaping of the access cavity and creation of the straight line access in all canal orifices, the gutta-percha points lie virtually parallel in the radiograph. If access were faulty, they would cross each other in the cavity.

Crown down preperation

The upper two-thirds of the canal are widened from coronally to apically (Fig 20-8). To be able to assess the length of the canal reliably, a precise analysis of the initial radiograph is essential. Instruments with descending diameter or decreasing conicity are used for the crown down technique. The use of rotary nickel-titanium (Ni-Ti) instruments is recommended. It is important to note that the canal lumen up to the particular penetration depth of the rotary instrument must have a diameter corresponding to ISO #20 (known as the "glide path", see below). Therefore, the canal definitely has to be scouted and might have to be pre-enlarged by hand.

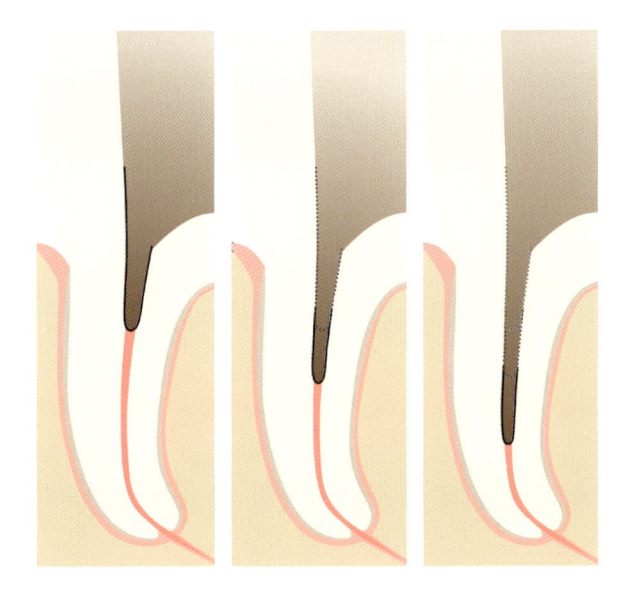

Fig 20-8 Schematic diagram of crown down preparation.

Endodontology

Delayed length measurement

The length measurement is only carried out after the crown down preparation. Thus the apical constriction can be felt in many cases. The working length measured endometrically with a third- or fourth-generation device in the wet canal (but without contact to metal) is verified radiographically (Fig 20-9 shows the Root ZX endometer from Morita as an example of these devices). A measuring radiograph should be carried out for forensic and practical reasons (optimum assessment of canal anatomy).

Apical patency

When measuring canal length, a #08 or #10 K-file (known as a "patency file") deliberately penetrates the apical foramen by about 0.5 mm (Fig 20-10). The selected working length (ie, the preparation length) is approximately 1 mm shorter. The patency file is repeatedly used, at least after every other root canal preparation instrument, to make sure no dentin accumulates. The apical foramen is not widened using the patency file – it merely serves to ensure apical patency. The apical foramen should be left as narrow as possible. (As a consequence of resorption or incomplete root growth, the apical foramen can be extended under certain circumstances.)

Glide path

Before the actual canal preparation can take place (with rotary Ni-Ti instruments), a glide path must be created. *All* rotary Ni-Ti instruments – even if the manufacturer claims otherwise – can only be safely used in the root canal when the root canal has been prepared beforehand by hand to a diameter corresponding to ISO #20. By this means, the path along which the canal is to be prepared is preset for the Ni-Ti instrument's pilot tip. This prevents the pilot tip from getting locked.

PathFiles® (Dentsply Maillefer) have recently become available for preparation of the glide path. These are fine, highly flexible rotary Ni-Ti instruments which display amazingly high fracture resistance (Fig 20-11). They are produced in sizes #13, #16, and #19 and provide a good alternative to the conventional preparation of the glide path. As previously, preparation must be done by hand up to #10.

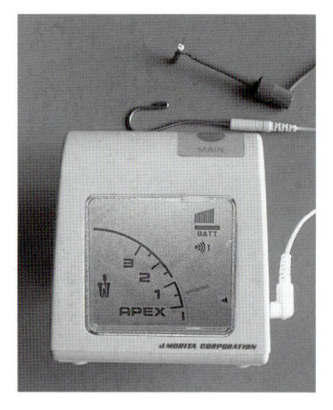

Fig 20-9 Device for electronic measurement of root canal length.

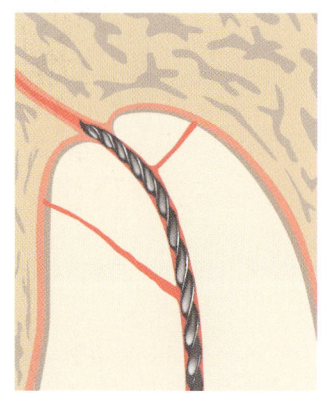

Fig 20-10 Schematic diagram of a patency file in the root canal.

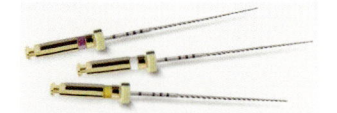

Fig 20-11 PathFiles® for creating the glide path.

Root canal preparation

Nowadays, root canal preparation is primarily carried out using rotary Ni-Ti instrumentation. Compared with conventional instrumentation by hand, these instruments create smoother canal walls with no irregularities, ideal shaping (conicity, respecting canal anatomy), and avoidance of ledge formation, as far as possible.

In very difficult situations, such as abrupt apical curvatures and S-shaped or corkscrew-type curvature of the root canal, it is advisable to prepare the tricky areas by hand, if in doubt. For this purpose, conventional K-files can be used, applying the balanced force technique (as described by Roane[8]) (Fig 20-14). Alternatively, the previously described Ni-Ti system can be used, either as rotary instruments by hand or using Roane's technique, depending on the product. Figure 20-12 shows industrially prefabricated ProTaper® hand instruments (Dentsply). Alternatively, instruments intended for use in a contra-angle handpiece can also be employed by hand, with or without a *Thomas* spanner key (Fig 20-13).

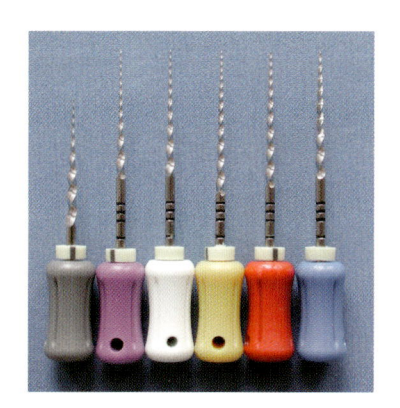

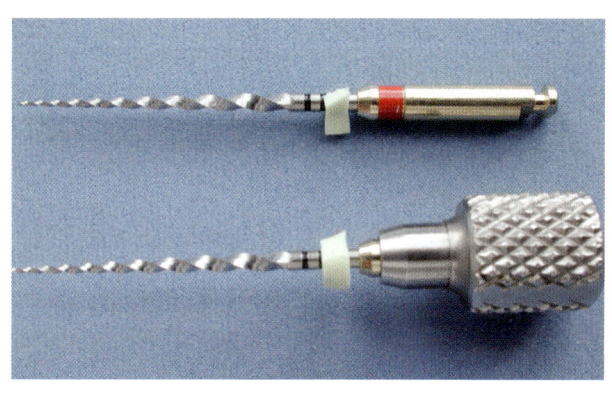

Fig 20-12 ProTaper® hand instruments for manual root canal preparation.

Fig 20-13 ProTaper® instruments can also be used for manual root canal preparation without a special handle or with a Thomas spanner key.

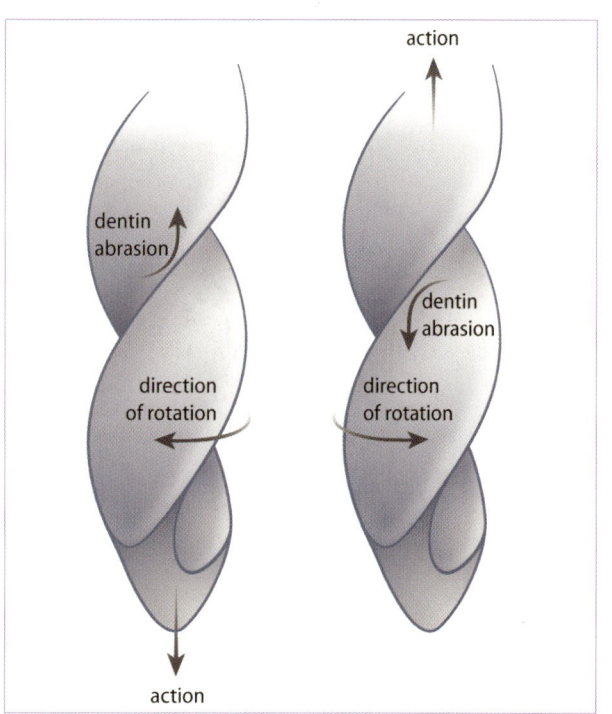

Fig 20-14 Schematic diagram of the working principle of the balanced force technique, according to Roane.[8]

Apical gauging

Depending on the pre-existing dimensions of the apical foramen and the planned obturation technique, the canal preparation must achieve a certain minimal apical size and conicity. The size and conicity of the preparation can be controlled by inserting K-files (eg, NiTiflex® K-files), probing up to the point in the canal at which they bind.

Figure 20-15 illustrates the principle: a canal was prepared up to size #25 with an instrument that has a conicity of 10%. The canal is correctly prepared when a file size #20 does not bind at working length, a file size #25 binds exactly at working length, a file size #30 binds 0.5 mm before the working length and a file size #35 would seize 1 mm short of working length (not shown).

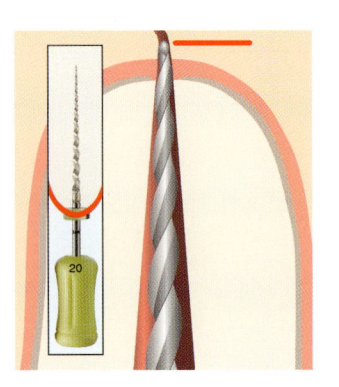

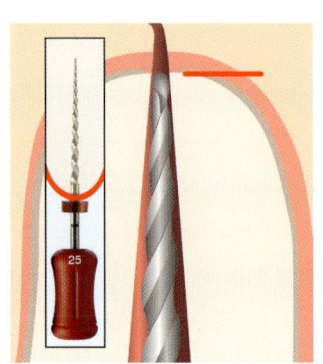

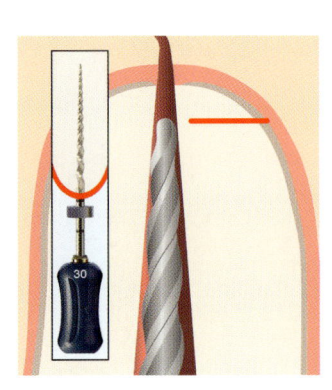

Fig 20-15 Schematic diagram of apical gauging.

Apical resistance form

Ni-Ti instruments such as GTX, ProTaper®, etc, guarantee a good apical resistance form (Fig 20-16) with appropriately high conicity in order to ensure subsequent hermetic obturation with the appropriate root filling techniques (absorption of hydraulic pressure).

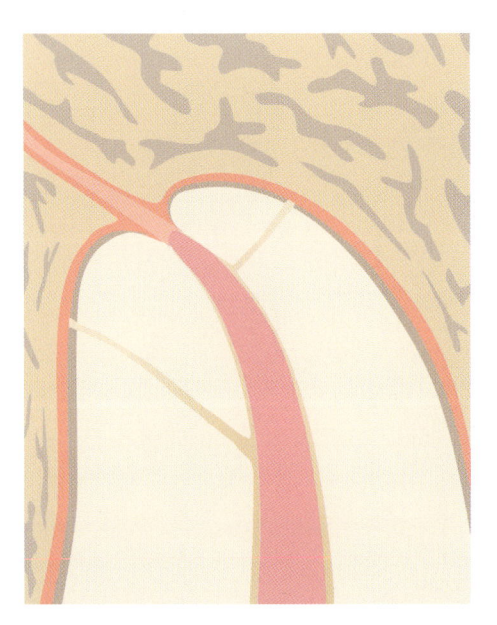

Fig 20-16 Schematic diagram of the apical resistance form.

Deep shape

Owing to the increased apical conicity of modern Ni-Ti instruments (see above), the apical foramen is left as small as possible, but directly coronal to the foramen a large volume is created (known as "deep shape", Fig 20-17) so that irrigation and disinfection can be carried out efficiently and root filling devices are able to reach the apical zone without any problems. Figure 20-18 shows a clinical example of deep shape.

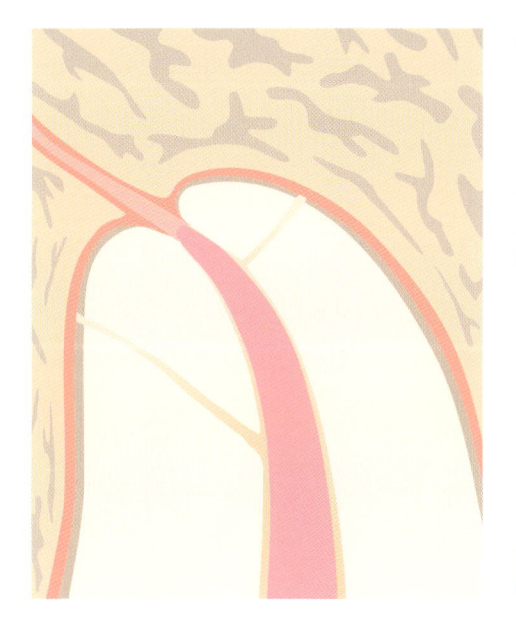

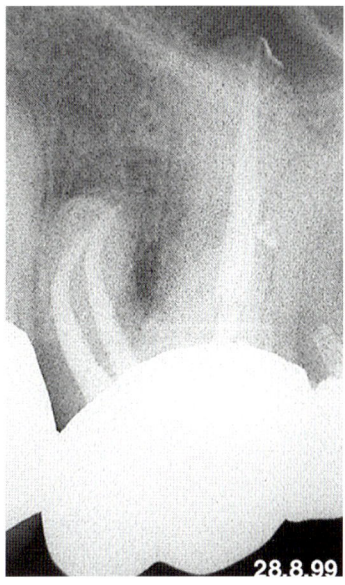

Fig 20-17 Schematic diagram of the deep shape.

Fig 20-18 Left maxillary first molar, after root filling. The properly shaped deep shape is clearly visible in the two mesial root canals.

■ Material properties of Ni-Ti root canal preparation instruments

All modern rotary root canal preparation systems work with instruments that are manufactured from a nickel-titanium alloy (Ni-Ti). This material is fundamentally different from conventional stainless steel, therefore it is important that practitioners familiarize themselves with the properties of the new material, finding out its advantages and disadvantages, to ensure error-free use of the instruments.

The alloy used for manufacturing root canal instruments comprises 56% nickel and 44% titanium. In addition, it contains traces of carbon, oxygen, iron, nitrogen, and hydrogen.[9] The material properties are optimized for use at body temperature. Ni-Ti is highly elastic and stress-resistant. These properties are the basic prerequisite for rotary instruments used in the root canal. The biocompatibility of the material is roughly comparable with that of stainless steel; and, as a rule, it does not pose a problem for people with a nickel allergy. As a result of the high titanium content, Ni-Ti is more corrosion-resistant than stainless steel.

Ni-Ti wire reacts with very strong elastic deformation, even under minimal stress. This is due to a kind of "shearing" of the crystal lattice structure, which is dependent on temperature (Fig 20-19). Irreversible (nonelastic) deformation only occurs at very high forces. Therefore, prebending of Ni-Ti instruments is very difficult and only limited bending is possible.

Endodontology

Fracture of Ni-Ti instruments can occur in the root canal because of two different mechanisms. First, excessive loading (torque) can cause a torsional fracture. Second, fatigue fractures are possible if the instrument is used too frequently or for too long. Both effects mutually foster each other. Fatigue of an instrument is dependent on the curvature angle and radius, on instrument thickness (size) and geometry, as well as working pressure and rotary speed (speed and feed). Fractures of Ni-Ti instruments can be avoided by using a motor with torque control, always keeping the instrument moving without changing the path of insertion, not forcing the instrument into the canal, and not shaping more than three teeth (= 12 canals) with the same instrument.

Instrument fatigue is dependent on
- Angle of curvature
- Radius of the canal curvature
- Instrument size
- Instrument design
- Working force (feed)
- (Speed)

How to avoid fractures
- Use motor with torque control
- Always keep instrument moving within the root canal
- Maintain the path of insertion
- Work without forcing
- Use instrument a maximum of three times (max 12 canals)

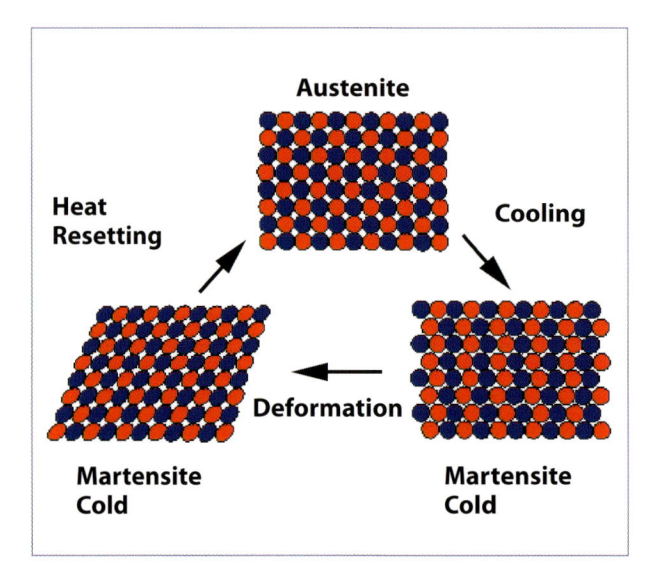

Fig 20-19 Different crystal lattice states in nickel-titanium alloys.

Techniques for root canal preparation

There are various possibilities in terms of root canal preparation. All the techniques follow the above principles, but have their own particular points of detail. For reasons of practicality, only the recently launched GTX system will be presented below. Using this system, which was presented by Dr Steve Buchanan in 2008,[1] canal preparations with very high anatomical accuracy and very low transportation effects can be achieved. Through basic modifications to instrument geometry and material properties, the system has been adapted to reflect the latest knowledge. A new Ni-Ti material known as "M wire" is used for the instruments.[3] The application technique for the GTX instruments is as follows[1] (reproduced with kind permission of Dr S. Buchanan).

All canals must be catheterized up to a K-file #15 – preferably in the presence of a lubricant – so that the pulp tissue is not compressed apically into small lateral canals. Ideally, an electronic apex locator (eg, Morita Root ZX®) should be used at the same time. When all the canals are catheterized and their lengths have been measured, the lubricant is washed out with an air/water syringe. The pulp cavity and canals are then irrigated with NaOCl solution (6%). The preparation is started with a 20.06-GTX file set to working length. The rotation speed and the torque limit are preselected (300 rpm and 1.7 Ncm).

The file should already be rotating before it touches the dentin (it should rotate during insertion, cutting, and withdrawal). As soon as the file is in contact with the dentin, pressure should be exerted very cautiously until it starts to move in an apical direction. A good sign is that the file is always moving into the canal (it takes some getting used to that feeling, but this familiarization is very important to the efficient use of the instruments). After 10 to 12 seconds the 20.06-GTX file usually will not move any further and has to be withdrawn and checked. Dentin debris between the blades indicates where the instrument is working. The file is cleaned, checked for deformation, and reinserted into the canal to start another working cycle.

In most canals this file will reach the working length in one or two working cycles. In this case the preparation can normally be completed in narrow canals with a 30.06-GTX file in a single cycle. If the 20.06 has not reached working length after two cycles, this can usually be completed successfully by using the 20.04-GTX file in one cycle. As a rule, once the 20.04 has reached working length the 20.06 can then be inserted up to working length. Preparation in this kind of canal is thereby completed. Medium-sized and wide canals are prepared up to the 30.08 or 40.08-GTX file unless there is severe curvature.

This gives an outline of the basic technique: one or two files for the preparation, minimal or no crown down preparation, and a greatly reduced fracture risk when new instruments are used.

Canals with apical obliterations or abrupt apical curvatures must be prepared in appropriate segments using GT hand files. For canals with a very large apical diameter, the preparation is finished with one of the 12 GT accessory files with a tip diameter of #50, #70, or #90. If slightly larger coronal widening is desired, a 40.10 file can be used in medium-sized or wide canals.

Another special feature of this new technique is "visual gauging". Previously, gauging by the tactile use of Ni-Ti K-files was recommended for checking for correct apical preparation. Based on his observations, Dr Buchanan believes that this step can often be omitted. With the first GTX file from the 20 series that reaches the working length, if the apical diameter of the canal is larger than 0.2 mm then no dentin residues will be found between the blades at the tip of the instrument. The preparation is then continued immediately with a 30-series file, without prior (tactile) gauging. If this file also does not show any dentin residues between the blades at the tip, the preparation is immediately continued with the 40 series. However, it is advisable to carry out tactile gauging before a gutta-percha point is tried in.

References

1. Buchanan LS. The new GT Series X rotary shaping system: objectives and technique principles. Dent Today 2008;27:70, 72, 74 passim.
2. Canadian Academy of Endodontics. Standards of Practice. 2006. URL: http://www.caendo.ca/about_cae/standards/standards_english.pdf
3. Johnson E, Lloyd A, Kuttler S, Namerow K. Comparison between a Novel Nickel-Titanium Alloy and 508 Nitinol on the Cyclic Fatigue Life of ProFile 25/.04 Rotary Instruments. J Endod 2008;11:1406–1409.
4. Peters LB. Präparation der endodontischen Zugangskavität und Darstellung der Kanäle I. Schneidezähne und Eckzähne. Endodontie 1992;1:57–64.
5. Peters LB. Präparation der endodontischen Zugangskavität und Darstellung der Kanäle II. Prämolaren. Endodontie 1992;1:141–149.
6. Peters LB. Präparation der endodontischen Zugangskavität und Darstellung der Kanäle III. Obere Molaren. Endodontie 1992c1:225–232.
7. Peters LB. Präparation der endodontischen Zugangskavität und Darstellung der Kanäle IV. Untere Molaren. Endodontie 1992;1:291–300.
8. Roane JB, Sabala CL, Duncanson MG Jr. The "balanced force" concept for instrumentation of curved canals. J Endod 1985;11:203–211.
9. Walia HM, Brantley WA, Gerstein H. An initial investigation of the bending and torsional properties of Nitinol root canal files, J Endod 1988;14:346–351.

21 Root canal irrigation

Stefan Hänni

■ Importance of irrigation

In 1894, Miller was the first to observe bacteria in the root canal. He speculated about a connection between these bacteria and the pathogenesis of apical periodontitis,[12] but the actual role of microorganisms in the etiology of apical periodontitis remained unresolved for many years. A connection was not demonstrated until the essential work done by Kakehashi and colleagues (1965) on rats and the confirmation of their findings in humans by Sundqvist (1976).[8,25]

> Infection of the endodontic system is the deciding etiological factor in the pathogenesis of apical periodontitis.

■ Where are the bacteria?

Vital pulp: The pulp tissue can defend itself against bacterial invasion by means of pulpitis. Infection only develops with increasing necrosis.[10]

Devitalized pulp with periradicular radiolucency: Bacteria are always present in the root canal.[8]

> Vital pulp is mostly free of microorganisms. In teeth with periapical periodontitis, bacteria are found throughout the canal system, but especially in the apical area, where they have optimum access to tissue fluid. The bacteria are able to colonize the dentin via open dentinal tubules. Apical granulomas are usually bacteria-free.

The bacteria occur in planktonic form, freely as clusters in the canal, adhered to the canal wall, or as structured biofilm. Colonization of the dentinal tubules and the formation of a biofilm make disinfection difficult.[26,29]

Bacteria can be found in the smear layer created by machining of the dentin on the canal wall and in the dentinal tubules. It is advisable to remove this smear layer.[7]

> Extremely thorough disinfection of the endodontium and prevention of reinfection are the keys to any successful endodontic treatment. These are predominantly achieved by thorough root canal irrigation.

■ Disinfection strategies

Aseptic treatment approach
Efforts at optimum canal disinfection are part of an overall aseptic approach.

> **Aseptic treatment approach**
> - Tooth isolation using rubber dam
> - Disinfection of the working field
> - Chemomechanical root canal preparation with sterile instruments
> - Intermediate disinfectant dressing
> - Bacteria-proof temporary filling
> - Bacteria-proof root canal filling
> - Tight restoration

Chemomechanical root canal preparation
The main functions of root canal preparation with instruments are mechanical debridement and the creation of space for efficient root canal irrigation (chemical debridement) and an adaquate root canal filling.

However, root canals cannot be rendered bacteria-free using mechanical preparation alone.[4] Owing to the complex anatomical conditions, nearly half of the canal wall surfaces are not touched, even with the best preparation technique.[18]

Maximum microbial reduction can only be achieved by chemomechanical root canal preparation; a combination of mechanical preparation and chemical disinfection ("*files shape – irrigants clean*"), in conjunction with a medicated dressing.[21]

Irrigants

Requirements for irrigants
- Disinfection (broad antibiotic spectrum with action against anaerobic and facultative anaerobic bacteria in biofilms)
- Inactivation of bacterial lipopolysaccharides (endotoxins)
- Dissolution of organic and inorganic root canal contents (tissue debris, smear layer)
- Removal of dentin chips
- Action as a lubricant for instruments
- Good tissue compatibility (periapical)
- Low cytotoxicity
- No adverse effects on the hard dental tissue (softening, discoloration)
- No negative effect on the root canal instruments (corrosion)
- No chemical interactions between the different irrigants used

■ Which irrigant?

Irrigants have a broad range of requirements, but these cannot be fully covered by any single disinfectant (Table 21-1).

Table 21-1 Comparison of irrigants (modified from Zehnder[32])

Irrigant	Effect against microorganisms	Dissolve tissue	Inactivate endotoxins	Dissolve smear layer	Toxicity	Allergy potential
NaOCl	++	+++	+	+	+*	+
CHX	++	–	+	–	–	+
H_2O_2	+	–	–	–	+*	–
EDTA	–	–	–	++	–	–
Citric acid	+	–	–	++	–	–
Iodine in aqueous potassium iodide	++	–	?	–	–	++
Alcohol	+	–	?	–	+	+
MTAD	+	–	?	++	?	+

*concentration-dependent

Sodium hypochlorite

Sodium hypochlorite (NaOCl) best fulfils the requirements.[4] Its tissue-dissolving effect[13] and its ability to neutralize microorganisms that are organized into biofilms or have migrated into dentinal tubules[16,24] make it the root canal irrigant of choice.

Its antimicrobial and tissue-dissolving activity are concentration-dependent. At the same time, its cytotoxicity also increases as the concentration rises.[23]

Authoritative authors recommend using a 1% solution, which balances the desired effect and toxicity.

Chlorhexidine

Chlorhexidine (CHX) is a potent disinfectant with a broad spectrum. Its efficacy is better against gram-positive than against gram-negative bacteria. CHX has an antifungal effect, especially against *Candida albicans*.[27] This is why it has been particularly recommended for revisions.[19] However, its efficacy has not been proven to be any better than that of sodium hypochlorite. Owing to the cationic structure of the molecule, binding to hydroxyapatite is possible, which causes an effect that lasts beyond the pure application time.[9] As CHX has little or no tissue-dissolving effect, it cannot be recommended as an irrigant on its own.

Ethylene diamine tetra-acetic acid

Ethylene diamine tetra-acetic acid (EDTA) is a chelating agent and was introduced for the preparation of narrow, calcified root canals.[15] It is capable of demineralizing dentin and removing the smear layer. EDTA is recommended as a lubricant by manufacturers of Ni-Ti root canal instruments. The liquid formulation proves to be more efficient than the gel form.[3]

Interactions – alternate rinses

None of the above-mentioned agents fulfils all the requirements for an irrigant. The obvious approach would be to combine the properties of the individual agents by direct mixing or by alternating the rinses. Unfortunately, the interactions in the mixtures are not always positive.

Mixing different irrigants can have adverse effects!

■ How to irrigate

The efficacy of irrigation is dependent on various parameters (Fig 21-1):

- Irrigant (concentration, temperature)
- Penetration depth of the irrigation, dependent on:
    - anatomy of the root canal system
    - root canal preparation (diameter, conicity, length)
    - method of application (cannula diameter, etc)
- Irrigant volume
- Turnover
- Exposure time

Apart from the anatomy of the canal system, all of these parameters, and hence the efficiency of the disinfectant measures, are in the hands of the practitioner!

Root canal irrigation

Table 21-2 Interactions – alternate rinsing

Irrigant 1	Irrigant 2	Interaction
NaOCl	EDTA	• Strong reduction of free chloride ions. NaOCl loses its antibacterial and its tissue-dissolving effect.[31] • Excessive alternate rinsing leads to marked erosion of the canal dentin and a decrease in dentin microhardness.[5]
NaOCl	CHX	Formation of a para-chloroaniline precipitate (toxic rust-brown precipitate)[2]
NaOCl	H_2O_2	Foaming effect due to O_2 evolved

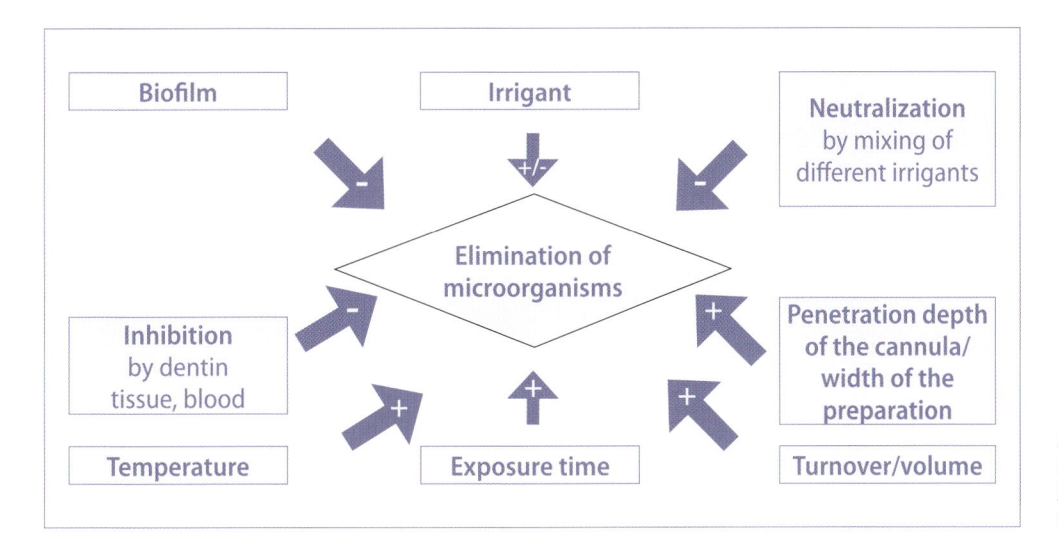

Fig 21-1 Factors that influence the elimination of microorganisms in the root canal (modified from Hecker et al[6])

Manual irrigation

Irrigation using a syringe and cannula as the form of application is hitherto the most widespread method.

It should be noted that the cannula usually cannot reach further than half-way into the canal. Furthermore, the irrigant does not penetrate further than 1 mm beyond the needle tip into the canal.[20]

Points to note during manual irrigation
- Intact or built-up cavity as an irrigant reservoir
- Pulp cavity/root canals after opening never dry, ie, always wetted with irrigant: exposure time↑, cutting performance of instruments↑, torsional forces↓
- Small irrigating syringes (5 to 10 ml): expenditure of effort↓, controllability↑, fatigue↓
- Irrigating needle configuration: small diameter (< 28 G, ideally 30 G), blunt rounded end, side vented (Max-i-Probe®)
- Bring cannula as close as possible to the working length (length marking), do not wedge it, always keep it moving, no excessive pressure
- After each instrument, 2 ml irrigant per root canal – at least 10 ml per root canal, at least 30 minutes' exposure time
- Regular use of a patency file

The ideal manual irrigation

The following options can be considered for improving the cleaning effect of manual irrigants:

- *Manual dynamic irrigation (MDI):*[11] This involves active movement of the fluid in the root canal using gutta-percha points. The irrigant is moved in the root canal by short up-and-down motions of a well-fitting gutta-percha point after root canal preparation.
- *Passive ultrasonic irrigation (PUI):*[28] After root canal preparation, energy is transferred to the irrigating medium using a noncutting file oscillating in the ultrasonic range. The results of the acoustic microstreaming thereby induced are:
  - better transportation of irrigant into the canal branches
  - better fluid exchange in the canal
  - heating of the irrigant
  - a significant reduction in the microbial count.[1]
- *Heating the irrigant:* The antimicrobial and tissue-dissolving activity is increased by heating the irrigant to 45 to 60°C.[22]

Alternative systems

As well as the different systems for application and activation of irrigants, such as the RinsEndo or the EndoVac system, there are some alternative approaches to disinfection:

- Direct application of laser light via fine glass fibers
- Photodynamic therapy (PAD) with diode laser
- Ozone
- Electrochemically activated water

However, none of these approaches can match simple NaOCl irrigation in terms of disinfection and especially with regard to tissue dissolution.

Irrigation protocol

```
Pulpitis          Necrosis          Retreatment
```

Intact access cavity, isolation with rubber dam

Instrument and irrigate
- regularly with NaOCl 0.5–3 % (min. 10 ml/canal, min. 30 minutes' exposure time)
- distribute the irrigant using the patency file and by manual dynamic irrigation (MDI)
- possibly passive ultrasonic irrigation (PUI)

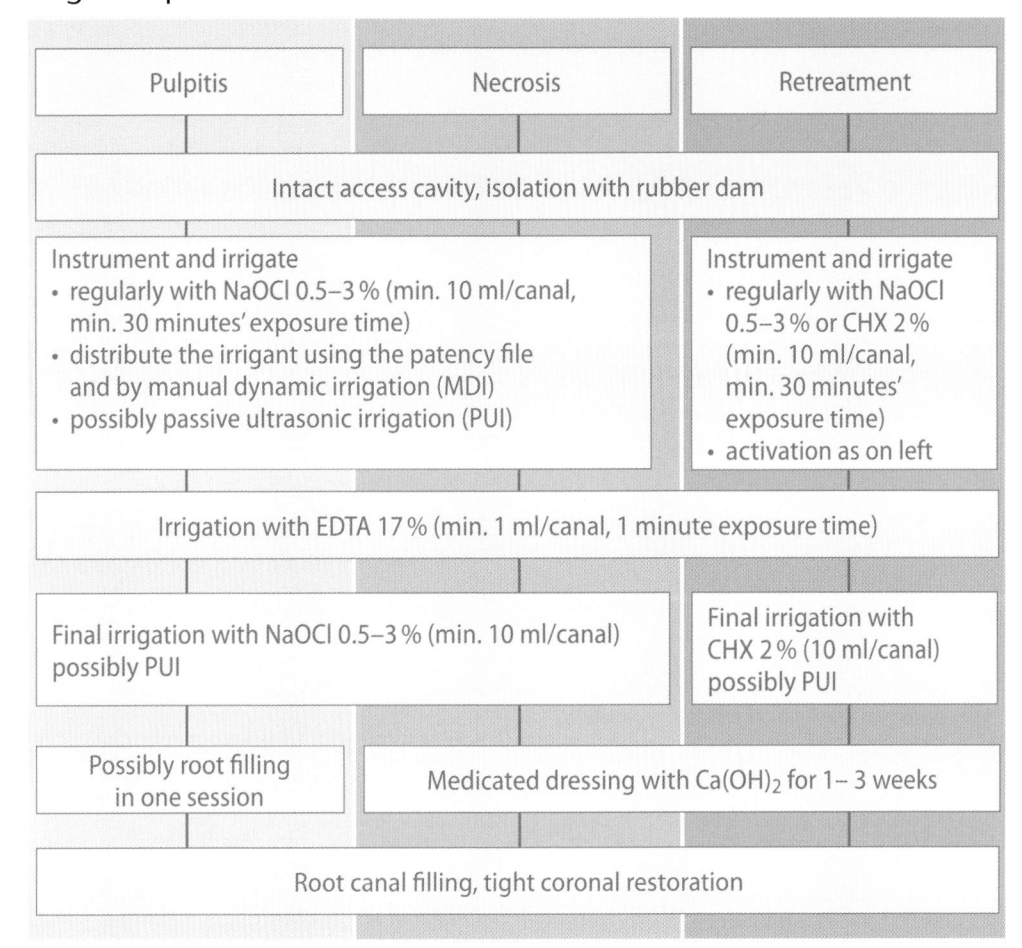

Instrument and irrigate
- regularly with NaOCl 0.5–3 % or CHX 2 % (min. 10 ml/canal, min. 30 minutes' exposure time)
- activation as on left

Irrigation with EDTA 17 % (min. 1 ml/canal, 1 minute exposure time)

Final irrigation with NaOCl 0.5–3 % (min. 10 ml/canal) possibly PUI

Final irrigation with CHX 2 % (10 ml/canal) possibly PUI

Possibly root filling in one session

Medicated dressing with Ca(OH)$_2$ for 1–3 weeks

Root canal filling, tight coronal restoration

Fig 21-2 Recommended irrigation protocol (based on Zehnder et al[30])

■ References

1. Ahmad M. Effect of ultrasonic instrumentation on Bacteroides intermedius. Endod Dent Traumatol 1989;5:83–86.
2. Basrani BR, Manek S, Sodhi RN, Fillery E, Manzur A. Interaction between sodium hypochlorite and chlorhexidine gluconate. J Endod 2007;33:966–969.
3. Boessler C, Peters OA, Zehnder M. Impact of lubricant parameters on rotary instrument torque and force. J Endod 2007;33:280–283.
4. Byström A, Sundqvist G. Bacteriologic evaluation of the efficacy of mechanical root canal instrumentation in endodontic therapy. Scand J Dent Res 1981;89:321–328.
5. Calt S, Serper A. Time-dependent effects of EDTA on dentin structures. J Endod 2002;28:17–19.
6. Hecker H, Amato M, Weiger R. Die Wurzelkanalspülung. Zahnmedizin up2date 2007;2:89–109.
7. Hülsmann M, Heckendorff M, Lennon A. Chelating agents in root canal treatment: mode of action and indications for their use – a review. Int Endod J 2003;36:810–830.
8. Kakehashi S, Stanley HR, Fitzgerald RJ. The effects of surgical exposures of dental pulps in germ-free and conventional laboratory rats. Oral Surg Oral Med Oral Pathol 1965 Sep;20:340–349.
9. Khademi AA, Mohammadi Z, Havaee A. Evaluation of the antibacterial substantivity of several intra-canal agents. Aust Endod J 2006;32(3):112–115.
10. Langeland K. Tissue response to dental caries. Endod Dent Traumatol 1987;3:149–171.
11. Machtou P. Irrigation investigation in endodontics. Paris VII University, Paris, France; Master thesis; 1980.

12. Miller WD. An introduction to the study of the bacterio-pathology of the dental pulp. Dental Cosmos 1894;36:505–528.
13. Naenni N, Thoma K, Zehnder M. Soft tissue dissolution capacity of currently used and potential endodontic irrigants. J Endod 2004;30:785–787.
14. Nair PN. Pathogenesis of apical periodontitis and the causes of endodontic failures. Crit Rev Oral Biol Med 2004 Nov 1;15:348–381.
15. Nygaard-Östby B. Chelation in root canal therapy. Odontol Tidskr 1957;65:3–11.
16. Orstavik D, Haapasalo M. Disinfection by endodontic irrigants and dressings of experimentally infected dentinal tubules. Endod Dent Traumatol. 1990;6(4):142–149.
17. Peters LB, Wesselink PR, Buijs JF, van Winkelhoff A.J. Viable bacteria in root dentinal tubules of teeth with apical periodontitis. J Endod 2001;27:76–781.
18. Peters OA, Barbakow F, Peters CI. An analysis of endodontic treatment with three nickel-titanium rotary root canal preparation techniques. Int Endod J 2004;37:849–859.
19. Portenier I, Waltimo T, Haapasalo M. Enterococcus faecalis– the root canal survivor and 'star' in post-treatment disease. Endodontic Topics 2003;6:135–159.
20. Ram Z. Effectiveness of root canal irrigation. Oral Surg Oral Med Oral Pathol 1977;44:306–312.
21. Schilder H. Cleaning and shaping the root canal. Dent Clin North Am 1974;18:269–296.
22. Sirtes G, Waltimo T, Schaetzle M, Zehnder M. The effects of temperature on sodium hypochlorite short-term stability, pulp dissolution capacity and antimicrobial efficacy. J Endod 2005;31:669–671.
23. Spangberg L. Kinetic and quantitative evaluation of material cytotoxicity *in vitro*. Oral Surg Oral Med Oral Pathol 1973;35:389–401.
24. Spratt DA, Pratten J, Wilson M, Gulabivala K. An *in vitro* evaluation of the antimicrobial efficacy of irrigants on biofilms of root canal isolates. Int Endod J 2001;34:300–307.
25. Sundqvist G, Bacteriological studies of necrotic dental pulps, PhD thesis, Umea, Sweden: Umea University, Odontology Dissertation (No. 7) (1976), pp. 1–94.
26. Svensäter G, Bergenholz G. Biofilms in endodontic infections. Endod Topics 2004;9:27–36.
27. Waltimo T, Haapasalo M, Zehnder M, Meyer J.Clinical aspects related to endodontic yeast infections. Endodontic Topics 2004;9:66–78.
28. Weller RN, Brady JM, Bernier WE. Efficacy of ultrasonic cleaning. J Endod 1980;6:740–743.
29. Wilson M. Susceptibility of oral bacterial biofilms to antimicrobial agents. J Med Microbiol 1996;44:79–87.
30. Zehnder M, Lehnert B, Schönenberger K, Waltimo T. Spüllösungen und medikamentöse Einlagen in der Endodontie. Schweiz Monatsschr Zahnmed 2003;113:756–763.
31. Zehnder M, Schmidlin P, Sener B, Waltimo T. Chelation in root canal therapy reconsidered. J Endod 2005;31:-817–820.
32. Zehnder M. Root canal irrigants. J Endod 2006;32:389–398.

22 Root canal filling

Stefan Hänni

■ Importance of root canal filling

The knowledge that thorough preparation and disinfection of the root canal is crucial to the success of a root canal treatment has now become accepted.[4,14] However, the literature does prove that there is also a direct correlation between the quality of the root canal filling and long-term success.[18]

Objectives of root canal filling
- To seal the link between mouth and apex (preventing recontamination).
- To isolate remaining microorganisms (entombment).
- To prevent fluid leakage from coronally and apically.

■ Quality of root canal filling

The quality of a root canal filling can usually only be assessed on radiographs. A radiologically satisfactory obturation shows a conical shape towards the apex which encompasses the original canal. It is homogeneous and continuous with the canal wall. It fills the canal system three-dimensionally as far as the defined working length.[9] Although the interpretation of a root canal filling on a radiograph is of limited informative value, we should nevertheless use it to help draw conclusions about the quality of the practitioner's disinfectant efforts.

■ Importance of coronal reconstruction

Bacteria-proof sealing of the root canal filling by a tight reconstruction is decisive in preventing reinfection with bacteria from the oral cavity. Some authors even attribute greater importance to this aspect than to the tightness of the root filling.[11] However, another study has failed to confirm this relationship.[13]

Furthermore, it is a fact that root-treated teeth fracture more frequently because of the substantial loss of dental tissue that often occurs and the lack of overload protection from pulpal mechanoreceptors.[12,10] In order to ensure long-term success, it is therefore advisable to treat such teeth – especially in the molar region – with an overlay or a crown covering the cusps.

Whereas in the past the definitive restoration was often postponed until a later date in order to await healing of the periapical tissues, nowadays the advice is to carry out definitive restoration as quickly as possible in order to minimize the risk of leakage.

■ When to fill?

Whether a root canal treatment should take place in one session, or in several sessions with an intermediate medicated dressing, is a matter of some debate.[2] While a single-visit treatment is generally accepted in cases of pulpectomy, an intermediate dressing is usually placed in nonvital cases. Before any root canal filling is carried out, the following conditions must always be met.

Requirements for root canal filling
- Preparation of the root canal must be completed and it must be thoroughly disinfected.
- The root canal must be dry and odor-free.
- The tooth should be free of symptoms.

■ What filling material?

Root filling materials

Requirements for an ideal filling material
An ideal filling material is:
- Biocompatible
- Easy to apply in the root canal
- Deformable (so that root canal irregularities can be properly filled)
- Not soluble in body fluids
- Sterilizable
- Not staining to the teeth
- Dimensionally stable (no shrinkage or expansion)
- Radiopaque
- Revisable (post insertion, retreatment)

To date, no single material has been able to fulfill all these requirements. This is why root canal fillings are performed as a combination of a volumetrically stable core material and a cement.

Core materials

Gutta-percha
The world's most widely used core material is gutta-percha. It is made from the rubber-like resin from the *Palaquium gutta* tree, with the addition of zinc oxide, waxes, and radiodense metallic salts.

Gutta-percha should always be used in combination with a root-filling cement (sealant).[19]

Resilon™
Resilon™ is a thermoplastic polymer introduced as a replacement for gutta-percha. A methacrylate is used as the sealant and a bonding agent is used to bond to dentine. Resilon can be worked like gutta-percha. Although assessments of the product were extremely positive after its introduction,[17] the judgment since then has proved to be far more cautious.[20]

Metal points
Metal pins (silver or titanium points) fall well short of the current requirements for a core material.

Root filling cements (sealants)
The above-mentioned criteria also apply when selecting the sealant to be used. Pastes with added medication, eg, N2 (Sargenti paste), do not meet today's standards because of a lack of biocompatibility and so they should be rejected.[9] There is some criticism of glass ionomer cements with regard to their solubility. Furthermore, their use for time-consuming or thermoplastic filling techniques is problematic because of the short setting time and their sensitivity to heat. The use of adhesively worked polymers should also be avoided for the time being because of the contradictory data currently available.[17,20]

With a view to the parameters of tissue compatibility, solubility, and wall tightness, sealers based on silicone, polyketone, zinc oxide-eugenol, and epoxide resin are suitable for clinical use. Among these, the epoxide resin-based root filling cements are the most commonly used and the most studied (Table 22-1).[15]

Table 22-1 Different root filling cements

Zinc oxide-eugenol-based	Synthetic resin-based	Silicone-based	Medicated pastes	Glass ionomer cements	Polyketone-based
TubuliSeal	AH26	RSA RoekoSeal Automix	Iodoform paste	Ketac-Endo	Diaket
Pulp canal sealer	AH Plus (2Seal)	GuttaFlow	Endomethasone		
			N2 (Sargenti paste)		

How to fill?

The range of filling techniques extends from pure cement/paste fillings, to the single-cone technique (paste filling with a central cone) and the cold lateral condensation technique, through to thermoplastic filling methods. The latter involve injecting warm gutta-percha or applying it with a carrier or by means of a condenser.

Paste fillings

Justified by the claim that disinfection of the complex canal system is too time-consuming and technically impossible, strongly toxic medicated pastes or cements have sometimes been applied into the canal – after minimal "preparation".

Pure paste fillings do not fulfill the current requirements for an adequate canal treatment.[9] In particular, they contradict the biological concept that, for long-term success, what you take out of the canal (disinfection) is more important than you what you put into it (obturation).

Problems of paste fillings
- Toxicity of the materials
- Shrinkage
- Solubility over time
- Difficult to control length
- Limited retreatability

Single-cone technique

In the single-cone technique, after preparation of an apical stop a single gutta-percha cone is cemented in the canal.[6] The single-cone technique is a simple and quick obturation method. The proportion of cement is relatively high, depending on the canal shape. With the advent of rotary nickel-titanium (Ni-Ti) instruments and matching gutta-percha points, use of the single-cone technique is again increasing. Filling with thinner and more homogeneous cement sealants is feasible due to the centered, more uniform preparation and the matching points and has been proven in laboratory studies.[3,8]

The single-cone technique should only be used where there is good congruence of form between the canal and the gutta-percha cone.

Problems of the single-cone technique
- Canal incongruencies can only be inadequately filled.
- Shrinkage.
- Solubility over time.
- Where points are conical throughout their length, the cone often binds in the cervical area rather than the apical area.

Lateral condensation

In lateral condensation, a gutta-percha cone that corresponds to the master file is inserted so that it binds at the apical stop. After it has been cemented, the master point is pressed against the root canal wall with a spreader. The resulting cavity is filled by pushing in an accessory point. A homogeneous root canal filling largely made up of gutta-percha is gradually achieved by repeated insertion of the spreader and by cold deformation.

The lateral condensation method is very widely used around the world and is generally regarded as the reference method.

Problems of the lateral condensation technique
- The filling technique is relatively complex and hence time-consuming.
- Improper condensation can lead to root fractures.[7]
- The technique is not ideal for root canals with a very oval cross-section, with abrupt changes of diameter (eg, in the case of internal resorption), or with open apices.

Thermoplastic filling methods

A suitable preparation geometry is a prerequisite for thermoplastic filling methods. The root canal preparation must be continuously conical and the apical foramen left as small as possible. Apically the aim is to achieve a so-called "resistance form," with a conicity of at least 8% in order to guarantee vertical condensation without substantial overfilling.[16] Such preparation forms can today be produced rapidly and predictably using rotary Ni-Ti instruments (see chapter 20).[5]

Warm vertical condensation technique[5]/continuous-wave technique[1]

In the warm vertical condensation technique, a suitable master cone is coated with sealant and inserted. The master cone is then melted using a warm plugger in several waves and condensed in an apical direction. This involves removing a gutta-percha increment from the canal every time until eventually a 4 to 5 mm long apical "plug" remains in the canal ("downpack").

In the continuous-wave technique, however, the downpack is performed in a single step. Using a gutta-percha injection gun, warm gutta-percha is applied to the apical seal in portions and condensed ("backfill"). The technique requires a relatively large amount of space in the root canal to be properly carried out. The dentin loss is thus relatively large. If the opening is not wide enough and consequently the pluggers do not get close enough to the root apex, the gutta-percha will be inadequately condensed and the technique only has the same effect as a single-cone filling in the sensitive apical area.

The warm vertical condensation technique is currently the best method for three-dimensional filling of the root canal system. The method is quick to use and versatile.

Problems of the warm vertical condensation technique
- A wide cervical preparation is required, which leads to relatively large dentin loss.
- The filling technique entails substantial equipment costs.

Carrier-based filling systems

The carrier-based systems involve heating the gutta-percha on a plastic carrier in a furnace, then placing it in the root canal. After cooling of the gutta-percha, the carrier is removed at the root canal orifice. Thermafil® is the best-known of these systems.

Carrier-based systems are widely used. They are especially efficient in long, curved root canals. Carrier-based fillings can be performed relatively quickly.

Problems of the carrier-based filling technique
- Overfilling of cement and gutta-percha cannot always be avoided.
- Genuine condensation and hence compensation for shrinkage during cooling is not possible.
- Preparation of the post space and retreatment of the filling are difficult to do.

Condenser-based technique (MicroSeal system)

This system combines the lateral condensation technique with thermoplastic filling. After a master cone has been fitted and cemented in place, as in lateral condensation, space for the warm gutta-percha is created using a spreader. The heated gutta-percha is picked up with a condenser clamped into the contra-angle handpiece and it is rotated into the cavity.

A three-dimensional root canal filling can be achieved with little time and effort.

Problems of the condenser-based technique
- The excessive overfilling of cement and gutta-percha cannot always be avoided.
- Instrument fractures can occur.

■ Conclusions

The literature does not provide any clear-cut statements on which root canal filling technique can guarantee the success of a root canal treatment over any other. Furthermore, as mentioned in the introduction, other factors such as careful preparation and conscientious disinfection contribute far more to the success of a treatment than the choice of material or method of root canal filling. Bearing this in mind, it may be justifiable to choose the filling method on the basis of individual, subjective criteria (Table 22-2).[21]

Table 22-2 Rating of different filling methods

Filling method	Tightness	Simplicity	Retreatability	Control of length	Toxicity	Costs
Paste fillings	O	++	O – ++	O	O – ++	O
Single-cone technique (gutta-percha, sealer)	+	++	O – ++	+	O	O
Lateral condensation technique (gutta-percha, sealant)	++	O	+ – ++	++	O	+
Warm vertical condensation technique (gutta-percha, sealant)	++	O	+ – ++	++	O	++
Carrier-based systems (Thermafil®)	+	+	O	O	O	++
Condenser-based systems (MicroSeal)	+	+	O – ++	O	O	+

O = none/minimal;   + = good/moderate;   ++ = very good/high

References

1. Buchanan LS. The continuous wave of condensation technique: a convergence of conceptual and procedural advances in obturation. Dent Today 1994;13: 80–85.
2. Figini L, Lodi G, Gorni F, Gagliani M. Single versus multiple visits for endodontic treatment of permanent teeth: a Cochrane systematic review. J Endod 2008;34:1041–1047.
3. Gordon MP, Love RM, Chandler NP. An evaluation of .06 tapered gutta-percha cones for filling of .06 prepared curved canals. Int Endod J 2005;38:87–96.
4. Haapasalo M, Endal U, Zandi H, Coil JM. Eradication of endodontic infection by instrumentation and irrigation solutions. Endod Topics 2005;10:77–102.
5. Hülsmann M, Peters OE, Dummer PMH. Mechanical preparation of root canals: shaping goals, techniques and means. Endod Topics 2004;10:30–76.
6. Ingle JI. A standardised endodontic technique using newly designed instruments and filling materials. Oral Surg 1961;14:83–91.
7. Lertchirakarn V, Palamara JEA, Messer HH. Load and strain during lateral condensation and vertical root fracture. J Endod 1999;25:99–104.
8. Ozawa T, Taha N, Messer HH. A comparison of techniques for obturating oval-shaped root canals. Dent Mater J 2009;28:290–294.
9. Qualitätsleitlinien in der Zahnmedizin. Handbuch. Schweizerische Zahnärzte-Gesellschaft SSO. 2005;105–118.
10. Randow K, Glantz PO. On cantilever loading of vital and non-vital teeth. An experimental study. Acta Odontol Scand 1986;44:271–277.
11. Ray HA, Trope M. Periapical status of endodontically treated teeth in relation to the technical quality of the root filling and the coronal restoration. Int Endod J 1995;28:12–18.
12. Reeh ES, Messer HH, Douglas WH. Reduction in tooth stiffness as a result of endodontic and restorative procedures. J Endod 1989;15:512–516.
13. Ricucci D, Bergenholtz G. Bacterial status in rootfilled teeth exposed to the oral environment by loss of restoration and fracture or caries – a histobacteriological study of treated cases. Int Endod J 2003;36:787–802.
14. Sabeti MA, Nekofar M, Motahhary P, Ghandi M, Simon JH. Healing of apical periodontitis after endodontic treatment with and without obturation in dogs. J Endod 2006;32:628–633.
15. Schäfer E. Wurzelkanalfüllmaterialien. Schweiz Monatsschr Zahnmed 2000;110:849–861.

16. Schilder H. Filling root canals in three dimensions. Dent Clin North Am 1967;11:723–744.
17. Shipper G, Ørstavik D, Teixeira FB, Trope M. An evaluation of microbial leakage in roots filled with a thermoplastic synthetic polymer-based root canal filling material (Resilon). J Endod 2004;30:342–347.
18. Sjögren U, Hägglund B, Sundquist G, Wing K. Factors affecting the long-term result of endodontic treatment. J Endod 1990;16:498–504.
19. Tagger M, Katz A, Tamse A. Apical seal using GPII method in straight canals compared with lateral condensation with or without sealer. Oral Surg Oral Med Oral Pathol 1994;78:225.
20. Tay FR, Pashley H. Monoblocks in root canals: a hypothetical or a tangible goal. J Endod 2007;33:391–398.
21. Withworth J. Methods of filling root canals: principles and practices. Endod Topics 2005;12:2–24.

23 Cracked tooth syndrome

Stefan Hänni and Adrian Lussi

■ Introduction

Dentin hypersensitivity is a common complaint. The following causes of pain, in descending order of prevalence, should be considered:
- Pain due to exposure of the dentin (dentin hypersensitivity)
- Pain due to cracks in the dentin and/or enamel (known as "cracked tooth syndrome")
- Pain following insertion of restorations

Dentin hypersensitivity mainly affects the canines, premolars, and molars. In various studies, between 4% and 57% of people questioned claimed to have at least one hypersensitive tooth.[2,3,5,6] The age of those affected is usually between 20 and 40 years. Later the formation of partly atubular secondary dentin is responsible for the fact that A-beta and A-delta fibers, which are significant for pain transformation, are not stimulated anymore.

Various active ingredients are recommended for the treatment of hypersensitive teeth:
- *Sealing the tubules*:
  - NaF varnish (22600 ppm F^-)
  - arginine (8%) with calcium carbonate.
- *Interrupting nerve conduction:*
  - dentifrice with potassium salts that contain 2% potassium ions as active ingredients. The most commonly used compounds are potassium nitrate (5%), potassium chloride (3.75%), and potassium citrate (5.5%).

The prevention of pain after insertion of restorations is based on using an adhesive system to seal the dentinal tubules exposed by acid (immediate dentin sealing, IDS; see chapter 17). This chapter explores the clinically challenging subject of cracked tooth syndrome.

Definition and etiology

The term "cracked tooth syndrome" covers all the symptoms associated with cracks in the dental tissue, which can range from a fine craze line through to complete splitting of a tooth.[1] Table 23-1 lists the five categories of possible cracks.

Teeth are capable of withstanding the masticatory forces that occur physiologically, therefore it is mainly nonphysiological stresses that lead to infractions (Table 23-2).

The individual risk of a crack or infraction of a tooth is influenced by a number of morphological factors; eg, pronounced intercuspidation, a large pulp cavity, premature contacts, and sharp contacts in the molar region in an open front bite or cross-bite. Loss of hard dental tissue of any origin (developmental anomalies, untreated carious lesions, erosion, abrasion, or attrition) can weaken teeth and make them susceptible to cracks.

However, it is dental procedures that have the greatest influence on the fracture risk (Table 23-3).

Table 23-1 Classification of cracked tooth syndrome

Craze line
Cracked tooth
Cusp fracture
Split tooth
Vertical root fracture (VRF)

Table 23-2 Etiological factors

Accidental trauma   Teeth impacting together as a result of an accident
Masticatory trauma   Unintentional biting onto a small hard object (the entire occlusal force is exerted on a small surface)
Occlusal trauma (parafunctions, oral habits, piercing)

Table 23-3 Iatrogenic factors

Cavity preparation   Dentin loss, undermining preparation   Vibrations due to rotary instruments, mechanical amalgam condensation
Underfilling   Lack of dimensional stability – washing out – wedging effect of unsupported restoration
Filling materials   Stress phenomena due to expansion or contraction of the material
Wedging effect when cementing inlays
Insertion of parapulpal pins, root canal posts, and screws
Placement of restorations/materials using acoustic or ultrasonic devices
Overloading of abutment teeth by fixed or removable dentures

■ Epidemiology

There are no precise figures on the epidemiology of individual fracture types.[10] While craze lines (enamel cracks) are relatively common and are found in 55% to 70% of all teeth,[12,16] infractions (cracked teeth) are generally seen as rare.[4,8] In his referral practice, Krell found infractions in only 9.7% of cases among more than 8,000 teeth.[9]

Cusp fractures are relatively common. The frequency of vertical root fractures and split teeth is not known.

Infractions are increasingly being observed nowadays. The life expectancy of patients is higher, teeth are being preserved longer and, not least, awareness of the problem among practitioners is gradually increasing, which leads to more diagnoses.

Only 10% to 15% of all teeth with vertical cracks will develop pains typical of infractions.[12,16]

■ Distribution

Depending on the cause, infractions can basically occur at any age. They are more common in people over the age of 40. The highest frequency is in the 40 to 50 years age group. Men and women appear to be equally affected.

■ Tooth type

The figures on the risk of cracked teeth for the different types of teeth are inconsistent. While Cameron described the mandibular second molar as the most susceptible tooth,[1] others regard the mandibular first molar as the most commonly affected.[16] Basically, the molars in the mandible seem to be more susceptible than the other teeth.[4,10] According to the data of Roh and Lee, however, the maxillary molars are the most commonly affected at 60%.[14]

Premolars are far less commonly affected than molars.[10] In the study by Veltmaat, the mandibular premolars seem to be markedly more resistant than the premolars of the maxilla.[16]

Essentially it can be said that the molars are more frequently affected by cracked tooth syndrome than the premolars.

Distribution of cracked tooth syndrome
Lower molars > upper molars > upper premolars >>> lower premolars

The mandibular molars are presumably the most severely affected because they are the longest in occlusion and because they are often extensively restored. The molars are also in the center of masticatory pressure and are hence the most strongly loaded.[12] Furthermore, the tooth inclination in mandibular molars is believed to predispose them to cracked tooth syndrome.[16] Another possible reason is a wedging effect of the prominent mesiopalatal cusps of the maxillary molars on the mandibular molars. In addition, the transverse crest might make the maxillary molars more resistant.

■ Restoration

The available data on the influence of restoration on the risk of a tooth becoming cracked are not very informative. There is a selected patient population in many of the studies, and some of the studies employ finite-element models whose clinical relevance is limited.

Nevertheless, the fact that filled teeth sustain fractures and cracks far more frequently than nonfilled teeth can be regarded as proven. The extent of the restoration is a crucial factor; in symptomatic cases in particular, the depth of the cavity seems to be more important than its width. Homewood[7] speculated that cracks starting from the transition between cavity floor and cavity wall run parallel to the direction of the forces acting on the relevant cusps. This would cause superficial cracks at the periphery in wide cavities and would tend to cause deep cracks running centrally in deep, narrow cavities.

Root-treated teeth are significantly more commonly affected.[16] The reason for this lies in very extensive loss of hard dental tissue in most of these teeth and in the lack of proprioception.[13]

However, restoration-free teeth can also display cracks or fractures. In the study by Roh and Lee,[14] 60% of the affected teeth had not been reconstructed.

■ Symptoms

Only about 10% to 15% of cracked teeth show symptoms typical of fractures.[12,16] The symptoms that originate from these teeth can be very varied and can therefore be confusing. Depending on severity, course, and extent, and depending on how long the symptoms have persisted, the patient will report a variety of symptoms. Nevertheless, there are some cardinal symptoms which should alert clinicians to the possibility of cracked teeth when diagnosing nonspecific complaints (Table 23-4).

Table 23-4 Cardinal symptoms of cracked tooth syndrome

Short, shooting pain on biting
Rebound pain
Increased sensitivity to thermal and/or osmotic stimuli
If the pulp is involved: • Symptoms of early or irreversible pulpitis
If the periodontium is involved: • Diffuse, dull pain combined with a narrow area of periodontal breakdown • Symptoms of a periodontal abscess
If pains have pre-existed for a long time: • Diffuse symptoms of chronic pain radiating into other areas (opposing jaw, temporomandibular jaw, ear, etc)

The pain typical of a cracked tooth is explained by the theory of hydrodynamic activation of A-beta and A-delta fibers in dentin. Fluid is moved rapidly in the tubules as a result of biting and, especially, relaxation of the bite, so that the nerve fibers in the plexus of *Raschkow* are stimulated.

■ Clinical picture

Table 23-5 Clinical picture, fracture paths

Cracked tooth
• Usually running vertically through the tooth
• Less commonly horizontal and oblique cracks also possible
• Usually originating from one or both marginal ridges in a mesiodistal direction
• Less commonly in the bucco-oral direction
Cusp fracture
• Often only one cusp affected
• Fracture line runs from the marginal ridge through the buccal and lingual fissure in a cervical direction
• Fracture line usually ends parallel to the gingiva or slightly subgingivally
Split tooth
• Usually a mesiodistal path
• Split runs through both marginal ridges
• Tooth is completely separated into two segments
Vertical root fracture
• Fracture starts in the root
• Fracture line usually runs in the bucco-oral direction
• Fracture line extends in a bucco-oral direction right through the root or the fracture is incomplete
• Vertical linear extension of the fracture line varies very widely

■ Diagnosis

Cracked teeth are relatively rare. The diversity of symptoms and the poor awareness among practitioners often result in misdiagnoses, delayed treatment, and ultimately tooth loss. It is impossible to diagnose what you are unaware of. Practitioners should therefore get to know about the symptoms and the clinical implications of cracked teeth. In all cases of unexplainable, puzzling chronic pain, the dentist should think of "cracked tooth syndrome".

During history-taking, clinicians should ask patients about their history of trauma and look for any signs of masticatory trauma, parafunctions, or oral habits. Repeated occlusal adjustment, repeated debonding of restorations, or unsuccessfully treated "cervical hypersensitivity" may provide evidence of the presence of cracked teeth. In addition to the general history-taking, a detailed record of the pain history should be taken.

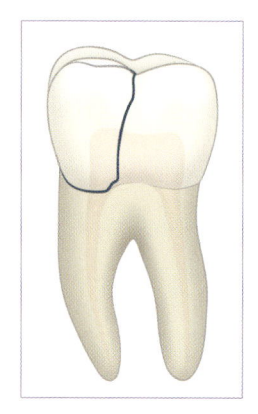

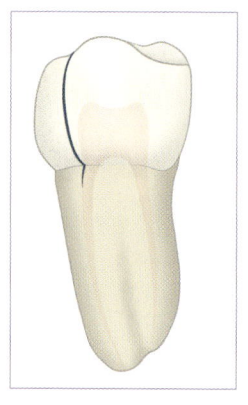

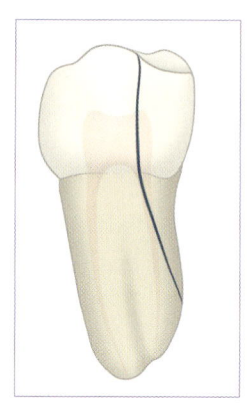

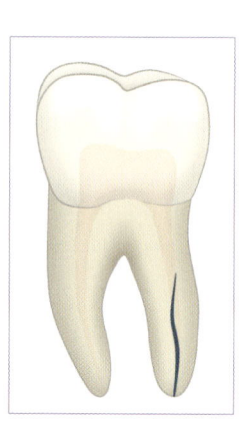

Fig 23-1 Typical fracture paths in cracked tooth syndrome.

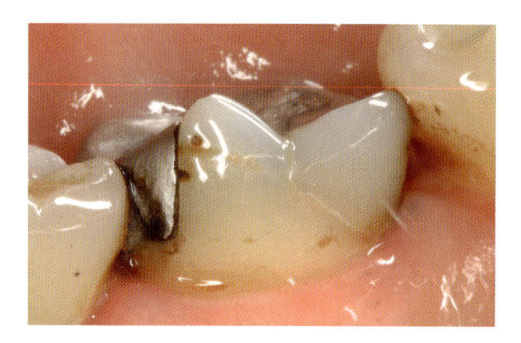

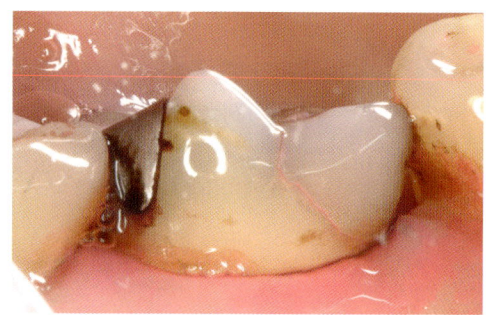

Fig 23-2 Visualizing the fracture line by staining with plaque revealer.

Clinical examination

The clinical examination first focuses on finding the tooth affected. Second, the exact location and path of the crack should be identified. Finally, it should be determined whether or not root canal treatment is necessary. Figure 23-1 shows typical fracture paths.

The possible elements of the clinical examination comprise the following:
- Visual inspection (on the dried and cleaned teeth; use a magnification aid):
  - examine the dentition for malocclusions which might shed light on inappropriate loading.
  - look for signs of oral habits (wear facets, linea alba, fractured reconstructions).
  - look for enamel cracks and fracture lines (staining with a plaque revealer makes them more clearly visible, Fig 23-2).
- Examination with a (perio-)probe:
  - look for atypical cracks in the teeth and between teeth and reconstructions.
  - look for isolated, narrow periodontal pockets.
- Examination using cotton roll or a special instrument (Crack Finder, Tooth Slooth):
  - conduct a bite test using a cotton roll to reproduce the reported pains and thus identify the tooth affected.
  - identify the cusp(s) affected by loading and unloading using the Crack Finder (Fig 23-3).
- Percussion test:
  - from occlusally often negative; sometimes lateral sensitivity.

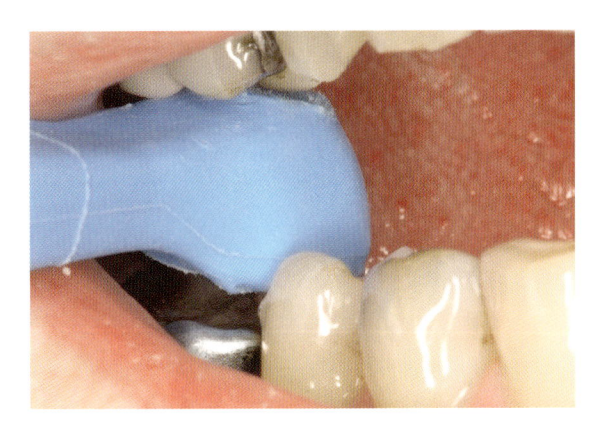

Fig 23-3 The Crack Finder can be helpful for diagnosis.

- Transillumination (using cold light probe; exceptionally using a curing light):
  - fractures that run through enamel and dentin will block the path of light.
  - by contrast, healthy dental tissue and enamel cracks do not block the path of light.
- Sensitivity test:
  - variable depending on the state of the pulp.
  - gives indication of whether root canal treatment is necessary.
  - an attempt can be made with a fine air syringe to reproduce thermal hypersensitivity.

Radiologic examination

Cracks can not usually be detected on radiographs. The image may provide indirect evidence in the case of vertical root fractures. A suspected diagnosis may be confirmed in the case of split teeth with dislocation of the fragments. Nevertheless a radiograph must always be taken if there are unexplained pains in order to exclude other pathologies.

Removal of a restoration or trial cavity

Given a strong enough suspicion, complete removal of the restoration is performed or, in the case of unfilled teeth, an occlusal cavity preparation is carried out in terms of extended fissure sealing, followed by examination of the cavity using a microscope or loupes. Staining with methylene blue or plaque revealers or brushing pumice powder into the cavity might be necessary for the best visualization of fractures. A rubber dam will increase the contrast and keep the cavity dry.

Treatment

There are indications in the literature that dental fractures are the third most common cause of dental loss in the industrialized societies. This is why it is important to raise awareness about cracked tooth syndrome.

In the case of cracked tooth syndrome, prevention still comes before treatment. The preventive measures include defect-related, minimally invasive preparation and early stabilizing treatment of teeth at risk of becoming cracked. A cusp-covering restoration is important, particularly for endodontically treated teeth with substantial loss of substance. Whenever possible, screws and posts should be dispensed with; parapulpal pins are obsolete. Treatment should be undertaken quickly if there are occlusal interferences and parafunctions.

Aims of treatment for symptomatic cracked teeth
- Stabilize the remaining hard dental tissue in order to prevent or at least slow down any further propagation of the fracture line.
- Relieve symptoms.
- Keep the pulp vital.

Based on the above goals, there are various therapeutic approaches to symptomatic cracked teeth. Possible forms of treatment are shown in Table 23-6. The clinical situation, the patient's needs, and the skills of the practitioner will dictate a pragmatic approach, which may differ from the proposed treatments listed below.

Traditional therapeutic approaches are usually based on a restoration with indirect reconstructions, especially with complete crowns. However, recent studies have questioned this approach. On the one hand, they prove that cracked teeth can be successfully treated for years with composite resin restorations.[11,15] On the other hand, it emerges that the compromised pulp of cracked teeth reacts to crowning with an increased rate of necrosis.[9]

Table 23-6 Forms of treatment and indications

Treatment	Indication	Advantages	Disadvantages
Banding	• Emergency treatment • Diagnosis	• Interim solution • Cost-effective	Interim solution
Composite resin restoration (with or without cuspal coverage)	Smaller defects	• Substance-sparing • Single session (no provisional)	
CEREC®	Extensive defects (supragingival)	• Single session (no provisional) • Life-span	• Loss of substance • Price
Ceramic restoration	Extensive defects (supragingival)	• Esthetics • Life-span	• Provisional necessary • Loss of substance • Price
PFM crown	Extensive defects (subgingival)	• Esthetics • Life-span	• Pulp vitality • Provisional necessary • Loss of substance • Price
Gold restoration	Extensive defects (subgingival)	• Life-span	• Esthetics • Loss of substance • Price
Extraction	When there are no alternatives	• Rapid freedom from pain • "Cost-effective"	Tooth loss

References

1. Cameron CE. Cracked-tooth syndrome. J Am Dent Assoc 1964;68:405–411.
2. Clark GE, Troullos ES. Designing hypersensitivity clinical studies. Dent Clin North Am 1990;34:531–544.
3. Docimo R, Montesani L, Maturo P, Costacurta M, Bartolino M DeVizio W, Zhang YP, Cummins D, Dibart S, Mateo LR. Comparing the efficacy in reducing dentin hypersensitivity of a new toothpaste containing 8.0 % arginine, calcium carbonate, and 1450 ppm fluoride to a commercial sensitive toothpaste containing 2 % potassium ion: An eight-week clinical study in Rome, Italy. J Clin Dent (Spec Iss) 2009;20:17–22.
4. Gher ME Jr, Dunlap RM, Anderson MH, Kuhl LV. Clinical survey of fractured teeth. J Am Dent Assoc 1987;114: 174–177.
5. Gysi A. An attempt to explain the sensitiveness of dentine. Br J Dent Res 1900;43:865.
6. Haywood VB. Dentine hypersensitivity: Bleaching and restorative considerations for successful management. Int Dent J 2002;52:376–385.
7. Homewood Cl. Cracked tooth syndrome – incidence, clinical findings and treatment. Aust Dent J 1998;43: 217–222.
8. Krejci I, Krejci D, Lutz F. Partial fracture of the molar. Treatment of a partial fracture of the molar using a composite for posterior teeth and a glass ionomer base filling. Schweiz Monatsschr Zahnmed 1988;98:260–263.
9. Krell KV, Rivera A. six year evaluation of cracked teeth diagnosed with reversible pulpitis: treatment and prognosis. J Endod 2007;33:1405–1407.
10. Löst C, Bengel W, Hehner B. Tooth infraction. Incomplete tooth fracture – a review of various aspects of the disease with case reports. Schweiz Monatsschr Zahnmed 1989;99:1033–1040.
11. Opdam NJ, Roeters JJ, Loomans BA, Bronkhorst EM. Seven-year clinical evaluation of painful cracked teeth restored with a direct composite restoration. J Endod 2008;34:808–811.
12. Pieper K, Betas J, Motsch A. Zur Prävalenz von Zahninfraktionen – eine Untersuchung mit der Kaltlichtsonde. Dtsch Zahnärztl Z 1994;49:822–824.
13. Randow K, Glantz PO. On cantilever loading of vital and non-vital teeth. An experimental clinical study. Acta Odontol Scand 1986;44:271–277.
14. Roh BD, Lee YE. Analysis of 154 cases of teeth with cracks. Dent Traumatol 2006;22:118–123.
15. Signore A, Benedicenti S, Covani U, Ravera G. A 4- to 6-year retrospective clinical study of cracked teeth restored with bonded indirect resin composite onlays. Int J Prosthodont 2007;20:609–616.
16. Veltmaat A, Gunay H, Guertsen W. *In vivo* study of the epidemiology of the cracked-tooth syndrome of restored posterior teeth. Dtsch Zahnärztl Z 1997;52:137.

24 Endodontology in the primary dentition

Markus Schaffner, Klaus Neuhaus, and Adrian Lussi

■ Introduction

Children with endodontic problems in the primary dentition often attend dental practices as emergency cases.[8,15,21] As a result of negative experiences during their emergency treatment, these children may develop a phobia of dentists which will make future treatments difficult or entirely impossible. When children with acute pain in the primary dentition come to the dentist for the first time, their anxiety is particularly high. This situation demands considerable psychological and therapeutic skill to avoid damaging the relationship of trust between child and practitioner.

This chapter deals with the diagnosis of endodontology problems in the primary dentition and examines treatment options – whether planned or emergency treatments.

A precise diagnosis needs to be made before any therapeutic measures are taken. Often, however, this is not straightforward with a child suffering from toothache. Not uncommonly the information from children proves to be inaccurate. They often keep quiet about pains in the hope of avoiding any treatment. Nevertheless the history-taking, the clinical examination, and the radiograph should lead to the correct diagnosis and treatment (Tables 24-1 and 24-2). As a rule, a radiographic image is actually indispensable in the primary dentition for diagnostic purposes. This is the only way to gain information about the proximity of a carious lesion or a restoration to the pulp, about physiological and non-physiological, internal and external resorptions, about periradicular or interradicular radiolucencies, and about the relationship of the permanent tooth germ to the roots of the primary tooth.

Table 24-1 History taking in children with toothache in primary teeth

Is the pain intermittent or constant? Does the child have pain during the night?
What irritant or stimulus triggers the pain? Is it cold or heat? Does the child have pain when chewing or eating sweet things?
Does the child have a bad taste in his/her mouth?
Does the child have a fever?
Have there been any previous injuries to the teeth?
What is the child's general medical condition? What medicines is the child taking or has he/she taken?
What medical or dental treatments have been carried out recently?

Endodontology

Table 24-2 Special features of the clinical examination

Caution is advisable during clinical examination because of particular aspects of some children's behavior. The following points should be looked for.
Is there any swelling of the face and/or lymph nodes?
Are there any intraoral swellings? Do these swellings fluctuate on palpation?
Can fistulous tracts be probed? Does any pus exude?
Is the painful tooth sensitive to percussion? What is the tap note like?
Are there any sore mucosal areas on palpation?
Is there mobility of the aching tooth?
If caries is present, the consistency and color of the carious material are of interest.
If pulp is opened, the size and location of the opened site as well as the extent and nature of the bleeding can provide valuable information about inflammation of the pulp.
The informative value of the CO_2 test is limited in small children because of the lack of cooperation and, for psychological reasons, it should therefore be used sparingly.

■ Reversible and irreversible pulpitis due to caries

Owing to the large pulp cavity and the minimal thickness of enamel and dentin, caries reaches the dentin close to the pulp after only a short time. Initial signs of inflammation in primary tooth pulp can be observed histologically soon after first contact of caries with dentin. At the beginning, this process is still reversible (reversible pulpitis). However, if the caries advances further, it will result in irreversible spread of the inflammation (irreversible pulpitis). These changes do not always involve severe pain. However, if a primary tooth causes persistent pain and/or pain in response to heat, this means the inflammation has spread to the entire pulp of the primary tooth. Sensitivity to percussion means the inflammation has reached the apical or interradicular periodontium. Clinically, it is often very difficult to distinguish between reversible and irreversible pulpitis, especially because the sensitivity test with cold is not very informative in children. In the same primary tooth, healthy, vital areas of pulp can be observed alongside severely inflamed to necrotic pulp segments (Fig 24-1).

■ Treatments for reversible pulpitis

Incomplete (stepwise) caries excavation

In the case of a vital, symptom-free primary tooth with profound caries, pulp opening can be prevented by incomplete caries excavation. Preparation and thorough excavation of caries close to the pulp are first performed. The carious residual dentin close to the pulp is left in place. The dentin wound is then cleaned and disinfected (eg, with Tubulicid or chlorhexidine). If disinfecting the cavity with hydrogen peroxide, it is important to make sure that polymerization of acrylic resin can be inhibited. After the carious residual dentin has been

Endodontology in the primary dentition

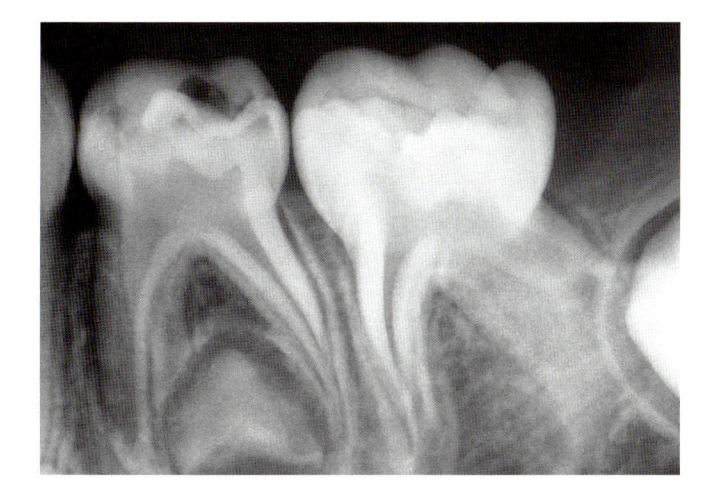

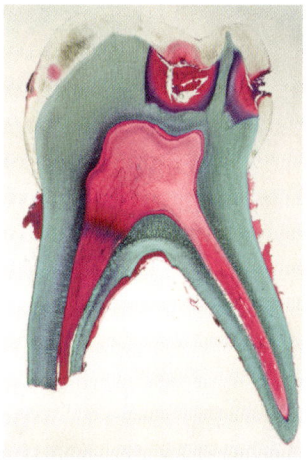

Fig 24-1 Reversible versus irreversible pulpitis

Left: coronal radiolucencies, but no interradicular or periapical radiolucencies, can be seen on the radiograph of the primary left mandibular first molar.

Right: in the histological section through the mesial area of the primary left mandibular first molar, apart from widening of the odontoblast border below the carious lesion and slight proliferation of the blood vessels, no inflammatory changes can be seen. Given appropriate treatment, these are reversible.

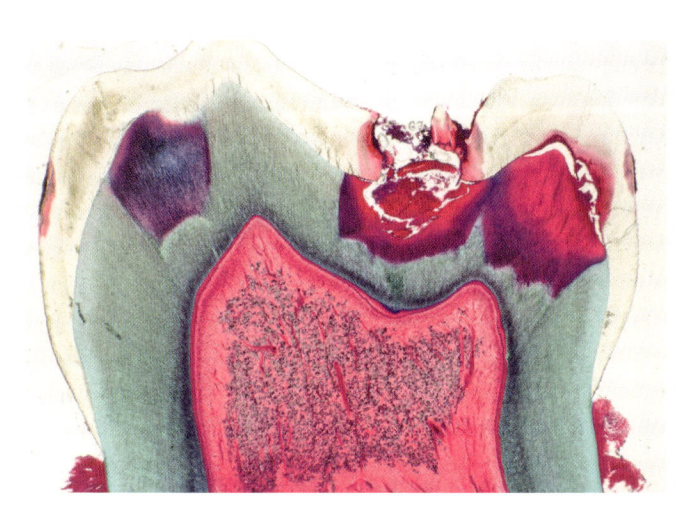

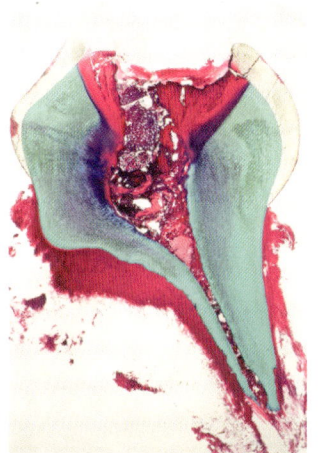

Left: in the histological section through the middle of the primary first molar, bacterial infiltrates and enlarged blood vessels are visible in the pulp. The entire pulp cavity in the area of the section shows pulpitis changes which are only partly reversible.

Right: the histological section through the distal area of the primary first molar shows massive pulp necrosis with opening of the pulp due to the carious process. The pulpal changes are irreversible.

covered with a glass ionomer cement cavity liner (eg, Vitrebond™), a tight seal is created using an adhesive system and composite resin. Various studies have shown that complete removal of caries is not necessary in deep carious lesions in order to prevent progression of the caries.[17] However, a tight restoration that isolates any bacteria remaining in the cavity is a prerequisite. Individual authors dispense with coverage of the carious residual dentin with a cavity liner.[13] Reopening of the cavity, as has been propounded for stepwise caries excavation, is therefore unnecessary for a symptom-free primary tooth where the restoration is intact.

Direct pulp capping

If the pulp is opened at points during caries removal from a symptom-free, vital primary tooth, direct pulp capping can be carried out. The opened pulp is covered with a calcium hydroxide material. This is followed by the application of a liner, then tight closure with a composite resin restoration. The use of mineral trioxide aggregate (MTA) is another option (though not very economical).

Direct capping procedure
1. Disinfection and drying of the cavity
2. Hemostasis with a sterile cotton pellet
3. Calcium hydroxide application (Calxyl or $Ca(OH)_2$ suspension)
4. Glass ionomer cement liner (eg, Vitrebond™)
5. Tight closure with adhesive system and composite resin

Pulpotomy

If more extensive pulp opening occurs during removal of caries from a symptom-free primary tooth then pulpotomy is the treatment of choice. Pulpotomy means removing the inflamed coronal pulp and leaving in place the root pulp that is still inflammation-free, under a calcium hydroxide covering. It has been shown that MTA is at least as effective as calcium hydroxide as a tight capping material for primary teeth.[18]

Pulpotomy is not indicated for total pulpitis of a primary tooth. Calcium hydroxide has no effect on tissue that is already inflamed. Therefore, failure is inevitable in the case of inflammation of the root pulp. Here the cardinal symptom is whether hemostasis of the root pulp can be achieved at the entrance to the root canal.

Pulpotomy procedure
1. Broaching the pulp cavity with a fine-grit spherical diamond
2. Visualization of the root canal entrances
3. Hemostasis; eg, by compression with a cotton pellet (possibly with 15.5 % iron sulfate solution)
4. Capping with calcium hydroxide or MTA
5. Glass ionomer cement cavity lining
6. Composite resin restoration

■ Treatment of irreversible pulpitis

Pulpectomy

Pulpectomy is indicated if the aching tooth displays no increased mobility or soft tissue infiltration in the area of the alveolar ridge, if radiographs show little or no visible periapical or interradicular osteolysis, or if hemostasis cannot be achieved. The root canals are prepared to about three-quarters of their length using fine instruments above ISO #40, then filled with calcium hydroxide, calcium hydroxide suspension, or iodoform paste (Vitapex®). The latter contains calcium hydroxide and iodoform. The primary tooth is preferably treated

Endodontology in the primary dentition

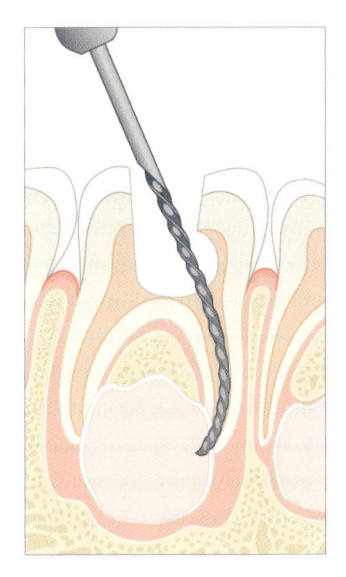

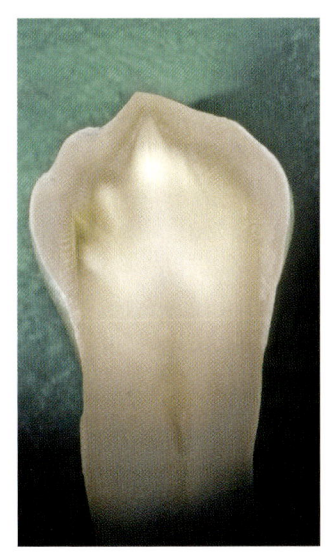

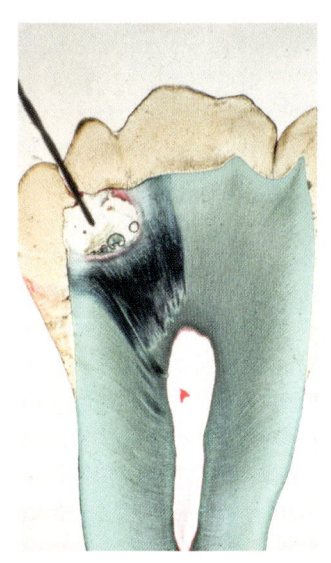

Fig 24-2 *(Left) Pulpectomy of a primary tooth. The root canals of the primary teeth must not be prepared right to the apex to ensure there is no injury to the permanent tooth germ.*

Fig 24-3 *Injury to the permanent tooth germ in pulpectomy of a primary molar. Left: in the section through an extracted premolar, local dentin destruction without the formation of enamel caries is identifiable. Right: in the histological section, the injury to the tooth from a root canal instrument can be reconstructed.*

initially with a provisional restoration. If this treatment does not provide any pain relief, or if soft tissue swelling or fistula formation occurs, the affected tooth will have to be extracted. Untreated total pulpitis of a primary tooth will develop into pulp necrosis.

If pulpectomy is performed on a primary tooth, the risk of injuring the permanent tooth germ with root canal instruments must be borne in mind. For this reason, the root canals must not be prepared down as far as the apex. Preparation should only be performed using instrument sizes ISO #40 and larger (Figs 24-2 and 24-3).

The following features must be considered when preparing primary tooth roots
- Irregular canal lumen
- Interradicular accessory root canals
- Severe root curvatures
- Physiological root resorptions
- Proximity to the tooth germ

Pulpectomy procedure
1. Root canal preparation to max. 3/4 of root length
2. Irrigation with chlorhexidine solution (2 %)
3. Drying of root canals
4. Root canal filling with calcium hydroxide or Vitapex®
5. Glass ionomer cement cavity lining
6. Provisional restoration, definitive composite resin restoration or steel crown

Treatment of pulp necrosis

Primary teeth with pulp necrosis – even though they are often symptom-free – should not be left untreated because of the risk of damage to the permanent tooth germ[20] or the risk of bacteremia. The affected primary tooth often has to be extracted. If a tooth absolutely needs to be preserved, an inlay and root filling with calcium hydroxide may be attempted.

For severely symptomatic primary teeth with pulp necrosis (pain, loosening, breath odor, possibly the start of an abscess), an inlay with Ledermix® and temporary closure might be necessary. Antibiotic coverage is indicated in the case of abscess formation with fever. After the acute symptoms have subsided, a decision on whether to preserve or extract the primary tooth must be taken.

Leaving asymptomatic, nonvital primary teeth open and treating with fluoride application should only be undertaken as a temporary measure if immediate extraction is not possible because of a lack of cooperation or if the tooth is to be left in place as a space maintainer. However, this treatment should definitely be regarded as a compromise because the cavities that are not fully accessible to tooth cleaning will act as a large reservoir for germs.

In the past, if there was a lack of cooperation, carious lesions in primary teeth were roughly excavated then etched with 50% silver nitrate and eugenol. This left behind black-discolored primary teeth. Nowadays, a 38% silver diamine fluoride solution is increasingly being used to control caries. This treatment is commonly used in developing countries where conventional rehabilitation of carious primary teeth is not possible or is prohibitively expensive. In the reaction of silver diamine fluoride with the hydroxyapatite of the tooth, calcium fluoride and silver phosphate are precipitated, which can halt the further spread of caries. The precipitated silver phosphate, like silver nitrate, causes dark discoloration of treated teeth. Furthermore, there is a metallic taste in the mouth which children can find unpleasant. It has been shown in trials that application of a 38% silver diamine fluoride solution (44,800 ppm fluoride) once or twice a year can stop the progression of caries. This treatment seems to be indicated especially for young children who are difficult to treat.[3]

As an alternative to silver diamine fluoride therapy, Duraphat (22,600 ppm fluoride) can be applied to the excavated and dried carious lesions. However, Duraphat application has to be repeated every 3 to 4 months in order to exert a caries-inhibiting effect.

Procedure for pulp necrosis
Extraction
or
Root canal treatment
1. Preparation as for irreversible pulpitis
2. $Ca(OH)_2$, Vitapex® or Ledermix® inlay
3. Provisional restoration
4. If symptom-free: root filling with $Ca(OH)_2$ or Vitapex® and definitive bacteria-proof closure

Endodontology in the primary dentition

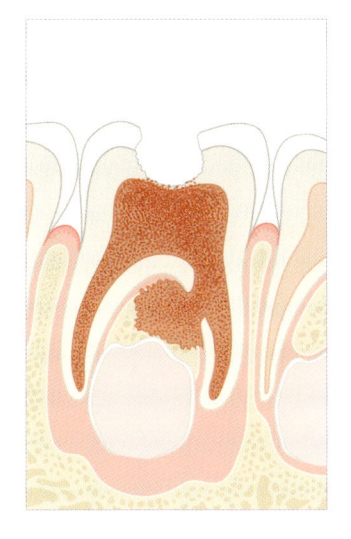

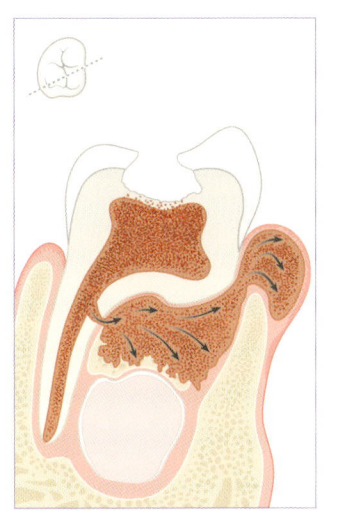

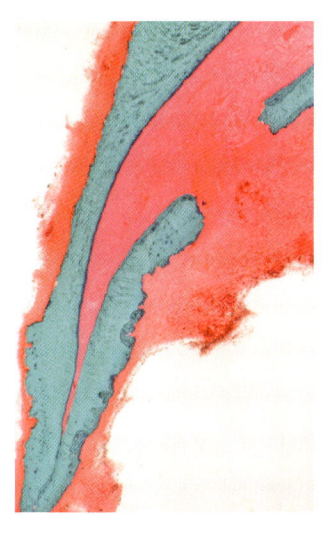

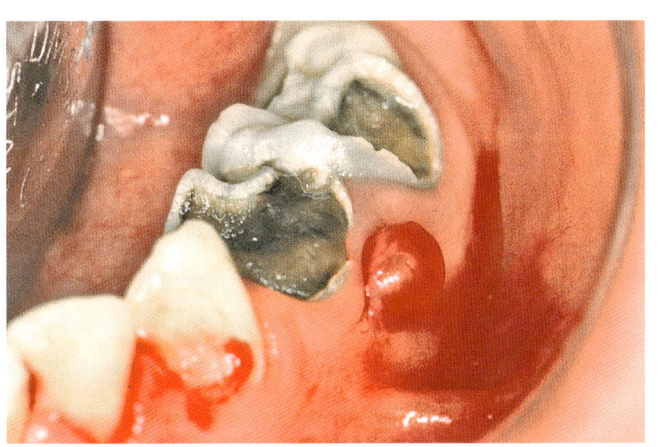

Fig 24-4 Interradicular periodontitis in primary molars.

Left: lateral canals encourage proliferation of bacteria and thereby allow inflammation to spread rapidly into the interradicular space. Interradicular periodontitis ensues.

Centre: from there the inflammation spreads in the direction of the gingival margin, so that abscess or fistula formation typical of primary molars occurs in the marginal area of the alveolar ridge.

Right: the histological section through a primary tooth root shows a lateral canal enlarged due to resorption, which enables bacteria to penetrate into the interradicular space and maintains inflammation there.

Fig 24-5 Fistula formation: a primary left mandibular first molar extensively destroyed by caries, with fistula formation in the marginal area of the alveolar ridge.

In primary molars, interradicular periodontitis is far more common than periapical periodontitis. This is due to the lateral canals of the pulp, which allow the rapid spread of inflammation into the interradicular space. From there the inflammatory process spreads in a marginal direction. The abscess or later the fistula therefore appears in the marginal area of the alveolar ridge (Figs 24-4 and 24-5). Sometimes the pus exudes directly through the periodontal space. This characteristic of the primary molars of allowing pulpal inflammation to spread into the interradicular area means that vital pulp remnants that are still bleeding might be present in the root canals, despite existing interradicular osteitis.[14]

Contraindications to root canal treatment in cases of pulp necrosis
- Time until exfoliation < 1.5 years
- Neglected dentition
- Build-up not possible
- Persistent fistula after medicated inlay
- Increasing osteolysis

Materials for endodontic measures in the primary dentition

A number of different materials and therapeutic approaches are recommended for endodontic measures in the primary dentition. The two best-known materials are formocresol and calcium hydroxide. In several studies, formocresol led to equivalent or better success rates in endodontic measures in the primary dentition in comparison with calcium hydroxide.[5,16,19] However, a different picture emerges if the biocompatibility or the toxicity of the two materials is compared. In *Buckley's* original formulation, formocresol contains approximately 19% formaldehyde. In order to reduce the toxicity, dilution of formocresol solution with distilled water at a ratio of 1:5 is proposed.[7] Nevertheless, the good clinical results of the formocresol technique must be seen alongside the greater reservations about the toxicity of substances containing formaldehyde. There is a variety of evidence of the cytotoxic, neurotoxic, allergenic, mutagenic, and carcinogenic effects of formaldehyde. However, it is not clear how much the quantities used for pulpotomy or pulpectomy of a primary tooth would have a toxic effect.[4,9] By contrast, calcium hydroxide is far less problematic in terms of biocompatibility. Admittedly, calcium hydroxide preparations frequently result in internal resorption.[10]

Mineral trioxide aggregate (MTA) has been available for a few years. In the endodontic studies on primary teeth so far conducted, the success rates of MTA are equal to or better than those of formocresol.[10,11,12,16] The biocompatibility of MTA seems to be good despite a certain proportion of heavy metal (5% Bi_2O_3).[2] MTA also rates better in comparison with other endodontic materials.[10,11] MTA is, however, very expensive for routine use in children. Medicinal Portland cement (available via www.medcem.ch) might be considered as a cheaper substitute.[1,6] Further studies will have to show whether medicinal Portland cement produces equally good results to those of MTA.

References

1. Abdullah D, Ford TR, Papaioannou S, Nicholson J, McDonald F. An evaluation of accelerated Portland cement as a restorative material. Biomaterials 2002;23:4001–4010.
2. Camilleri J, Pitt Ford TR. Mineral trioxide aggregate: a review of the constituents and biological properties of the material. Int Endod J 2006;39:747–54.
3. Chu CH, Lo EC. Promoting caries arrest in children with silver diamine fluoride: a review. Oral Health Prev Dent 2008;6:315–321.
4. Cortés O, Fernandez J, Boj JR, Canalda C. Effect of formaldehyde on rat liver in doses used in pulpotomies. J Clin Pediatr Dent 2007;31:179–182.
5. Coser RM, Gondim JO, Aparecida Giro EM. Evaluation of 2 endodontic techniques used to treat human primary molars with furcation radiolucency area: A 48-month radiographic study. Quintessence Int 2008;39:549–557.
6. Islam I, Chng HK, Yap AU. Comparison of the physical and mechanical properties of MTA and Portland cement. J Endod 2006;32:193–197.
7. Ketley CE, Goodman JR. Formocresol toxicity: is there a suitable alternative for pulpotomy of primary molars? Int J Paediatr Dent 1991;1:67–72.
8. Lygidakis NA, Marinou D, Katsaris N. Analysis of dental emergencies presenting to a community paediatric dentistry centre. Int J Paediatr Dent 1998;8:181–190.

9. Milnes AR. Is formocresol obsolete? A fresh look at the evidence concerning safety issues. Pediatr Dent 2008;30:237–246.
10. Moretti AB, Sakai VT, Oliveira TM, Fornetti AP, Santos CF, Machado MA, Abdo RC. The effectiveness of mineral trioxide aggregate, calcium hydroxide and formocresol for pulpotomies in primary teeth. Int Endod J 2008;41:547–555.
11. Ng FK, Messer LB. Mineral trioxide aggregate as a pulpotomy medicament: an evidence-based assessment. Eur Arch Paediatr Dent 2008;9:58–73.
12. Noorollahian H. Comparison of mineral trioxide aggregate and formocresol as pulp medicaments for pulpotomies in primary molars. Br Dent J 2008;204:E20.
13. Ribeiro CC, Baratieri LN, Perigao J, Baratieri NM, Ritter AV. A clinical, radiographic and scanning electron microscopic evaluation of adhesive restorations on carious dentin in primary teeth. Quintessence Int 1999;30:591–599.
14. Schaffner M, Lussi A. Die Behandlung akuter Beschwerden im Milchgebiss. Schweiz Monatsschr Zahnmed 1994;104:310–319.
15. Sheller B, Williams BJ, Lombardi SM. Diagnosis and treatment of dental caries-related emergencies in a children's hospital. Pediatr Dent 1997;19:470–475.
16. Sonmez D, Sari S, Cetinbas T. A comparison of four pulpotomy techniques in primary molars: a long-term follow-up. J Endod 2008;37:950–955.
17. Thompson V, Craig RG, Curro FA, Green WS, Ship JA. Treatment of deep carious lesions by complete excavation or partial removal: a critical review. Evid Based Dent 2008;9:71–72.
18. Tuna D, Olmez A: Clinical long-term evaluation of MTA as a direct pulp capping material in primary teeth. Int Endod J 2008;41:273–278.
19. Waterhouse PJ, Nunn JH, Whitworth JM. An investigation of relative efficacy of Buckley's formocresol and calcium hydroxide in primary molar vital pulp therapy. Br Dent J 2000;188:32–36.
20. Wetzel W E. Folgen apikaler Milchzahnerkrankungen auf Mineralisation und Durchbruch bleibender Zähne. Dtsch Zahnärztl Z 1986;41:179–181.
21. Wilson S, Smith GA, Preisch J, Casamassimo PS. Nontraumatic dental emergencies in a pediatric emergency department. Clin Pediatr 1997;36:333–337.

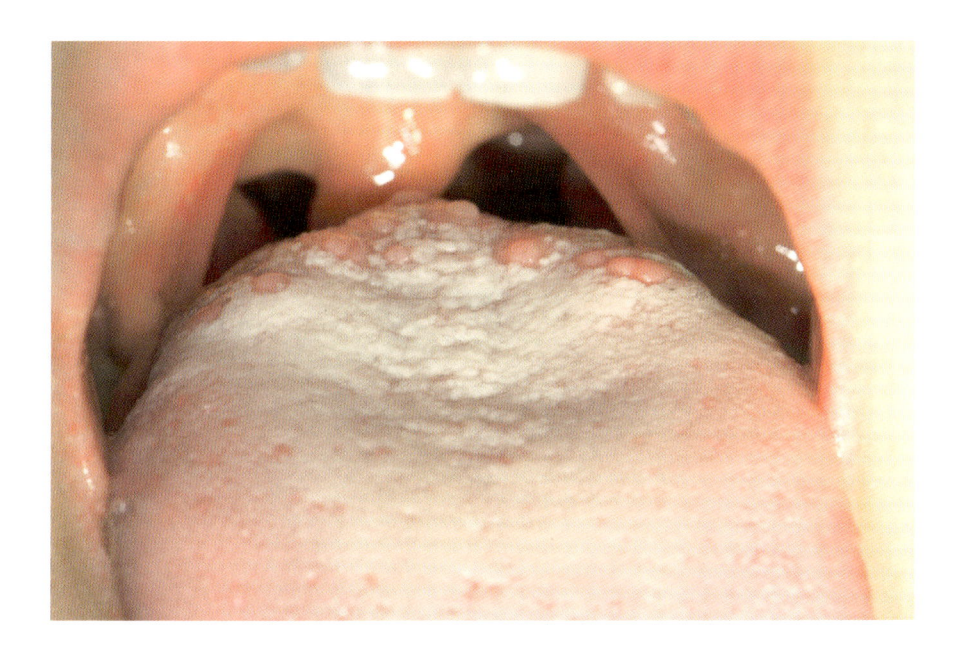

Halitosis

X

25 Halitosis

Rainer Seemann and Karin Kislig

■ Forms and prevalence

Strictly speaking, the term "halitosis" denotes an unpleasant odor of breathed air, whereas an odor originating in the oral cavity is known as "fetor ex ore". However, this distinction has ceased to be applied consistently in recent literature. Instead, the term "halitosis" is used for all forms of oral malodor and various subforms are defined. Another distinction is between genuine halitosis and pseudohalitosis.[20] Within genuine halitosis, a further differentiation is made between oral and extraoral forms, depending on the source of the odor. Pseudohalitosis is understood to mean that a patient believes he or she has bad breath while no oral malodor is actually perceptible. This problem will be described in more detail later.

Bad breath can develop into a serious psychological and social problem for those affected. The problem of "halitosis" has attracted more public interest in recent years and hence awareness has been raised among dental practitioners. As a result, an increasing number of epidemiological studies have been conducted. In one of our studies we found that 31% of 400 randomly selected subjects from the city of Berne were suffering from oral malodor discernible by organoleptic examination.[1] The same measurement was carried out in a Chinese study,[6] which reached the conclusion that 27.5% of subjects had bad breath. In the Berne study, measurements with a Halimeter revealed that 27.9% of those tested exceeded a threshold of 75 ppm. This threshold was exceeded by 35.4% in China[6] and by 23% in Japan.[8] These studies show that around a third of the population suffers from breath odor to a variable degree.

The source of bad breath can most commonly be found in the oral cavity (in about 90% of cases). This is why the diagnosis and treatment of halitosis belongs in the hands of dental practitioners.

Table 25-1 Forms of halitosis, their characteristics and possible causes (from Yaegaki and Coil[10], modified by Schüz and Seemann[14])

Form of halitosis	Characteristics and sources (or causes) of odor
Genuine halitosis	Pronounced fetor beyond a socially tolerable level.
– Oral source	• Fetor due to coating of the tongue, modified by pathological conditions (eg, periodontal diseases, xerostomia). • Fetor due to pathological process inside the oral cavity – poor hygiene and infections (eg, stomatitis, gingivitis, periodontitis, candidiasis), neglected dentures, overhanging crown margins, open root canals, pemphigus, Behçet's disease, erythema exudativum multiforme, abscesses, ulcerating and disintegrating tumors).
– Extraoral source	• Fetor from the ENT area (eg, tonsillitis, sinusitis, pharyngitis, diphtheria, glandular fever, Vincent's angina, foreign bodies, abscesses, stage 3 syphilis, chronic rhinitis (ozaena), postnasal drip, ulcerating and disintegrating tumors in the nasal, paranasal or laryngeal cavities). • Fetor from the respiratory and the upper digestive tract (eg, purulent bronchitis, pneumonia, foreign bodies, abscesses (lungs), gangrene of the lung, Wegener's granulomatosis, diverticula, esophagitis, gastrointestinal diseases, diabetes mellitus, precomatose states and coma (uremia, hepatic coma), yellow fever, medications (eg, dimethyl sulfoxide), trimethylaminuria, ulcerating and disintegrating tumors.
Pseudohalitosis	• The patient complains of bad breath although this cannot be detected by other people. • Situation is improved by education of the patient with the aid of literature and discussion of the test results (pseudohalitosis). • Patient is still not convinced that there is no fetor despite thorough education and discussion of the test results (somatoform / imagined halitosis or halitophobia).

■ Causes and sources of odor

If the source of the unpleasant odor lies in the mouth, it may be assumed that the cause is bacterial metabolism, which mainly gives rise to volatile sulfur compounds (VSCs: hydrogen sulfide, methyl mercaptan, and dimethyl sulfide)[17] through the bacterial breakdown of proteins (Fig 25-1).[5] Food remnants left in the mouth, cell debris, shed epithelial cells, as well as blood constituents and host secretions such as saliva and gingival crevicular fluid act as organic substrates.[3,17]

Bacterial coating on the dorsal area of the tongue is the most common intraoral source of odor.[21,2] The special morphology of the tongue, which is characterized by fissures and papillary areas, offers perfect conditions for the retention of food constituents and bacteria (Fig 25-2). As well as microorganisms, the coating on the tongue comprises desquamated epithelial cells, leucocytes, and other blood constituents as well as food remnants.[21] The composition of the tongue coating is subject to several modifying influences. These cofactors – eg, reduced salivary flow, dehydration, excessive drinking of coffee, smoking, and long-term medication, as well as poor oral hygiene – also increase the tendency to form a coating on the tongue.[21] Table 25-1 summarizes factors that can lead to furring of the tongue or which are themselves possible sources of odor that cause bad breath.

Generally speaking, there is some justification for stating that bacterial plaque and deposits are the main cause of bad breath. A more subtle distinction, however, would be

Peptides/Proteins (blood, saliva, epithelial rests, etc)
↓ bacterial proteolysis
Amino acids (cysteine, cystine, methionine, tryptophan, ornithine, lysine)
↓ bacterial aminolysis
Putrefaction products (VSC, indole, skatole, cadaverine, putrescine)

VSC = Volatile sulfur compounds

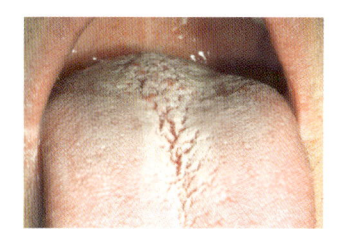

Fig 25-1 Left: breakdown of protein-rich substrate into volatile, foul-smelling compounds (from Kleinberg and Codipilly[4]).

Fig 25-2 Right: papillary structure of the tongue with coating in the dorsal area.

Oral cavity as an ecosystem

bacteria-bacteria, bacteria-host interactions ↕ stable biofilm ↑

substrate supply, exogenous bacteria, hygiene ↓↓↓ environmental influences ↓

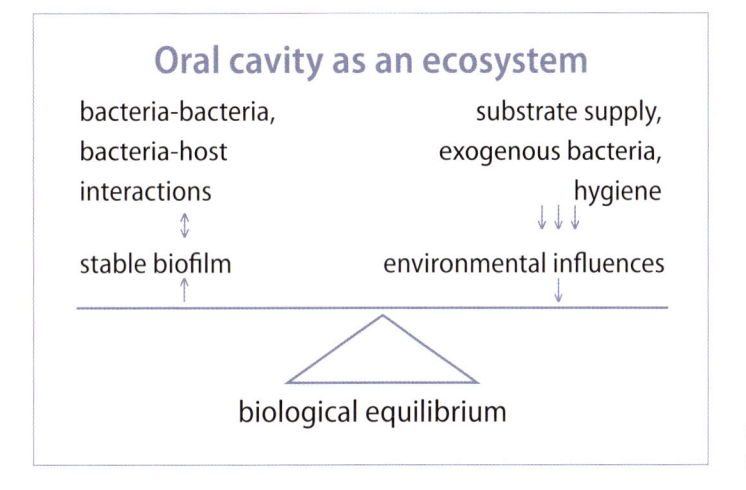

biological equilibrium

Fig 25-3 Bacterial homeostasis (from Marsh[7]).

that these odor-causing biofilms are merely the source of the odor. The actual causes are the factors that promote the growth and metabolism of the coatings.[14] According to Marsh and Bradshaw[7] a stable biofilm is shaped and kept in balance by a suitable supply of substrate and environmental influences, thus following ecological principles. With respect to bad breath, depending on environmental influences and substrate supply, the ecosystem of the mouth therefore contains higher or lower numbers of odor-producing microbes or provides space for more or less pronounced metabolic activity of these microorganisms (Fig 25-3).

An impressive example in support of this hypothesis is presented in Figs 25-4 and 25-5. The patient in question had unpleasant bad breath that was noticeable from several meters away. A heavily coated tongue had clearly been identified as the source of the odor, so that intensification of oral hygiene, including tongue cleaning, seemed to be indicated. The cause of the tongue coating, however, was a roughly pea-sized piece of impression material which had inadvertently got into the patient's nose 6 years earlier through an incompletely closed cleft palate during the course of fabrication of an anterior partial denture. The induced formation of nasal secretion led to severe posterior rhinorrhoea resulting in massive coating of the tongue. Once the foreign body had been removed from the nose, the coating of the

Fig 25-4 Clinical situation of a patient with cleft palate. The patient displayed a strong oral malodor and massive coating of the tongue.

Fig 25-5 Impression material which was removed from the nose of the patient in Fig 25-4 after about 6 years in place.

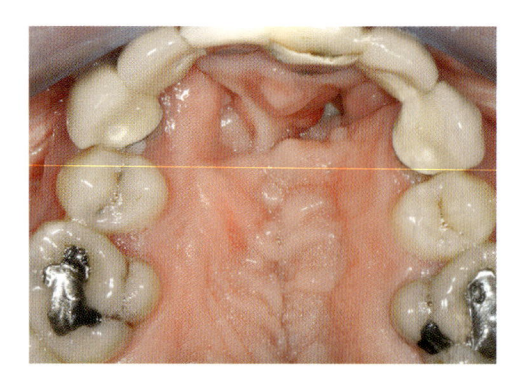

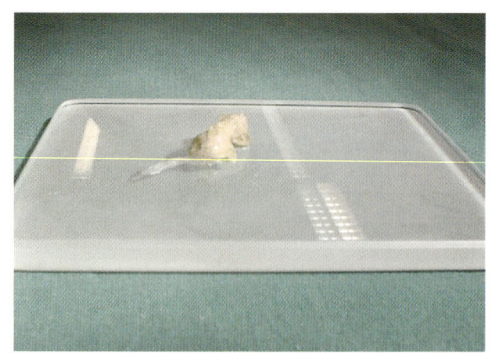

tongue and the bad breath disappeared spontaneously. Other factors that trigger posterior rhinorrhoea are likely to have a similar effect of varying severity (eg, chronic sinusitis or chronic rhinitis).

While the source of an unpleasant odor is usually easy to identify, its causes are often difficult to determine. It is conceivable that, in terms of a multifactorial etiology, several factors may combine to result in the formation of unpleasant-smelling tongue coatings. For instance, overhanging, uncleanable crown margins provide ideal environmental conditions for the growth of anaerobic microorganisms. If this situation coincides with poor oral hygiene and nocturnal snoring, which leads to drying of the oral cavity, bad breath due to a coating on the tongue can arise. If possible, the source of the odor and potential causes should be considered when making the diagnosis.

■ Diagnostic procedure

The first step in a systematic examination for bad breath is to find out whether mouth odor actually exists. This advice seems paradoxical, but it is extremely important because an appreciable number of patients who attend their doctor complaining of the condition do not have oral malodor at all. These patients with pseudohalitosis require a different procedure from patients who have objectively detectable bad breath (see "Dealing with pseudohalitosis patients").[16]

We recommend the following procedure:
1. Patient history in relation to mouth odor
2. Organoleptic examination to establish whether bad breath is present and isolate the source of the odor
3. Instrumental odor diagnosis to complement the organoleptic examination
4. Dental examination to identify possible causes and cofactors
5. If necessary, repeat investigations to confirm the diagnosis

Patient history

The history of bad breath complements the history generally taken in a dental practice to record general and dental diseases, by focusing on the patient's oral hygiene behavior as well as his or her attitudes and observations on the subject of mouth odor. The questions specifically targeted at the problem of oral malodor that we use in the questionnaire for our clinic are detailed below. These have been formulated over the course of time and we do not claim that they are exhaustive. The medical history forms should be tailored to the specific structures and needs of the particular practice. Space for comments and notes enable the practitioner to note additional factors that are not covered by the questionnaire so that the specific case details can be clearly viewed more easily at follow-up examinations.

General

- Why are you attending the breath odor clinic?
- How did you find out about our breath odor clinic?

Patients will sometimes regard the first question as redundant. You will usually have no problems with those patients. However, the answer to this question can reveal a lot. Answers such as, "Because you are my last hope" or "Because at long last I really need the opinion of an expert" give some impression of the patient's suffering and expectations.

The answer to the second question can provide valuable information about the effectiveness of the practice's marketing.

Personal and other people's perception

- Have you noticed yourself that you have bad breath? (Since when? How often?)
- Have other people noticed that you have bad breath?
- Has your partner talked to you about your bad breath?
- Have other people (eg, colleagues) talked to you about your bad breath?
- Do you notice other people's reactions to your bad breath?
- Is your life influenced by your bad breath? (private or working life)
- Do you have a bad taste on your tongue?
- Is your tongue coated?

With the aid of these questions, it is possible to assess how long the patient has been suffering from the problem and how badly. Comparison of the person's own perception with those of other people might give some indication of the presence of pseudohalitosis. The findings from our clinic show that patients with pseudohalitosis state with significantly higher frequency that they have not been talked to about bad breath by a partner or a person they trust, even though their own perception is that oral malodor is definitely present.[15,16]

Cofactors and diet

The following questions can help in the identification of possible cofactors that encourage the development of oral malodor. As a rule, these are concomitant circumstances which have a negative effect on saliva production. The questions provide an indication of whether or not it would be helpful to measure the patient's salivary flow rate.

The dietary history is deliberately kept short. As there are no reliable data on the influence of dietary habits on oral malodor, we limit ourselves to asking whether patients drink enough fluids, whether they stick to regular mealtimes and whether they have an unbalanced diet.

- Do you suffer from a dry mouth?
- Do you have to talk a lot and for long periods? (eg, on the telephone, lecturing)
- Do you have a lot of stress?
- Do you snore?
- Can you breathe sufficiently through your nose?
- Do you smoke?
- Do you drink alcohol? (How much?)
- Are you regularly taking any medication? (What medication? What for?)
- How many times a day do you eat?
- How much and what do you drink per day?
- Do you avoid certain foods?
- Do you suspect that certain foods make the problem worse?

Experience of medical professionals

- Have you consulted any of the following doctors about bad breath?:
  - general practitioner
  - specialist in internal medicine
  - ear, nose and throat (ENT) doctor
- What were you treated for?
- Was there an improvement?
- Did any of the doctors assess the strength of the odor?

These questions complement the medical history and provide information about relevant previous illnesses or diseases excluded by previous diagnostic investigations. The last question helps us to judge whether, despite extensive diagnostic efforts, oral malodor might not be present in the patient. It is possible that, apart from the patient's own perception, no assessment of oral malodor has ever been carried out. Analysis by our breath odor clinic revealed that such an assessment is only done very rarely and therefore diagnostic and therapeutic measures that are often unnecessary are carried out.[12]

Oral hygiene

- Do your gums bleed?
- Do you see a hygienist regularly for tooth cleaning?
- How often do you clean your teeth?
- Do you use dental floss?
- Do you use dental sticks?
- Do you use interdental brushes?
- Do you use mouthwash or a rinsing solution?
- Do you clean your tongue?
- Do you use chewing gum to conceal bad breath?
- Do you use sweets to conceal bad breath?

The basic aim of the oral hygiene history is to find out whether interdental hygiene and regular professional tooth cleaning sessions take place. Some patients use chewing gum or eat peppermint sweets excessively in order to conceal their bad breath. It is essential to restore these habits to a normal level.

Organoleptic examination

An organoleptic examination refers to odor diagnosis using the examiner's own sense of smell. The basis for the examination is that the patient feels he or she is being taken seriously and has come to trust the person performing the examination. This is achieved by thoroughly discussing the history questionnaire completed by the patient while in the waiting room.

Most of the organoleptic measuring methods described in the literature stipulate that an examiner assesses the strength of an odor at a defined distance from the source of the odor and locates it on a scale of defined odor strengths. The scale can include up to nine severity levels, but a scale of six levels is frequently used. A disadvantage of these methods is that the examiner needs to be trained to be able to make distinctions in a reproducible way; in addition, describing the odor's strength can cause problems when communicating with the patient. It does not sound very motivational to the patient if they are told that they have improved from category 6 (extremely foul-smelling) to category 3 (moderate). This is why for routine practice we recommend a method that merely differentiates whether or not an unpleasant odor can be perceived. When evaluating the strength of an existing odor, assessments are made at predefined distances from the patient. For the first assessment, the patient is asked to count loudly backwards from "999" to "990". If an odor is perceptible from a distance of 1 meter, this is equivalent to severity level "3", 30 cm distance corresponds to severity level "2", and 10 cm to level "1". If no odor can be perceived from a distance of only 10 cm, this equates to a severity of "0" (Fig 25-6).[14,15]

If no oral malodor can be detected, the assessment should definitely be repeated at a different time. This will help to clarify whether the patient is suffering from pseudohalitosis (see "Dealing with pseudohalitosis patients") or the odor only occurs at certain times.[15]

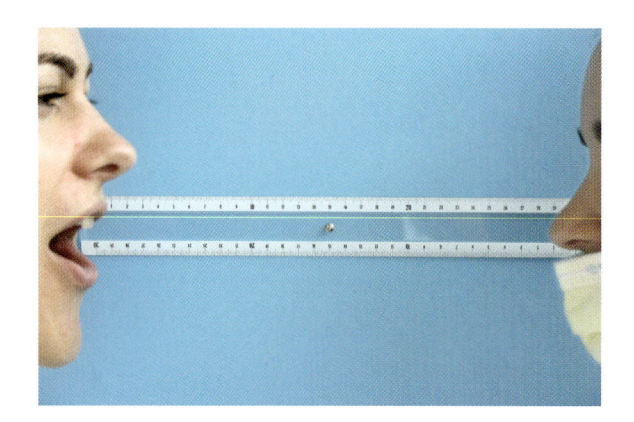

Fig 25-6 Organoleptic examination to assess the presence of an odor at defined distances between examiner and patient.

Table 25-2 Organoleptic assessment of air from different areas and isolating the source of the odor

	Findings when locating the source of odor in		
	Mouth	Nose	Lungs
Oral air Patient counts from "999" to "990" or breathes out through the mouth	+	–	+
Nasal air Patient breathes out slowly through the nose	–	+	+
Lung air Patient breathes out forcibly through the nose	–	–	+

Isolating the source of odor

In order to isolate the source of the odor, a separate assessment of the oral, nasal, and lung air is undertaken, as per Table 25-2. The method described above can also be used for this purpose. If the source lies in the mouth, it is the practitioner's responsibility to treat it; if the source is in the nose, the patient should be referred to an ENT specialist; finally, if the source is in the area of the lungs, thorough internal medical investigations must be carried out.

Instrumental odor diagnostics

A measuring device to assess oral malodor may be helpful, but it is no substitute for the organoleptic examination. One device used in practice is the Halimeter® (Interscan Corporation, Chatsworth, CA). The device is able to measure the concentration of volatile sulfur compounds (VSCs) directly at the chairside without any appreciable time delay. However, no distinction is made between different sulfur compounds.

For measuring, the opening of a replaceable mouthpiece (usually a simple plastic drinking straw) is inserted about 4 cm into the mouth and the patient is asked to continue breathing gently through the nose. Air is fed to an electrochemical sensor by means of a pump integrated into the device. The Halimeter determines the total concentration of VSCs in parts per billion (ppb) and shows this on a digital display (Fig 25-7).[9,10] At first there is typically a rapid increase until a peak value is reached. This peak is actually the measurement of interest and is noted. The baseline "0" is reached again a few seconds after the mouthpiece has been removed from the mouth. It is advisable to obtain an average of two or three measurements

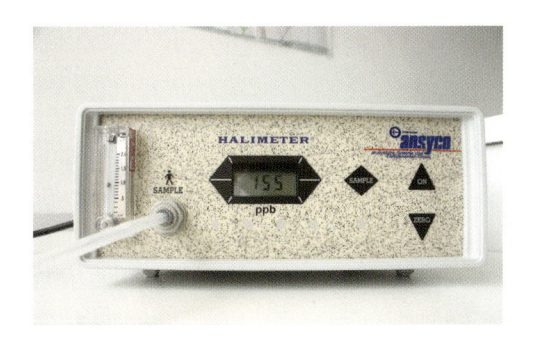

Fig 25-7 Halimeter® for measuring oral concentrations of volatile sulfur compounds.

because small fluctuations will repeatedly occur. Use of the Halimeter is easy to learn and can be done by staff members who have been familiarized with the device. The patient should not talk and should keep his or her mouth closed for a few minutes before the measuring process.

A major reported disadvantage of the Halimeter is that it cannot distinguish between different sulfur-containing components. The total VSCs are generally known to comprise hydrogen sulfide (H_2S), methyl mercaptan (CH_3SH), and dimethyl sulfide (($CH_3)_2S$). As already stated by Yaegaki and Sanada, the concentrations of methyl mercaptan and hydrogen sulfide vary considerably in relation to each other.[21] The sensitivity of the Halimeter to hydrogen sulfide is increased, being twice as high as for methyl mercaptan. By contrast, the human nose has a three times higher perception threshold for hydrogen sulfide (0.5 ng/10 ml for methyl mercaptan and 1.5 ng/10 ml for hydrogen sulfide).[18] This can result in discrepancies between objectively detectable oral malodor and Halimeter readings. Thus it may be found that patients with low readings have strongly perceptible fetor and vice versa. In view of this problem, it is difficult to stipulate a threshold above which objectifiable oral malodor exists. Values between 70 and 140 ppb sulfur equivalent are given as the normal range.[11] This is why the Halimeter should not be regarded as a substitute for organoleptic measurement but as a useful complementary tool.

When being examined for the intimate problem of "bad breath", the patient is more likely to trust a practitioner using the Halimeter. In addition, the Halimeter provides an objective method of monitoring progress. If a chosen form of treatment shows some effect, the Halimeter baseline readings will decrease markedly, which means reassurance for the practitioner and helps the patient to regain some confidence in interactions with other people. Furthermore, the device helps to convince patients suffering from pseudohalitosis that in fact they are not producing any unpleasant mouth odor and that the actual problem must be sought elsewhere.

Although the Halimeter only measures the concentration of VSCs, it is easy to operate and is a helpful adjunct to the organoleptic examination in dental practices. However, a measuring device is not absolutely necessary for assessing oral malodor.

Halitosis

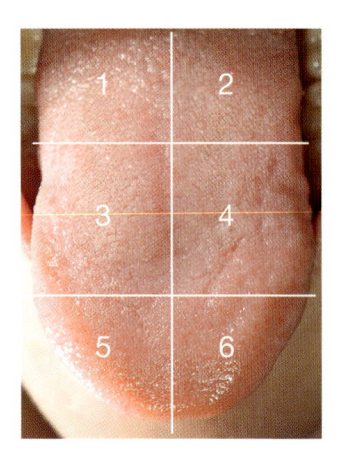

Fig 25-8 Winkel tongue coating index.[19] The tongue is divided into six segments and the coating of the tongue is rated for each segment.

Other investigations

During the dental examination, oral hygiene and mucosal, dental, and periodontal findings are recorded. These examinations are used to identify the source of the odor (coating of the tongue, interdental plaque, etc) and causal diseases (periodontitis, mucosal changes, tonsillitis, posterior rhinorrhoea, etc). The recording of these findings will not be explored here in detail because these findings form part of routine work in dental practices.

In addition, an assessment of the tongue is carried out, because bacterial tongue coating is the most commonly encountered source of malodor. The Winkel tongue coating index[19] is used for the purpose (Fig 25-8). This index involves dividing the tongue into sextants and assessing the thickness of the coating in each sextant (0 = no coating, 1 = slight coating, 2 = thick coating). The tongue coating index is obtained by adding together the individual scores. All the findings are recorded on an assessment form.

■ Treatment in the dental practice

Treatment of oral malodor should focus on the identified cause; therefore, treatment options are as heterogeneous as the causes themselves (Tables 25-3 and 25-4). If there are obvious bacterial retention sites, eg, massively overhanging margins of prosthetic restorations or periodontal pockets, these must be removed. If the patient has severe periodontitis, this must be treated systematically, which can prove time-consuming. If the cause is in the area of the tonsils, the patient must be referred to an ENT specialist, who will take the necessary steps. Treatment of all the possible diseases will not and cannot be explored further here and readers are advised to consult the relevant textbooks.

Table 25-3 Description of forms of treatment (from Yaegaki and Coil[20], modified by Schüz and Seemann[14])

Treatment	Description
T 1	Explanation of what causes halitosis, instruction on oral hygiene and support in implementing the oral hygiene measures, including tongue cleaning
T 2	Professional tooth cleaning and treatment of oral diseases (eg, periodontitis)
T 3	Referral to a doctor with the appropriate specialism (eg, ENT specialist)
T 4	Detailed and repeated description and explanation of the recorded examination findings; continuing professional instruction to endorse the fact that there is no oral malodor present
T 5	Referral to a psychologist or psychiatrist

Table 25-4 Overview of possible forms of treatment (from Yaegaki and Coil[20], modified by Schüz and Seemann[14])

Form of halitosis	Recommended form of treatment
Genuine halitosis	
Oral source	T1 and T2
Extraoral source	T1 and T3
Pseudo halitosis	T1 and T4, possibly T5

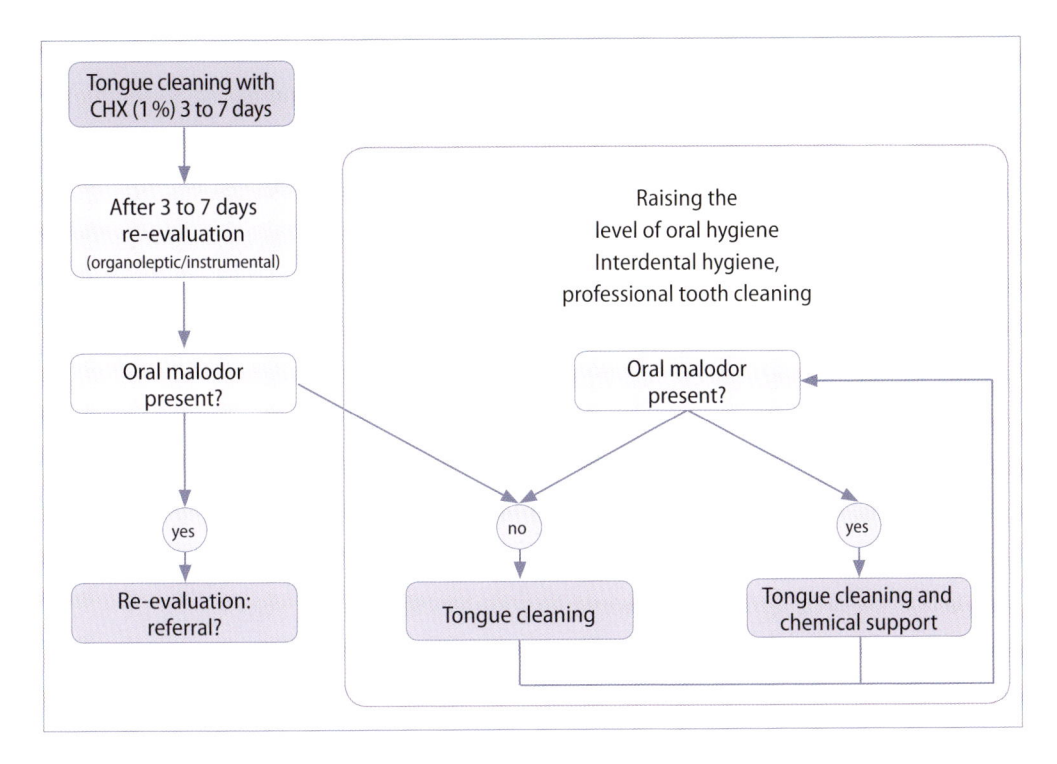

Fig 25-9 Schematic diagram of the treatment of oral malodor where the odor source is "tongue coating".

In most cases, some degree of oral hygiene improvement is required in order to treat oral malodor. As well as dental and interdental hygiene, this also extends to the area of the tongue.

Symptomatic treatment

A proven initial therapeutic approach when locating the source of the odor in the mouth is illustrated in Fig 29-9. The patient receives brief instruction on oral hygiene and a tongue cleaner together with around 3 ml 1% chlorhexidine gel (eg, Corsodyl or Blend-a-med gel) filled into a disposable syringe. The patient is instructed to clean his or her tongue morning and evening after meals, then apply the chlorhexidine gel to the tongue. For this purpose we recommend a tongue cleaner that has a brush element, which can be used to apply a small, but adequate, amount of gel to the tongue (Fig 25-10).

After application, the patient should spit out excess gel, but no more than that. The patient is given the additional instruction to ask a person he or she trusts whether there has been any improvement. After a week the patient is called in for an individual preventive session and the oral malodor is reassessed. If the diagnosis was correct, the bad breath will usually have receded noticeably. If the odor persists, either the diagnosis was incorrect or the patient has not carried out the recommended measures correctly. After tooth cleaning and specific instruction on interdental care have taken place, the patient is told just to carry out purely mechanical tongue cleaning. Under ideal circumstances and provided the patient is able to maintain oral hygiene at a high level, purely mechanical cleaning of the tongue is enough to keep the patient free of oral malodor.

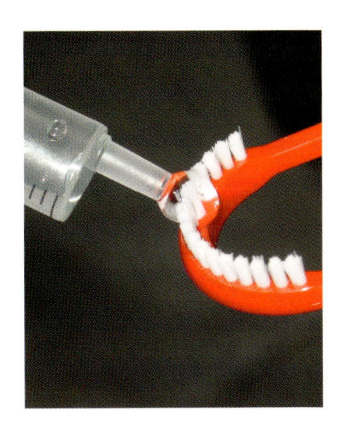

Fig 25-10 Application of chlorhexidine gel to a tongue cleaner.

> Achieving a high level of oral hygiene is the basis for successful eradication of the most common forms of oral malodor.

Nevertheless, the success of these efforts should always be monitored after 1 or 2 weeks, or the patient should receive appropriate feedback from someone at home. If purely mechanical cleaning of the tongue is not sufficient, various antibacterial products which are designed for daily use (eg, Meridol® Halitosis, Halita®, Retradex, Listerine®) may be tried. They should be used according to the principle "as much as necessary, as little as possible". If the patient has managed to get the problem under control, the oral malodor is checked regularly during recall appointments.

If the symptomatic treatment works, possible causes and cofactors may be further investigated at the same time. If these can be eliminated, the degree of symptomatic treatment required can be drastically reduced (see "Causes and sources of odor").

Delegation of services

Many of the above tasks can be performed by a preventive dental nurse or dental hygienist. The dentist can be consulted if any questions arise. However, despite this possible delegation of work, the dentist should perform the first examination and should closely monitor the treatment steps so that rare serious causes, eg, carcinomas of the oral mucosa, are not overlooked.

> **Caution:** Many of the steps can be delegated, but the dentist should definitely perform a thorough initial examination so that serious illnesses are not overlooked.

Mechanical tongue cleaning

The large number of tongue cleaners available on the market raises the question of what to recommend. Tongue cleaners can basically be divided into three different groups. A distinction is made between brushes (Fig 25-11), scrapers (Fig 25-12), and combinations of both (Fig 25-13).

Which product most effectively removes deposits from the tongue is impossible to answer based on the studies published to date. In the context of clinical trials, our study group analyzed the impact of different tongue cleaners on the concentration of VSCs. It was found that the combination of scraper and brush achieved a slightly more prolonged reduction of VSC levels. However, generalized recommendations cannot be deduced from these results because the differences found were negligible. The same result is achieved if professional tongue cleaning is performed in the dental practice using a special ultrasonic attachment.[14] Compared with a simple scraper, there were no appreciable differences when ultrasound was used. As yet there is no proof of the benefit of professional tongue cleaning with the aid of rotary minibrushes. However, excessive mechanical working carries a risk of injury to the mucosa of the tongue.

Halitosis

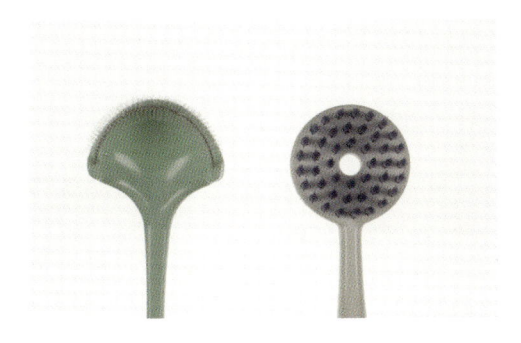

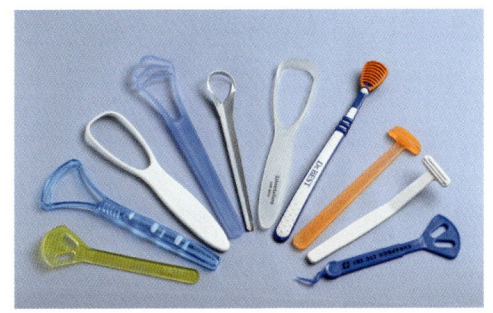

Fig 25-11 Examples of tongue brushes.

Fig 25-12 Examples of tongue scrapers.

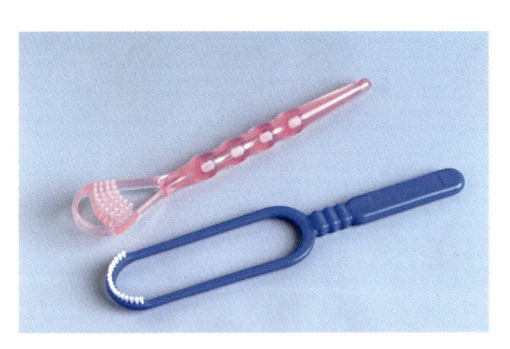

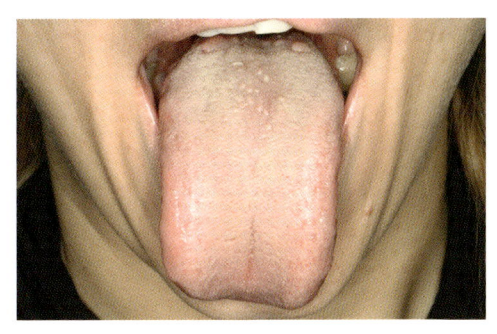

Fig 25-13 Examples of combinations of scraper and brush.

Fig 25-14 No mechanical tongue cleaning should take place beyond the vallate papillae in the posterior part of the dorsum of the tongue.

Therefore the general advice is to recommend a tongue cleaner that the patient gets on well with. The cleaner should not have any sharp edges in order to avoid injuries. Correct use of the cleaner should definitely be practiced with the patient. If professional tongue cleaning is required, this can be used as a demonstration for the patient. It should therefore be carried out using the tongue cleaner recommended to the patient.

Practical aspects of tongue cleaning

As most people in our culture are unfamiliar with the idea of cleaning their tongue, it is essential to give instruction on the correct procedure. The tongue should be streched out of the mouth as far as possible. It may be helpful to hold it with a face-cloth or a gauze pad. The cleaner is then placed on the dorsum of the tongue and moved forwards while applying slight pressure. Any material sticking to the cleaner should be rinsed off under running water. It is essential to ensure that the tongue is not cleaned posterior to the vallate papillae in order to avoid injuries (Fig 25-14).

Instruction on correct use of a tongue-cleaning aid is more important than the choice of cleaner. In all cases it is important to ensure that the tongue cleaner has no sharp edges which might injure the mucosa of the tongue.

If tongue cleaners are used correctly, they are unlikely to have any side effects. There are hence no objections to their preventive use as part of daily oral hygiene, provided that a high-quality product is used. No mechanical cleaning of the tongue should extend posterior to the vallate papillae.

Dealing with pseudohalitosis patients

If no oral malodor can be detected in a patient, this should first be reported factually to the person concerned, followed by a consultation. No form of treatment should ever be started without oral malodor being measured.[16] A negative odor finding may have several causes:
- The patient only suffers occasionally from malodor.
- The examiner's sense of smell on the day of the examination is impaired, or the odor concerned is generally not perceived as unpleasant by the examiner.
- The patient does not have oral malodor (pseudohalitosis).

The measurement should be repeated in order to find out which of the above reasons is responsible for the discrepancy between the patient's perception and that of the examiner. To do this, it is advisable to choose a time of day when the patient firmly believes to have oral malodor (eg, at the end of a working day or in the morning immediately after getting up). If possible, another person should also be called in to make an additional odor assessment.

It can be very helpful to ask the patient to bring along their partner or a close friend to the consultation. This person could either confirm that there is normally no unpleasant oral odor or provide important evidence of on what occasions and how often the malodor occurs. If it is not possible for the patient to bring an accompanying person to the next examination, by the following appointment they should ask people who they think are bothered by their bad breath whether their suspicions are correct. If a patient can bring themselves to do this and learn from the people they ask that there is no oral malodor, this usually gives them renewed self-confidence in their interactions with other people. If the person affected does not dare to talk openly to other people, a repeat examination in a breath odor clinic might bring about a similar result. The effect of this procedure is usually backed up by instrumental measurement of oral odor. In this instance, the examination also forms part of the treatment. Experience from our breath odor clinic shows that patients who have pseudohalitosis often have a long history of disease. In fact, it is an extremely pleasant task for a dental professional to be able to give these patients back their quality of life by the simple measures described above.

> With pseudohalitosis patients, repeated examinations and measurements of oral malodor together with feedback from others gathered by the patient might be sufficient treatment.

Typically, patients with halitophobia (somatoform or imagined halitosis) fail to ask other people about their bad breath, as requested, or the accompanying person they have promised to bring along does not appear at the appointment because of circumstances arising at short notice. Even when no unpleasant odor is established in repeated examinations, the sufferers of halitophobia stick to their view that they have bad breath. As a rule, the recommendation to seek psychological or psychiatric help is categorically declined and usually leads to a breakdown in the patient-practitioner relationship, which in turn means the patient fails to attend again.

■ How do I tell my patient?

Given the circumstances outlined above, the diagnosis and treatment of halitosis belongs in the hands of dental practitioners. This often means that the dental practitioner is not only the first point of contact for the halitosis patient but should also be responsible for informing patients who suffer from halitosis. As bad breath is a taboo subject, it can be very difficult for dental practitioners to indicate the problem tactfully to their patients.

> The long-term aim must be to remove the taboo from the subject of oral malodor. After all, to whom should a patient turn if not the dental practitioner?

If the taboo around the subject of oral malodor could be overcome, a dental practitioner would be able to talk openly to a patient about oral malodor, just as he or she would do, for instance, when discussing oral hygiene findings or the discovery of caries. However, given that this ideal situation has not yet been achieved, it remains necessary to approach the subject gently. There is some justification for not informing patients directly that they have halitosis, but rather to tell them, for instance, that they have a heavily coated tongue and that this in turn can lead to oral malodor. Addressing the subject indirectly this way, the patient should feel encouraged to ask questions.

Another frequently used option is to include a question about the subject of oral malodor on the medical history questionnaire of the dental practice. If the patient ticks the box indicating that he or she occasionally has problems with bad breath, this will open up the possibility of an open discussion.

■ References

1. Bornstein MM, Kislig K, Hoti BB, Seemann R, Lussi A. Prevalence of halitosis in the population of the city of Bern, Switzerland: a study comparing self-reported and clinical data. Eur J Oral Sci 2009;117:261–267.
2. Bosy A, Kulkarni GV, Rosenberg M, McCulloch CA. Relationship of oral malodor to periodontitis: evidence of independence in discrete subpopulations. J Periodontol 1994;65:37–46.
3. De Boever EH, Loesche WJ. Assessing the contribution of anaerobic microflora of the tongue to oral malodor. J Am Dent Assoc 1995;126:1384–1393.
4. Kleinberg I, Codipilly M. The biological basis of malodour formation. In: Rosenberg M, editor. Bad breath. Research perspectives. 2nd ed. Tel Aviv: Ramot Publishing; 1997. p. 13–41.
5. Kleinberg I, Westbay G. Salivary and metabolic factors involved in oral malodor formation. J Periodontol 1992:63: 768–775.
6. Liu XN, Shinada K, Chen XC, Zhang BX, Yaegaki K, Kawaguchi Y. Oral malodor-related parameters in the Chinese general population. J Clin Periodontol 2006;33: 31–36.
7. Marsh PD, Bradshaw DJ. Physiological approaches to the control of oral biofilms. Adv Dent Res 1997;11:176–185.

8. Miyazaki H, Sakao S, Katoh Y, Takehara T. Correlation between volatile sulphur compounds and certain oral health measurements in the general population. J Periodontol 1995;66:679–684.
9. Rosenberg M, Kulkarni GV, Bosy A, McCulloch CA. Reproducibility and sensitivity of oral malodor measurements with a portable sulphide monitor. J Dent Res 1991a;70:1436–1440.
10. Rosenberg M, Septon I, Eli I, Bar-Ness R, Gelernter I, Brenner S, Gabbay J. Halitosis measurement by an industrial sulphide monitor. J Periodontol 1991b; 62:487–489.
11. Seemann R. Halitosis 2: Diagnostik und Therapie. Zahnärztl Mittlg 2000;90: 644–648.
12. Seemann R, Bizhang M, Höfer U, Djamchidi D, Kage A, Jahn KR. Ergebnisse der Arbeit einer interdisziplinären deutschen Mundgeruchsprechstunde. Deutsche Zahnärztl Zeitschr 2004;59:514–517.
13. Seemann R, Kison A, Jahn KR. Reduzierung oraler Schwefelverbindungen nach Anwendung eines Unltraschall-Zungenreinigers. Oralprophylaxe und Kinderzahnmedizin 2004; 27:56–59.
14. Seemann R. Halitosismanagement in der Zahnärztlichen Praxis. 1 ed. 2006: Spitta Verlag, Balingen.
15. Seemann R, Bizhang M, Djamchidi C, Kage A, Nachnani S. The proportion of pseudo-halitosis patients in a multi-disciplinary breath malodour consultation. Int Dent J 2006;56:77–81.
16. Seemann R, Bornstein M, Lussi A. Umgang mit Pseudohalitosispatienten in der zahnärztlichen Praxis. Prophylaxe Impuls 2009;13: 6–10.
17. Tonzetich J. Direct gas chromatographic analysis of sulphur compounds in mouth air in man. Arch Oral Biol 1971;16:587–597.
18. Tonzetich J, Ng SK. Reduction of malodor by oral cleansing procedures. Oral Surg Oral Med Oral Pathol 1976;42:172–181.
19. Winkel EG, Roldan S, Van Winkelhoff AJ, Herrera D, Sanz M. Clinical effects of a new mouthrinse containing chlorhexidine, cetylpyridinium chloride and zinc-lactate on oral halitosis. A dual-center, double-blind placebo-controlled study. J Clin Periodontol 2003;30:300–306.
20. Yaegaki K, Coil JM. Examination, classification, and treatment of halitosis; clinical perspectives. J Can Dent Assoc 2000; 66:257–261.
21. Yaegaki K, Sanada K. Volatile sulfur compounds in mouth air from clinically healthy subjects and patients with periodontal disease. J Periodontal Res 1992; 27:233–238.

Index

A

abrasion 176, 185
accessory canals 12–13
acellular afibrillar cementum (AAC) 11
acellular extrinsic fiber cementum (AEFC) 11
acid attack 26–27
acidic drinks 185, 186
adhesive luting agents, classification 120–121
adhesive systems 115–121
adjacent tooth damage 97–103
　aids to prevent 99–102
　consequences 98
　origin 97–98
air abrasion 105–107
air-polishing technique 106
aluminum oxide 105–107, 130
amalgam restoration repairs 139
amelogenesis 5
anorexia nervosa 183, 184
antibacterial agents, topical application 53–57
antibacterial approaches 53
　limitations 59
apical periodontitis, etiology 207
aseptic treatment approach 208
attrition 176, 185

B

bacteria
　metabolism 15, 33, 59, 246
　where found 207–208
balanced force technique 201
Basic Erosive Wear Examination (BEWE) 177–178
Bevelshape file 100–101
bifidobacteria 40, 41
bioactive glass 50, 106
bleaching 163–171
　home 165–167, 170–171
　household products 170
　in-office 169
　mechanism 164–165
　over-the-counter products 170
　procedure 165
　walking bleach technique 133, 167–168, 170
bulimia nervosa 183, 184

C

c-factor 127
calcium content, of drink or food 185
calcium fluoride (CaF2) 30–31
calcium hydroxide 79, 235–240
canal inlay 155, 156
carbon posts 144
caries 14–15, 65–83
　activity 76–77
　antibacterial agents for prevention 53–60
　approximal 71–74
　CPP-ACP use in prevention 47
　diagnosis 65–78
　fluorescence measurement 68–70
　incomplete (stepwise) excavation 234–235
　measures to combat vertical transmission 57–58
　minimally invasive treatment 90–92
　noninvasive treatment techniques for initial lesions 80–83
　pit and fissure 66–68, 70–71, 79
　prevention of progression 79–83
　in primary dentition 233–240
　probiotics and 42–43
　protective and promoting factors 25
　risk assessment (CRA) 76–78
　root 74–76
　selective removal of dentin 109–110
　smooth surface 65–66
　understanding 20
Carisolv 109–110
carrier-based filling systems 220, 221
caseins 45–46
　see also CPP-ACP
Cavishape file 100
cellular intrinsic fiber cementum (CIFC) 11
cellular mixed stratified cementum (CMSC) 11
cementum 11
　types 11
ceramic restoration repairs 138
CEREC system 151–159
　case studies 153–159
　aftercare 159
　amalgam replacement 153–155
　anterior rehabilitation with veneers 157–158
　endo-crown 155–157
　preparation guidelines for ceramic restoration fabrication 152–153
cheek retractors 125
chemochemical excavation 109–110
chlorhexidine (CHX)
　in caries prevention 54–55, 57–58
　in root canal irrigation 210
　in tongue cleaning 255
Clearfil SE Bond 117
CO_2 laser 107, 108
CoJet system 137, 138, 139
compomers 124
composite resin materials 123–124
　see also direct restorative technology

261

composite resin restoration repairs 137–138
condenser-based technique 220, 221
continuous-wave technique 219
core materials 217
coronal reconstruction, importance 215–216
correlation method 158
CPP-ACP 46–49, 185
cracked tooth syndrome 223–230
    clinical examination 228–229
    clinical picture 227
    definition 224
    diagnosis 227–229
    distribution 225
    epidemiology 225
    etiology 224
    radiologic examination 229
    restoration and 226, 229
    symptoms 226–227
    tooth type 225–226
    treatment 229–230
    trial cavity 229

D

demineralization 118
    inhibition
        by condensed phosphates 49
        by fluoride 29
        by metallic ions 49
dental erosion 175–188
    Basic Erosive Wear Examination (BEWE) 177–178
    case studies of progression 181
    CPP-ACP for 48–49, 185
    diagnosis 175–176
    etiology 182–185
    incidence 178
    localization in dentition 179–180
    nutritional factors 185
    occupation and leisure activities and 186
    patient-related factors 182–185
    prevalence 178
    prevention 186–188
    risk assessment 186

denticles 12–13
dentin 8–11
    chemical properties 26
    dysplasias 7–8
    selective removal 109–110
dentin hypersensitivity 223
development of teeth 3–5
DIAGNOdent pen (DD pen) 69–70, 71, 73, 74
diet, and halitosis 250
diode laser 107, 108
direct pulp capping 235–236
direct restorative technology 123–135
    clinical application 125–131
        auxiliary instruments 126–127
        final finishing and polishing 130–131, 134–135
        layering techniques 127–129
        light polymerization 129–130
        optimal operating field creation 125–126
    composite resin materials 123–124
    composite resin restoration fabrication procedure 132–135
discoloration, etiology 164
disinfection
    alternative approaches 212
    see also root canal irrigation
Duraphat 29, 31, 238

E

eating and drinking habits 182–183
ecological plaque hypothesis 39
electronic apex locator 205
enamel 5–8
    chemical properties 26
    dysplasias 7–8
    paraplasias 7
    structural defects 7
Er:YAG laser 107–109
Er,Cr:YSGG laser 107, 108
erosion see dental erosion
etch-and-rinse luting agents 120, 147
etch-and-rinse systems 115–117, 118, 132, 147–148

etching, enamel 117
ethylene diamine tetra-acetic acid (EDTA) 210
extension for prevention principle 97

F

fetor ex ore 245
fiber-optic transillumination (FOTI) 71, 73
fiber posts 143, 144, 145, 146
Filtek Silorane 124
finishing 130–131, 134–135
fluorapatite (FAP) 25, 26, 29
fluorescence measurement 68–70
fluoridated hydroxyapatite (FHAP) 26, 27–28, 29
fluorides 25–31
    adsorbed 30
    demineralization inhibition by 29
    and dental erosion 187
    incorporated 30
    remineralization promotion by 27–28
    usage recommendations 31
    see also calcium fluoride
formaldehyde 240
formocresol 240
four-step adhesive systems 116

G

Galilean loupes 88
gastroesophageal reflux 181, 183–184, 187
glide path 200
gold-cast cores 143, 144, 145
GT hand files 205
GTX system 205–206
gutta-percha 217

H

Halimeter 252–253
halitophobia 259
halitosis 245–259
    causes of odor 246–248
    cofactors 250
    diagnostic procedure 248–254

forms 245–246
informing patient 259
patient history 249
prevalence 245
pseudohalitosis 245, 248, 249, 258–259
sources of odor 246–248, 252
treatment in dental practice 254–258
hand instruments 102
HEMA 119, 128
Hertwig's epithelial root sheath 3–5
hybrid layer 118, 119
hydrofluoric acid 138, 157, 158
hydroxyapatite (HAP) 26, 27
hypersalivation 184
hyposalivation 188

I

iatrogenic damage 97–98
ICDAS system 67
incomplete caries excavation 234–235
infiltration technique 80–81, 83
Intensiv Margin Shaper 100–101
iodoform paste 209, 236
IPS e.max CAD ceramic 155, 156, 158, 159
irreversible pulpitis 234, 235
treatment 236–237

K

K-files 201, 202, 206
Kepler loupes 88

L

lactobacilli 40, 41, 42–43, 75
laser preparation 107–109
lateral condensation technique 219, 221
layering techniques 127–129
light polymerization 129–130
loupes 87, 88

M

M wire 205
magnification aids 87–92, 102

manual dynamic irrigation (MDI) 212
matrices 99, 126–127, 132
metal matrices 99
metal points 217
metal posts 143, 145
metal restoration repairs 139
microbial homeostatis 59
microscopes, operating 87, 89
MicroSeal System 220, 221
milk proteins 45
mineral trioxide aggregate (MTA) 235, 236, 240
minimally invasive preparation 97
minimally invasive restorations 90–92

O

odontogenesis 3
odor diagnostics, instrumental 252–253
one-step adhesive systems 116, 117
operating microscopes 87, 89
Optibond FL 117, 132
oral hygiene
action 21–22
and halitosis 248, 249, 255–256
motivation 19–21
overcoming implementation deficits 22–24
practical implications for dental team 24
see also teeth cleaning
oral infections 39
organoleptic examination 251–252
ormocers 124
oscillating instruments 99–102
Oswald maturation 156
Owen, lines of 8

P

passive ultrasonic irrigation (PUI) 212
paste fillings 218, 221
patency file 200, 211
PathFiles 200
pellicles 185

periodontitis
etiology 207
probiotics and 42–43
understanding 20
phosphate content, of drink or food 185
photodynamic therapy (PDT) 212
planning, oral hygiene 22–23
polishing 130–131, 134–135
post-and-core restoration 143, 148
post systems 143–149
povidone iodine (PI), in caries prevention 55–56, 57–58
Prepcontrol system 100–101
prevention of extension approach 97
primary dentition, endodontology in 233–240
clinical examination 234
history taking 233
materials for endodontic measures 240
see also irreversible pulpitis; pulp necrosis; reversible pulpitis
primary-primary prevention 57–58
prismatic loupes 88
probiotics 39–43
ProTaper instruments 201
proton pump inhibitors 187
Proxoshape file 100
pseudohalitosis 245, 248, 249, 258–259
pulp 12–13
devitalized, with periradicular radiolucency 207
vital 207
zones 12
pulp necrosis, treatment 238–239
pulpectomy 236–237
pulpitis 15–16
pulpotomy 236

Q

quantitative laser fluorescence (QLF) 70

R

radiography, in caries diagnosis 71–73, 75
Raschkow, nerve plexus of 12
remineralization 45
    promotion
        by bioactive glass 50
        by CPP-ACP 46–48
        by fluoride 27–28
        by milk proteins 45
replacement therapy 41
Resilon 217
resin patch 82, 83
restoration repairs 137–140
Retzius, lines of 5
reversible pulpitis 234, 235
    treatments 234–236
rinsing 31
root canal filling 215–221
    importance 215
    materials 216–217
    quality 215
    rating of methods 221
    requirements 216
    techniques 218–220
root canal irrigation 207–213
    alternate rinsing 210, 211
    choice of irrigant 209–210
    disinfection strategies 208–209
    efficacy 210
    heating of irrigant 212
    importance 207
    manual 211–212
    protocol 213
    requirements for irrigants 209
root canal preparation 193–206
    anatomy of root canals 196–197
    chemomechanical 208
    modern principles 198–203
        apical gauging 202
        apical patency 200
        apical resistance form 202, 218
        crown down preparation 199
        deep shape 203
        delayed length measurement 200
        glide path 200
        inlay-shaped access cavity 198
        instrumentation 201
        straight line access 198–199
    Ni-Ti instrument properties 203–204
    for post placement 145–147
    risk analysis 193–195
    techniques 205–206
root filling cements 217
root filling materials 216
rotary Ni-Ti instruments 199, 200, 201, 202–203
    fractures 204
    material properties 203–204
rubber dams 125–126

S

saliva, protective actions 185
sealants 217
sealing 79–83
    conventional 80, 83
self-adhesive luting agents 120–121, 147
self-etch luting agents 120, 147
self-etch systems 116, 117, 118–119, 147–148
self-observation 23
separating rings 126–127, 133
silanization 108, 138, 139, 146, 147
silicatization 147
siloranes 124
silver diamine fluoride (SDF) 53, 57, 61, 238
single-cone technique 218, 221
sodium hexametaphosphate 49
sodium hypochlorite (NaOCl) 146, 209, 212–213
SONICflex airscaler 101–102
stannous fluoride 187
stepwise caries excavation 234–235
streptococci 33, 34, 36, 40–42, 57, 75
subjective perception, scientific evidence vs. 87–88
Syntac classic 117

T

teeth cleaning
    and dental erosion 185, 187
    and rinsing 31
    see also oral hygiene
tetracycline 9, 11
Thermafil 220, 221
thermoplastic filling methods 219
Thomas spanner key 201
TiF4 187
tongue
    assessment 254
    cleaning 255–258
    morphology 246
triclosan, in caries prevention 56
two-step adhesive systems 119

V

visual gauging 206
volatile sulfur compounds (VSCs) 246, 252–253, 256
vomiting 183, 184, 187
von Ebner, lines of 8

W

walking bleach technique 133, 167–168, 170
warm vertical condensation technique 219–220, 221
wedges 88, 89, 126, 132
Weil, zone of 12
white spot lesions, CPP-ACP in treatment 47–48
white teeth 163
Winkel tongue coating index 254

X

xerostomia 188
xylitol, role in caries prevention 33–37, 57–58
    clinical evidence 34
    clinical guidelines 37
    cost-benefit perspective 35–36
    doses 34, 35
    patients benefiting 36
    products 36–37
    side effects 34

Z

zirconium posts 143, 144–145